Handbook
of Palliative Care
in Cancer

Handbook of Palliative Care in Cancer

Alexander Waller, M.D.
Acting Medical Director, Tel Hashomer Hospice
Tel Hashomer, Israel

Nancy L. Caroline, M.D.
Adjunct Professor of Critical Care Medicine,
University of Pittsburgh School of Medicine, Pittsburgh;
and Medical Director, Hospice of the Upper Galilee
Metulla, Israel

Butterworth–Heinemann
Boston   Oxford   Melbourne   Singapore   Toronto   Munich   New Delhi   Tokyo

Butterworth–Heinemann

R   A member of the Reed Elsevier group

Every effort has been made to ensure that the drug dosage schedules within this text are accurate and conform to standards accepted at time of publication. However, as treatment recommendations vary in the light of continuing research and clinical experience, the reader is advised to verify drug dosage schedules herein with information found on product information sheets. This is especially true in cases of new or infrequently used drugs.

 Recognizing the importance of preserving what has been written, Butterworth–Heinemann prints its books on acid-free paper whenever possible.

Library of Congress Cataloging-in-Publication Data
Waller, Alexander.
    Handbook of palliative care in cancer. / Alexander Waller, Nancy L. Caroline
        p.   cm.
    Includes bibliographical references in index.
    ISBN 0-7506-9744-X
        1. Cancer—Palliative treatment.   I. Caroline, Nancy L.   II. Title.
    [DNLM: 1. Neoplasms—therapy.   2. Pain, Intractable—therapy.
    3. Palliative Care.   QZ 266 W198h 1996]
RC271.P33W34   1996
616.99'406--dc20
DNLM/DLC
for Library of Congress   95-52215
                                                                        CIP

British Library Cataloguing-in-Publication Data
A catalogue record for this book is available from the British Library.

The publisher offers discounts on bulk orders of this book.
For information, please write:

Manager of Special Sales
Butterworth–Heinemann
313 Washington Street
Newton, MA 02158-1626

10   9   8   7   6   5   4   3   2   1

Printed in the United States of America

In memory of my parents, Bola-Bluma Waller and Dr. Shmuel Waller, who survived the liquidation of the Warsaw ghetto, and in tribute to my father's work as surgeon of the Jewish Hospital in the ghetto.

To my wife, Janine, and my daughters, Dahlia, Myriam, Emmanuelle, and Iris, for their love and support.

A.W.

To Dr. Gerald Baum, Dr. John F. Burke, and Dr. Eric J. Cassell, who personify all that is best in the practice of Medicine and from whom I am still learning.

N.L.C.

Contents

GASTROINTESTINAL AND ABDOMINAL

RESPIRATORY

URINARY

NEUROLOGIC AND NEUROPSYCHIATRIC

Preface

The physician who sees his role only as the curer of disease or the battler against death is often helpless; the physician who knows that his function is to help the sick to the limit of his ability is almost always able to offer something. In his care the sick are protected from helplessness, fear, and loneliness, agonies that are worse than death.

ERIC J. CASSELL, *THE HEALER'S ART*, 1976, CHAPTER 7

What This Book Is About

Each subspecialty of medicine stakes out a certain territory—an organ system, a group of illnesses—and thereby defines itself. In the established specialties, the territories have been relatively clearly defined: The cardiologist deals with diseases of the cardiovascular system; the rheumatologist deals with illness that manifests itself in mostly inflammatory changes in the connective tissues of the body. The physician entering the relatively new specialty of palliative medicine, however, immediately encounters a problem of self-definition: What precisely *is* palliative medicine? At what point in the treatment of a patient with cancer does care become palliative and therefore fall within the purview of the palliative care specialist rather than, say, the oncologist?

It can be argued that *all* care of the cancer patient in fact constitutes palliative care, in that so few cancers are amenable to cure. The continuum of treatment of the patient with cancer may therefore be viewed as one in which solely palliative measures assume an ever larger proportion of the patient's management:

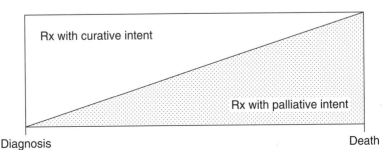

Rx with curative intent

Rx with palliative intent

Diagnosis

Death

Ideally, then, the specialist in palliative medicine should enter the picture, as a consultant in the wings, early in the patient's illness, to provide advice to the attending physician—usually an oncologist—in the management of difficult symptoms. Patients who are still relatively healthy and are undergoing oncologic therapy have as their first priority cure of their disease or at least prolongation of life. In the pursuit of that priority, patients in the early stages of cancer are generally willing to tolerate a considerable degree of discomfort. While every effort must be made to minimize that discomfort, top priority of treatment in early cancer—for the patient and the medical team—must remain prolongation of life.

As the patient nears the end of the road, however, the intervention of a palliative care specialist becomes more and more important. Gradually, the patient's priorities shift. Cure seems less and less likely, and increasing debility from the cancer saps the patient's strength and will to fight the illness. Control of symptoms—of pain, nausea, vomiting, and a host of other problems that can make a misery of the patient's last days—assumes more and more importance.

The transition from active to palliative care is not something that happens in a single point in time; it is a process, and its dynamics are different in every patient. Still, the specialist in palliative medicine must define his or her turf, and this book must define its subject matter. If we look again at the continuum of care, we can at least delimit the universe of medicine with which this book will deal:

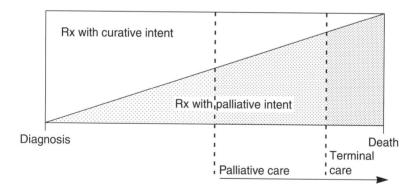

Our primary focus in this handbook will be on care in the *terminal* phase of cancer; we shall also provide information on therapeutic interventions that may be useful earlier in the palliative care process. Thus, for example, when we consider the problem of cerebral metastases, which most usually signal advanced malignant disease, we shall consider different alternatives of palliative management according to the performance status of the patient (which is simply another way of labeling the x-axis of the continuum shown above). But our principal concern is with the last weeks and months of life.

General Principles of Palliative Care in Advanced Cancer

Certain general principles govern the care of patients with advanced cancer. Most of those principles are simply matters of good medical practice, but they bear particular emphasis in the context of palliative care:

- **Listen to the patient.** He is the most credible source of information about distressing symptoms, and the alleviation of those symptoms is your principal task.
- **Make a diagnosis before you treat.** Palliative medicine is a medical discipline and follows the method of a medical discipline: history taking, physical examination, laboratory investigation where warranted, formation of a working diagnosis, and only then treatment. If the discipline of Medicine is neglected in palliative care, the enterprise will fail. Reflex prescription of an antiemetic to every patient with nausea and vomiting, for example, will not benefit the patient who is vomiting because of fecal impaction or because of hypercalcemia.
- **Know the drugs you use, and know them well.** That is, know the pharmacology of the drug, its usual dose range, its indications and contraindications, its possible interactions with other drugs the patient may be taking, its expectable side effects (and ways to ameliorate them). Appendix 1 of this book is intended to provide detailed information about the majority of medications used in palliative care. Before prescribing any drug with which you are not entirely familiar, consult Appendix 1 or other sources to learn the characteristics of the drug, lest untoward drug reactions or interactions aggravate the patient's suffering. The informed and judicious use of pharmacologic agents is the cornerstone of palliative medicine.
- **Whenever possible, use portmanteau medications,** that is, medications that will accomplish more than one objective. For instance, a patient suffering from itching will need an antipruritic agent. If that patient also has pain, nausea, and insomnia, it makes sense to use hydroxyzine as the antipruritic and to exploit its analgesic,

antiemetic, and sedative properties at the same time—rather than prescribe one drug against itching, another for nausea, a third for sleep, and yet another for adjuvant treatment of pain.

- **Keep treatment regimens as simple as possible.** A medication that can be given only once or twice daily is to be preferred over an equivalent medication that requires dosing every 4 to 6 hours. Use low-technology comfort measures, such as hot water bottles, before turning to more complicated and more intimidating devices.
- **Not everything that hurts can be treated with analgesics.** When a patient's symptoms resist amelioration by conventional drug regimens, consider the role of emotional distress in the patient's symptoms. Try to find out what is worrying the patient. Look for signs of anxiety and depression. Morphine does not relieve existential pain.
- **Palliative care is intensive care.** It requires the same attention to detail as intensive care, the same careful dose titration, the same continual reassessment. Like genius, palliative care is an infinite capacity for taking pains.
- **Learn to enjoy small accomplishments**, and teach that skill to patients and their families. It is not always possible to eradicate every symptom, but it is usually possible to bring some degree of relief. In a patient whose bowel is obstructed, for example, it may not be possible to eliminate vomiting altogether, but the amelioration of nausea and the reduction of vomiting to only once or twice a day is usually achievable.
- The phrase "There is nothing more that can be done" does not exist in the lexicon of palliative medicine. **There is always something that can be done,** even if it is simply to sit beside the patient and hold her hand and offer a few words of comfort and solidarity.
- **Learn something new from every patient.** Physicians, especially physicians who treat the dying, enjoy an unparalleled privilege in being allowed intimate access—physical and emotional—to strangers in their most vulnerable moments. To earn that privilege, the physician who cares for the dying has an obligation to learn something from every patient he or she treats, so that a future patient may benefit.

Acknowledgments

In writing a book about caring for patients—the very heart of the medical vocation—the authors have inevitably been influenced by many teachers, colleagues, and friends far too numerous to mention in a few pages. Each of us would like, though, to cite those whose help has been especially important in the creation of this book.

Dr. Alexander Waller gratefully acknowledges the contribution of

Dr. Marian Rabinowitz, Director of Geriatric Medicine, Chaim Sheba Medical Center, Tel Hashomer, who introduced palliative care in Israel and who was my teacher;

Dr. Rami Adunsky, Chief of Geriatric Medicine, Chaim Sheba Medical Center, Tel Hashomer, who schooled and encouraged me in the scientific approach to palliative medicine.

Dr. Nancy Caroline gratefully acknowledges the help of

Dr. Thomas Tichler, Deputy Director of the Department of Oncology, Chaim Sheba Medical Center, Tel Hashomer, who taught me all I know of oncology;

Mrs. Amira Morag, Chief Nurse of the Oncology Ward at Chaim Sheba Medical Center, Tel Hashomer, and her entire nursing staff, whose expert and compassionate care of patients with cancer has been a source of education and inspiration;

Both of us, in addition, wish to acknowledge our shared debt to

The interdisciplinary team of the Tel Hashomer Hospice, for their friendship and their devotion to excellence;

Our patients and their families, who have played such an important part in our lives.

Introduction to Palliative Care

Historic Background of Hospice and Palliative Care

Palliative care is a direct outgrowth of the hospice movement, and hospice has its earliest roots in fourth century Byzantium, in the Christian institutions that were established to welcome travelers. In Greek, those institutions were called *xenodochia*, or refuges for the stranger. When, in the course of time, xenodochia spread into the Roman Empire, they took on the Latin name *hospitium*, derived from the word *hospes*, or host; and until today, the concept of hospitality and welcome is integral to the hospice idea. Hospices proliferated widely during the Crusades in the Middle Ages, and many hospices sprang up in the Holy Land along the routes of pilgrims. Furthermore, by medieval times, hospices were giving care not only to travelers but also to the destitute, the sick, and the dying. With the coming of the Reformation, hospices virtually disappeared from Europe and from the pilgrimage routes and were not seen again until the nineteenth century, when hospices specifically for the care of the dying were founded in Dublin, Ireland and Lyons, France. Similar hospices, of various Christian denominations, soon followed. It was at one of those hospices, St. Luke's in London, that a social worker named Cecily Saunders came to work as a volunteer nurse in the late 1940s. There, Saunders observed the special methods the sisters employed in caring for the dying, such as the practice of giving analgesics around the clock rather than waiting for the patient to complain of pain. After completing a medical degree, Cecily Saunders took up a post as medical officer at St. Joseph's Hospice in London; and in 1967 she founded the first modern hospice, St. Christopher's, in Sydenham, London, whose aim was to combine the tradition of compassion that characterized the medieval hospice with the achievements of modern medicine—in the service of relieving the suffering of terminally ill patients and their families.

At around the same time that Cecily Saunders founded St. Christopher's, the psychiatrist Elisabeth Kübler-Ross, working in Chicago, was exploring the psychological stages through which a person passes after learning that he or she has a terminal illness. The writings and lectures of Kübler-Ross (1969) brought the heretofore taboo subjects of death and dying out of the closet and placed them firmly in the mainstream agenda of the American middle class—at precisely the time when that middle class was demanding greater participation in decisions about their own health care. Thus the ground was prepared for the introduction of the hospice concept to the American continent.

The first hospice in America, the Connecticut Hospice, was established in 1974, to provide supportive care to terminally ill patients in their own homes. The following year, Balfour Mount opened the Palliative Care Service in the Royal Victoria Hospital in Montreal, and in so doing brought the term *palliative care* into the lexicon as a synonym for supportive or hospice care.

The 1970s through the 1990s saw a rapid proliferation of supportive care units—700 hospices in the United Kingdom, 1500 in the United States, and scores of others in Europe and elsewhere, including the Third World. International congresses were convened to share experiences and research findings in the developing field of palliative care, while national and international organizations—such as the National Hospice Organization in the United States, the European Association for Palliative Care, and the Israeli Palliative Care Association—were established to bring together the growing number of people from various disciplines involved in this type of care. By 1994, only 27 years after St. Christopher's Hospice opened its doors, there were at least five journals being published in the field of palliative care (two of them, *Palliative Medicine* and *Journal of Palliative Care*, listed in *Index Medicus*), and a comprehensive textbook—*Oxford Textbook of Palliative Medicine* (1993)—had been issued. Furthermore, chairs in palliative medicine had been established at universities in Canada, Australia, and the United Kingdom.

Nearly two millennia after the establishment of the first hospices of Byzantium, then, hospices are once again flourishing throughout the world and providing comfort to travelers on their last journey. We have more sophisticated measures today for relieving the symptoms of terminal illness—those measures are the subject of this book—but the concept of *caring* unites twentieth century palliative care with its fourth century predecessors.

Important Concepts and Definitions

The Terminally Ill Patient

- The terminally ill patient is one whose treatment has shifted from a regimen with curative intent to one with supportive intent.
- The patient, his family, his friends, the medical team, and society as a whole consider him to be terminally ill.
- The patient's life span is relatively short (by Medicare's definition, less than 6 months).
- Because there is no longer a prospect of cure, it is the right of the terminally ill patient not to incur suffering from medical investigations or treatment.
- For the terminally ill patient, time has a special meaning because it is rationed, limited, and therefore emotionally laden.
- In the terminal period, the patient tries to close the circles—familial, social, psychological, spiritual—and asks questions about the meaning of existence.

Palliative Care

The World Health Organization (1990) defines *palliative care* as "the active total care of patients whose disease is not responsive to curative treatment." According to the WHO definition, the goal of palliative care must be the best possible quality of life for the patient and his family, so symptom control and attention to the whole patient—in his psychological, social, and spiritual dimensions—have primacy. WHO (1990) further defines palliative care by its characteristic principles, as care that

- Affirms life and regards dying as a normal process.
- Neither hastens nor postpones death.
- Provides relief from pain and other distressing symptoms.
- Offers a support system to help patients live as actively as possible until death.
- Offers a support system to help the family cope during the patient's illness and in their own bereavement.

Hospice is not a building and not a model but a supportive *approach*. The methods and models of palliative care can change from place to place, but certain basic characteristics are common to every hospice program everywhere. In every hospice, there is

- A concerted, meticulous, and **ongoing effort to control** the patient's **symptoms**.
- Continuous attention to **helping the patient cope** with fear of death, loneliness, and the many losses that attend advanced illness (loss of control over one's body and one's destiny, loss of self-image, loss of self-esteem, loss of role in family and society, anticipated loss of loved ones).
- Maximum **regard for the patient and family as partners** in identifying the sources of distress and shaping the treatment program.
- High priority to the **support of the patient's family**, emotionally, socially, and in their practical and financial problems.
- A commitment to offering a place of **security and** tranquil **refuge** to the patient and family—a place where patients and families can feel at home and where they can receive personal attention.
- Absolute **availability** of the palliative care team **around the clock**, including weekends and holidays. This is one of the most important prerequisites for the success of a palliative care program.
- **Continuity of care and caregivers**, especially in the transfer of the patient to a palliative care facility.
- Emphasis given to establishing **relations of full trust** between the patient and family and the palliative care team. That is the reason why it is impermissible in palliative care to lie to the patient about his condition; dishonesty is immediately sensed and destroys trust. The task of the palliative care team is to convey honest, existential hope rather than unrealistic hope of cure.

The degree to which a palliative care program is able to achieve the tasks and objectives described above will depend in part upon putting together all the elements of a full-fledged hospice. Those elements include

- An inpatient service.
- Home care.
- Day care.
- An information center.
- A program of volunteers.
- Bereavement services.

Depending on the institutional context, a hospice may also include a consultation service, pain clinic, and follow-up clinic.

In summary, the task of the palliative care team is to see the patient and family through the physical and emotional stages of terminal illness and to ease their burden along the way—to **walk alongside**, not to give orders from above; to **be there** when symptoms arise, when hard questions have to be faced, when fear and loneliness threaten; and to apply to the care of the dying the same high standards of clinical analysis and decision making as are demanded in the care of patients expected to get well.

The Interdisciplinary Team

The interdisciplinary team comprises individuals from different professional spheres, each responsible for decision making within his or her area of competence. An *inter*disciplinary team is not the same as a *multi*disciplinary team, the latter being the model that is more familiar throughout the health care system:

Multidisciplinary Team	*Interdisciplinary Team*
Individuals are known first by their professional identities and only secondarily by their team affiliation.	The identity of the team supersedes individual professional identities.
Team members share information via the medical record (where each charts his own observations separately and reads the observations charted by others).	Team members share information through discussion and work together to formulate goals.
Leadership resides in the highest-ranking member of the team (usually the physician).	Leadership is assumed by different team members depending on the task at hand.
Because the team is not the primary vehicle for action, the interactional process within the team is irrelevant.	Because the team is the vehicle of action, the interactional process is vital for success.

Adapted from Ajemian (1993).

The work of the interdisciplinary team, therefore, is based on negotiation and discussion and requires that each member of the team be willing to consider the viewpoint of the others.

Why is the interdisciplinary team so important in palliative care?

Cecily Saunders (1978) developed the concept of "total pain," that is, the idea that pain has a physical, mental, social, and spiritual component. In a similar vein, Eric Cassell (1991) distinguishes between *pain*, a thing that the body experiences, and *suffering*, which only a *person* can experience. And because suffering is experienced by the person, it cannot be mitigated without knowing something of what constitutes that person: his body, his personality, his past, his life experiences, his family, his cultural background, his roles and relationships, his regular behaviors, his perceived future. The physician alone cannot easily know all those things about a person; nor can the nurse, nor the social worker, nor the psychologist, nor the physiotherapist, nor the volunteer who comes to chat. But working together, and sharing information, those members of the interdisciplinary team can form a good composite picture of the person whose care they have undertaken and can thereby provide the kind of holistic treatment that hospice requires.

The Role of the Physician in the Interdisciplinary Team

From the earliest times, the role of the physician has been to relieve suffering and, where possible, to restore health. Until very recently, the stress was on relief of suffering (palliation), since restoration of health (cure) was rarely feasible; the physician followed the patient through the course of the disease and did whatever was possible to ease the patient's distress along the way. It was perhaps the discovery of penicillin by Alexander Fleming, and the subsequent successes of antibiotics, that fostered the illusion in our own time that it is possible in almost every case to cure disease or at least to prevent death. And with the establishment of intensive care units, starting in the 1960s, came the widespread impression (not by any means limited to the lay public) that if a patient died, it was because of a failure of the physician at some stage of treatment.

The reality is that the role of the physician has not changed since ancient times: The physician must relieve suffering and also try to restore health. But owing to the often invasive and aggressive nature of modern diagnostic and treatment methods, the duty to palliate and the duty to cure are apt to come into conflict. For that reason, the physician must continually reevaluate the patient's situation and the likelihood of gain from diagnostic and therapeutic interventions. And as the patient's disease worsens, the physician must be able to shift treatment goals toward minimizing painful procedures and ensuring comfort. At that stage, the whole atmosphere around the patient must become therapeutically quieter, removed from the tumult of x-rays and scans and blood tests and chemotherapy. But at the same time, the physician must maintain the analytic approach to the patient's problems that is the hallmark of the medical discipline. The method of clinical decision making does not change when the patient is beyond cure; that method is simply applied to a different set of problems—to the investigation and alleviation of distressing symptoms.

The roles and obligations of the physician as a member of the interdisciplinary team reflect both the roles traditionally ascribed to the profession and those that derive from the special nature of hospice care:

- The physician must have a **comprehensive knowledge of symptom control** in general and pain control in particular, with emphasis on drug treatment and understanding of the pharmacology of every medication prescribed.
- Only a physician may **prescribe drugs**, particularly opioids and other controlled substances.
- The physician will be regarded by the patient and the patient's family, and in many cases by the other team members, as the **leader of the interdisciplinary team**; for that reason the physician must have specialized skills in communication and respect for the professional contribution of other members of the team.
- It is the physician's task to brief the patient, the family, and the team about the patient's illness, condition, and prognosis.
- The physician must be involved in mobilizing resources from the community, working with volunteers, and designing the physical arrangements of the hospice.
- One of the most important and special roles of the physician as part of the interdisciplinary team is **to build consensus** between the patient, the family, and the professional caregivers—for every decision concerning the patient's supportive care. There is no value to any treatment proposal if the patient, family, and professional team do not support it wholeheartedly. This point cannot be overemphasized, for it is the outstanding feature of palliative medicine and the feature that distinguishes palliative care from care given on general medical wards or even care by *multi*disciplinary teams in rehabilitation or geriatric units.

There is a widespread impression among both the lay and medical public that in the terminal stages of illness, it is appropriate that care be handed over entirely to the nursing staff. We believe, however, that palliative medicine—in that it *is* a discipline within medicine—requires the guidance of skilled and experienced physicians no less than any other branch of clinical medicine. The interdisciplinary team, that is, should be medically directed and nurse centered.

The Question of Euthanasia

The subject of euthanasia evokes strong feelings among the general public and the medical profession and involves religious, philosophic, psychological, ethical, and medicolegal considerations. We cannot in this discussion address ourselves to all those aspects of the subject or go into the academic classification of types of euthanasia, all of which have been considered at great length elsewhere. For our purposes here, what is important to explain is how the hospice movement in general looks upon euthanasia.

One of the pioneers of palliative care, Robert Twycross, defines euthanasia as an action whose intention is to shorten life. That is to be distinguished from the inadvertent shortening of life through actions taken to relieve suffering. The distinction is explained by Latimer (1991) through the "principle of double effect": that is, an action whose *intention* is to do good may be taken ethically even though it may cause damage.

The Israeli scientist and philosopher Yeshayahu Leibowitz insisted that euthanasia (as in the definition by Twycross) could not be justified as a measure to ease severe suffering or to release a person from a life that was no longer worthwhile either to himself or to society. According to Leibowitz, life is not a value that can be weighed or measured; it is a fact, a given:

> For not of thy will were you formed and not of thy will were you born and not of thy will do you live and not of thy will shall you die and not of thy will shall you give an account and reckoning before the King of the king of kings, the Holy One, Blessed be He.
> *Pirke Avoth (Sayings of the Fathers), Talmud*

Life, according to this view, *includes* different values, but life itself cannot be assigned a value, and therefore it is invalid to shorten life on the grounds that life has lost its value. We must instead work to ease the suffering of the patient and the family and thereby to enable them to pass through the important experience of the terminal phase with dignity and solace. It is the conviction of those involved in palliative care that euthanasia is ethically inadmissible and that there are better answers to the problem of suffering at the end of life—answers that good palliative care can help to provide.

Future Directions of Palliative Care

For almost 30 years, palliative care has been in a state of expansion, but there is still much to be achieved.

- We need to define the optimal model for delivering palliative care.
- Progress is needed in research on alleviating such symptoms as anorexia, cachexia, and weakness at least to the same degree as we are now able to relieve pain.
- Palliative care must be integrated into the management of the patient with cancer much earlier in the disease course, even at the point of diagnosis, and should become part of routine care in general medical wards and in the community.
- Subjects relating to supportive care must be introduced into the curricula in schools of medicine, nursing, psychology, social work, and physiotherapy.
- Hospices in wealthy countries must undertake the support of hospices in poor countries.
- And with all that, we must be wary that the successful establishment of palliative care as part of the mainstream of medicine does not suppress the creativity, flexibility, and pioneering spirit that have given the hospice movement its special importance.

Summary

Palliative care has its roots in ancient Christianity. In modern times, palliative care began as a grassroots movement of the middle class in Anglo-Saxon countries. As palliative care has spread throughout the world, it has been characterized by flexibility and adaptability to local religions, philosophies, conditions, and needs. In the future, palliative care needs to become an integral part—the innovative and humanizing part—of academic medicine and of the health care system as a whole.

References and Further Reading

Ajemian I. The Interdisciplinary Team. In Doyle E, Hanks GWC, MacDonald N (eds). *Oxford Textbook of Palliative Medicine*. New York: Oxford University Press, 1993, p. 18.

Cassell EJ. *The Healer's Art*. Philadelphia: Lippincott, 1976.

Cassell EJ. *The Nature of Suffering and the Art of Medicine*. New York: Oxford University Press, 1991.

Corr CA, Corr DM. *Hospice Care: Principles and Practice*. New York: Springer, 1983.

Doyle E, Hanks GWC, MacDonald N (eds). *Oxford Textbook of Palliative Medicine*. New York: Oxford University Press, 1993.

Kübler-Ross E. *On Death and Dying*. New York: Macmillan, 1969.

Latimer EJ. Personal decision-making in the care of the dying and its applications to clinical practice. *J Pain Symptom Manage* 6:329, 1991.

Saunders C (ed). *The Management of Terminal Disease*. London: Edward Arnold, 1978, p. 194.

Siebold C. *The Hospice Movement: Easing Death's Pains*. New York: Twayne, 1992.

WHO Expert Committee. *Cancer Pain Relief and Palliative Care*. Geneva: World Health Organization, 1990, p. 11.

Symbols and Abbreviations Used in This Book

Symbols

Symbol	Indicates
→	"Leads to" *or* "Followed by" *or* "Therefore" depending on context
>	Greater than
<	Less than
↑	Increased
↓	Decreased
±	With or without
×	For a duration of, *or* Times

Abbreviations

Abbreviation	Signifies
ac	Before meals (*ante cibum*)
ACE	Angiotension-converting enzyme
ACTH	Adrenocorticotropic hormone
AMI	Acute myocardial infarction
AMP	Adenosine monophosphate
ARF	Acute renal failure

continued

Abbreviation	*Signifies*
ATP	Adenosine triphosphate
bid	Twice a day (*bis in die*)
BP	Blood pressure
BPH	Benign prostatic hypertrophy
BUN	Blood urea nitrogen
Ca^{2+}	Calcium
CBC	Complete blood count
CCT	Creatinine clearance
CHF	Congestive heart failure
CK	Creatine kinase
cm	Centimeter
CNS	Central nervous system
COPD	Chronic obstructive pulmonary disease
CR	Controlled-release
Cr	Creatinine
CSF	Cerebrospinal fluid
CT	Computed tomography
CTZ	Chemoreceptor trigger zone
D/C	Discontinue
DJD	Degenerative joint disease
D5/NS	5% Dextrose in normal saline
DTIC	Dacarbazine (5-[3,3 dimethyl-1-triazeno]-imidazole-4-carboxamide)
DTRs	Deep tendon reflexes
D5W	5% Dextrose in water
ECF	Extracellular fluid
ECG	Electrocardiogram
ECOG	Eastern Cooperative Oncology Group
FEV_1	Forced expiratory volume in 1 second
5-FU	5-Fluorouracil
GFR	Glomerular filtration rate
GI	Gastrointestinal

Abbreviation	Signifies
gm	Gram
gtt	Drops
GU	Genitourinary
Gy	Gray (=100 rads)
h	Hour
Hb	Hemoglobin
Hg	Mercury
h/o	History of
H_2O_2	Hydrogen peroxide
hr	Hour
hs	At bedtime (*hora somni*)
hx	History
Hz	Herz (cycles per second)
ICF	Intracellular fluid
ICP	Intracranial pressure
IM	Intramuscular, intramuscularly
I&O	Intake and output
IV	Intravenous, intravenously
K^+	Potassium
KCl	Potassium chloride
kg	Kilogram
L	Liter
LDH	Lactate dehydrogenase
LES	Lower esophageal sphincter
LFTs	Liver function tests
LLQ	Left lower quadrant of the abdomen
LUQ	Left upper quadrant of the abdomen
MAO	Monoamine oxidase
mg	Milligram
µg	Microgram
Mg^{2+}	Magnesium
min	Minute

continued

Abbreviation	*Signifies*
ml	Milliliter
mm	Millimeter
MMEF	Maximal mid-expiratory flow
mmol	Millimoles
MRI	Magnetic resonance imaging
MTX	Methotrexate
N/A	Not available
Na^+	Sodium
N/V	Nausea and vomiting
NE	Norepinephrine
NG	Nasogastric
NS	Normal saline
NSAID	Nonsteroidal anti-inflammatory drug
OTC	Over the counter
p	After
PA	Posterior/anterior
pc	After meals (*post cibum*)
PCO_2	Partial pressure of carbon dioxide (in arterial blood)
PE	Physical examination
PO	By mouth (*per os*)
PO_2	Partial pressure of oxygen (in arterial blood)
PR	Per rectum
prn	As needed (*pro re nata*)
PT	Prothrombin time
PTH	Parathyroid hormone
PTT	Partial thromboplastin time
PUD	Peptic ulcer disease
q	Every (*quaque*)
qam	Every morning
qd	Every day (*quaque die*)
qhs	Every night
qid	Four times a day (*quater in die*)

Abbreviation	Signifies
qXh	Every [X] hours
RBC	Red blood cell
RLQ	Right lower quadrant of the abdomen
RT	Radiation therapy
RUQ	Right upper quadrant of the abdomen
Rx	Therapy, treatment
SCLC	Small cell lung cancer
SGOT	Serum glutamic-oxaloacetic transaminase
SGPT	Serum glutamic-pyruvic transaminase
SIADH	Syndrome of inappropriate antidiuretic hormone
SQ	Subcutaneous, subcutaneously
stat	Right away, immediately
SVC	Superior vena cava
Sx	Symptom
tab	Tablet
TB	Tuberculosis
tbsp	Tablespoon
TCC	Transitional cell carcinoma
TENS	Transcutaneous electrical nerve stimulation
tid	Three times a day (*ter in die*)
TMP/SMZ	Trimethoprim-sulfamethoxazole
tsp	Teaspoon
U/A	Urinalysis
UGI	Upper gastrointestinal
UTI	Urinary tract infection
WBC	White blood cell
Zn	Zinc

Pain Control

1 General Considerations

Physical pain is not a simple affair of an impulse traveling at a fixed rate along a nerve. It is the resultant of a conflict between a stimulus and the whole individual.

RENE LERICHE, *SURGERY OF PAIN*

Definition

According to the International Association for the Study of Pain, pain is an unpleasant sensory and emotional experience associated with actual or potential tissue damage, or described in terms of such damage. **Pain is always subjective**.

- The severity of pain is not in linear relation to the amount of tissue damage.
- Many factors influence a person's perception of pain, including
  - Fatigue.
  - Depression.
  - Anger.
  - Fear and anxiety.
  - Feelings of helplessness and hopelessness.

Cecily Saunders (1978) introduced the concept of "**total pain**," comprising several components:
- Physical.
- Mental.
- Social.
- Spiritual.

Incidence of Pain in Patients with Cancer

- Moderate to severe pain occurs in 30% of cancer patients receiving treatment and in **60% to 90% of patients with advanced disease**.
- The prevalence of pain increases as disease progresses.
- **Sources of pain** in patients with cancer (Twycross and Fairfield, 1982):
  - The cancer itself (61%).
  - Related to cancer or debility, for example, muscle spasm or constipation (12%).
  - Related to treatment, for example, surgical incision pain or mucositis (5%).
  - Concurrent disorder, for example, arthritis (22%).
- A given patient with advanced cancer is likely to suffer several types of pain, and adequate treatment will depend on identifying the source of each.
- Pain can be completely relieved in 80% to 90% of patients, and an acceptable level of relief can be achieved in most of the rest.

Pathophysiology of Pain and Pain Control
Anatomic Considerations

Afferent Pathways

- Specialized receptors that respond only to noxious stimuli (**nociceptors**) are distributed in all tissues except the CNS. →
- Pain afferents enter the spinal cord via the **dorsal root**, where they have their cell bodies, and synapse in the substantia gelatinosa of the **dorsal horn**. →
- Nociceptive stimuli reaching the dorsal horns activate
  - Interneurons within the dorsal horn (which play a central role in "gate control" mechanisms).
  - The ascending nociceptive system in the spinothalamic, spinocervical, and spinoreticular tracts.

Efferent Pathways

- Antinociceptive descending tracts originate in the somatosensory cortex, periaqueductal gray matter in the midbrain, and other areas → lateral posterior columns of the spinal cord.
- Descending pathways modulate nociceptive transmission.
- The descending pathways may be activated centrally by morphine and other opioids, which mimic the activity of endogenous **endorphins**.
- Many descending inhibitory pathways are **serotonergic** → may account for analgesic action of tricyclic antidepressant drugs (which inhibit reuptake of serotonin and thus lead to increased serotonin levels in the CNS).

Opioid Receptors

- Opioids exert their effects by interacting with specific receptors that are distributed
  - In the nociceptive cells of the dorsal root ganglia.
  - Throughout the nervous system.
  - In various locations outside the nervous system (e.g., within joints, probably in the lung).
- Opioid receptors important in mediating analgesia are classified as mu (μ), kappa (κ), and delta (δ):

Receptor	Prototypical Stimulator	Effects of Stimulation
Mu_1	Morphine	Supraspinal and spinal analgesia
		Feelings of well-being
Mu_2		Respiratory depression
		↓GI tract motility
		Urinary retention
		Miosis
		Bradycardia
		Physical dependence
Kappa	Dynorphin	Spinal analgesia
		Dysphoria
		Psychotomimetic effects
		Slight miosis and respiratory depression (less than from mu activation)
Delta	Enkephalin	Spinal analgesia
		Respiratory depression
		May act synergistically with mu receptors

▪ Different opioid drugs have different receptor affinities and are divided into four principal categories according to their receptor affinities:
  • **Agonists:** stimulate receptor sites to produce analgesia.
  • **Partial agonists:** stimulate receptor sites to less than the maximum possible.
  • **Antagonists:** occupy receptor sites without producing stimulation and thereby block the action of opioid agonists (of these, naloxone is the only true competitive antagonist).
  • **Mixed agonist-antagonists:** opioids whose attachment to certain receptors produces analgesia, while their attachment to other receptors has analgesic blocking actions.
    – Type I (e.g., buprenorphine): mu antagonists only at high dosage.
    – Type II (e.g., nalorphine): mu antagonists at all dosages.

▪ A given opioid can be an agonist at one or more receptor types and an antagonist at another type of receptor:

Activity at Different Receptors

Opioid	Mu	Kappa	Delta
Morphine	A	a	a
Fentanyl	A	a	a
Methadone	A	—	A
Levorphanol	A	—	A
Pentazocine	pA	A	Ant
Buprenorphine	pA	Ant	A
Nalorphine	Ant	a	a
Naloxone	Ant	Ant	Ant

A = strong agonist; a = weak agonist; pA = partial agonist; Ant = antagonist; — = negligible activity.

▪ Clinical implication: A patient who has been treated with a pure agonist such as morphine should *not*
  • be switched to an agonist-antagonist.
  • be given an agonist-antagonist in addition to morphine lest withdrawal be precipitated.

Classification of Pain by Pathophysiologic Mechanism

It is useful to classify pain in cancer patients according to the presumed pathophysiologic mechanism:

Category	Characteristics	Examples	Response to Opioids
N Somatic pain **O** **C**	Dull, aching, throbbing, or gnawing. Well localized.	Bone pain Incisional pain Myofascial and musculo- skeletal pain	Excellent
I Visceral pain **C** **E** **P** **T** **I** **V** **E**	Originates from injury to sympathetically inervated organs. Caused by infiltration, compression, distention, or stretching of thoracic/ abdominal viscera. Poorly localized, deep, dragging, squeezing, or pressure-like. When acute, may be colicky and associated with auto- nomic symptoms (nausea, vomiting, sweating, tachy- cardia). Often referred to cutaneous sites remote from the lesion (e.g., shoulder pain of hepatic origin).	Bowel obstruc- tion Stretching of liver capsule	Good
Neuro- pathic pain	Results from injury to pe- ripheral and/or central nervous system, by tumor compression or infiltra- tion or damage from sur- gical, radiation, or chemo- therapy. Superficial burning, stinging, sometimes with superim- posed lancinating, electric shock–like pain.	Brachial/ lumbosacral plexopathies Postherpetic neuralgia Vincristine or cisplatin neuropathy Diabetic neuropathy	Poor

continued

Category	Characteristics	Examples	Response to Opioids
Neuro-pathic pain *cont.*	Often associated with sensory changes. There may also be associated muscle atrophy, autonomic changes, and trophic changes in the skin.		

Drugs Used to Control Pain in Patients with Advanced Cancer

Nonopioid Analgesics

- All nonopioid analgesics (see Table 1.1) have a **ceiling effect**, that is, after a certain dosage, further increases of dosage do not produce increasing analgesia.
- Addition of a nonopioid drug to opioid analgesia may have a **dose-sparing effect** and permit lower dosages of the opioid.
- Two general categories:
  - Nonsteroidal anti-inflammatory drugs (NSAIDs), including aspirin.
  - Simple analgesics: acetaminophen.
- **Nonsteroidal anti-inflammatory drugs (NSAIDs):**
  - Site of action: entirely on the injured tissue itself (not central).
  - Presumed mechanism: block synthesis of prostaglandins.
  - Effective against *slow, prolonged tissue damage* and its pain:
    - Pain from **pancreatic cancer** (aspirin uniquely effective); head and neck cancers.
    - **Bone metastases**, periostitis, paraneoplastic osteoarthropathy.
  - Do not produce tolerance or physical/psychological dependence.
  - **Side effects**
    - **Gastroduodenal irritation** and bleeding are the most important and serious side effects and the most likely to require discontinuation of treatment. Try to reduce the incidence of NSAID-induced peptic ulcer by
      - Giving NSAIDs with less gastric toxicity (e.g., ibuprofen).
      - Giving prophylactic **misoprostol, 100 to 200 μg PO bid to qid** to **high-risk patients** (e.g., patients taking both NSAIDs and corticosteroids).
    - Interference with platelet activity → **bleeding** tendency (aspirin).
    - Renal effects
      - Can increase sodium/fluid retention → **edema**, hypertension.

- ○ Can decrease renal blood flow in susceptible individuals →
  renal failure.
- ▪ **Acetaminophen (paracetamol)**:
  - • No anti-inflammatory activity.
  - • Site of analgesic action unknown.
  - • Equianalgesic with aspirin.
  - • No gastric side effects, but potential liver toxicity after overdose or
    after therapeutic doses given to alcoholic patients.

TABLE 1.1   Nonsteroidal Anti-Inflammatory Drugs and Acetaminophen

Drug	Starting Dose*	Maximum Dosage (mg/day)	Comments
Acetaminophen/ paracetamol (Tylenol)	650 mg q4–6h	6000	Scant if any anti-inflammatory action. For headache due to brain metastases. Overdose → hepatotoxicity.
Aspirin	650 mg q4–6h	6000	GI toxicity. ↓Platelet function → bleeding.
Choline magnesium trisalicylate (Trilisate)	1500 mg × 1, then 1000 mg q12h	4000	Minimal GI toxicity. Less effect on renal blood flow than other NSAIDs. No effect on platelet function.
Choline salicylate (Arthropan)	870 mg q3–4h		
Diclofenac (Voltaren)	25 mg q6–8h	200	Usually well tolerated. Useful in renal/biliary colic.
Diflunisal (Dolobid)	1000 × 1, then 500 mg q6h	1500	Salicylate with less GI toxicity than aspirin.
Fenoprofen (Nalfon)	200 mg q6h	3200	
Flurbiprofen (Ansaid)	50–100 mg bid	200	May be useful for detrusor instability, to reduce urinary urgency and frequency. Requires only twice-daily dosing.

continued

TABLE 1.1 Nonsteroidal Anti-Inflammatory Drugs and Acetaminophen
continued

Drug	Starting Dose*	Maximum Dosage (mg/day)	Comments
Flurbiprofen *cont.*			Occasional massive fluid retention. Causes diarrhea in some patients.
Ibuprofen (Motrin)	400 mg q6–8h	4200	Available OTC. Less GI toxicity than other NSAIDs.
Indomethacin (Indocin)	25 mg q8–12h	200	Not recommended because of high probability of severe GI toxicity. Likely to produce headaches in dose >100 mg/day.
Ketoprofen (Orudis)	50 mg q8h	300	
Ketorolac (Toradol)	30–60 mg IM × 1, then 15–30 mg IM q6h or 10 mg PO q6h	150 mg IM on day 1; then 120 mg IM	For short-term use only. The only NSAID available for parenteral administration. Coverage with misoprostol advisable. IM administration has same GI toxicity as PO. Can be given by SQ infusion (separate syringe).
Magnesium salicylate (Magan, Mobidin)	650 mg q4–6h		
Meclofenamate (Meclomen)	50 mg q6–8h	400	
Mefenamic acid (Ponstel)	500 × 1, then 100 mg q6–8h	1000	Best to use < 1 week. Diarrhea occurs in >10% of patients.
Naproxen (Naprosyn)	250 mg q12h	1000	Preferred in many palliative care units because it requires only twice-daily dosing.
Naproxen sodium (Anaprox)	275 mg q6h	1100	
Sulindac (Clinoril)	150 mg q12h	400	Less renal toxicity than other NSAIDs.

*All doses are given orally unless otherwise specified.

Opioid Analgesics

- The term *opioids* includes **all drugs with morphine-like actions** on endogenous opioid receptors, irrespective of chemical structure (see Table 1.2).
- It has been customary to subdivide opioids into two general categories:
  - **Weak opioids** (e.g., codeine, propoxyphene).
  - **Strong opioids** (e.g., morphine, methadone, hydromorphone).
- The WHO *Revised Method for Relief of Cancer Pain* (1994) recommends a different classification:
  - Opioids for mild to moderate pain.
  - Opioids for moderate to severe pain.
- It is likely that the former classification will remain in general use because of the very different connotations, for the general public and the medical profession, of treatment with codeine and treatment with morphine.
- Opioid analgesia is mediated through central opioid receptors (see above).
- Opioid analgesics have **no ceiling effect** → dosage may be increased virtually without limit.
- Side effects of opioids are detailed in Chapter 2.

Adjuvant Drugs with Secondary Analgesic Effect

- Adjuvant drugs (see Table 1.3) are those that were developed for clinical indications other than pain relief.
- Adjuvant drugs may be used at all steps of the analgesic ladder (see Chapter 2).

Other Modalities of Pain Management in Advanced Cancer

Treatment with analgesic drugs will be sufficient to manage the vast majority of pain problems in cancer patients, but in about 10% of cases, other modalities (discussed on pages 16 to 22) are required in addition.

TABLE 1.2 Opioid Analgesics

Drug	Equianalgesic Dosage (based on 10 mg of morphine IM) Oral	Equianalgesic Dosage (based on 10 mg of morphine IM) Parenteral	Dosing Interval	Comments
Weak Opioids				
Codeine + aspirin or acetaminophen	180–200 mg	130 mg	q3–4h	Codeine doses > 65 mg usually not useful because of diminishing incremental analgesia with ↑ dosage but continuing increase in side effects (nausea, constipation).
Propoxyphene napsylate (Darvon)	270–300 mg	N/A	q6h	No advantages over other weak opioids. Can cause seizures with overdose. May cause adverse reactions in patients taking carbamazepine.
Strong Opioids: Pure Agonists				
Morphine	30 mg	5 mg IV 10 mg IM 15 mg SQ	q3–4h	Standard of comparison for opioids.
Controlled-release morphine (MS Contin)	30 mg	N/A	q8–12h	No parenteral formulation. Tablet should not be cut, crushed, or chewed. May be given rectally.
Fentanyl transdermal system (Duragesic)	N/A	Not certain	q48–72h	Patches deliver 25 µg/hr, 50 µg/hr, 75 µg/hr, and 100 µg/hr. Starting dose in µg/hr = dose of MS Contin in mg/12 hr. Slow onset of action → must use additional analgesic for several days at onset of Rx. Slow decrease in effect after removing patch. Expensive.

Drug	Oral dose	Parenteral dose	Interval	Comments
Hydrocodone (Lorcet, Lortab, Hycodan)	30 mg	N/A	q3–4h	Available only in fixed combination with acetaminophen, which limits upward titration. Used principally as an antitussive rather than an analgesic.
Hydromorphone (Dilaudid)	7.5 mg	1.5 mg IM / 3 mg PR	q3–4h	By spinal route, causes less pruritus than morphine.
Levorphanol (Levo-Dromoran)	4 mg	2 mg IM	q6–8h	Long half-life (12–15 hours) → drug accumulates after starting or increasing dose. May be unsuitable in the elderly. Causes less nausea/vomiting than morphine.
Meperidine (Demerol) Pethidine	300 mg	75 mg IM	q3–4h	NOT recommended for cancer pain: Short duration of action → frequent dosing is necessary. Repeated administration → accumulation of toxic metabolite (normeperidine) → CNS toxicity (tremor, confusion, seizures). No antitussive properties. Produces less pupillary constriction → harder to monitor for overdosage. Contraindicated in patients taking MAO inhibitors.
Methadone (Dolophine)	20 mg	10 mg IM	q6–8h	Requires close monitoring because of risk of delayed toxicity (half life = 15–57 hours). Should not be used in the elderly or debilitated. Should not be used in hepatic/renal failure. Use best confined to patients attending pain clinics.
Oxycodone	15 mg	N/A	q3–4h	For moderate pain. Dosage of combined drug (aspirin or acetaminophen) may be limiting.

continued

TABLE 1.2   Opioid Analgesics *continued*

| Drug | Equianalgesic Dosage (based on 10 mg of morphine IM) | | Dosing Interval | Comments |
	Oral	Parenteral		
Oxycodone *cont.*				Switch to morphine when requirement exceeds 15 mg of oxycodone q3h.
Oxymorphone (Numorphan)	N/A	1 mg IM 5–10 mg PR	q3–4h q4–6h	Morphine analog. No oral formulation.
Partial Agonists				
Buprenorphine (Buprenex)	0.4 mg (SL)	0.3 mg	q4–6h IM	Alternative to morphine in low to middle part of morphine's dose range (up to around 180–300 mg/day). Analgesic ceiling around 3–5 mg/24 hr. Sublingual form not available in United States. Can precipitate withdrawal. Very high doses of naloxone are required to reverse effects.
Opioid Agonist-Antagonists				
Pentazocine (Talwin)	180 mg	60 mg IM	q3–6h	NOT recommended for cancer patients: Analgesic ceiling. Unpleasant psychotomimetic effects (dysphoria, hallucinations). Risk of precipitating withdrawal in opioid-dependent patients.
Butorphanol (Stadol)	N/A	2 mg	q3–4h	As for pentazocine.
Nalbuphine (Nubain)	N/A	10 mg IM	q3–4h	As for pentazocine, but psychotomimetic effects less severe.

N/A = not available.

TABLE 1.3   Adjuvant Analgesic Drugs

Class	Drug	Comments
Anticonvulsants		Used to manage neuropathic pain. Serum levels should be monitored.
	Carbamazepine	Useful for lancinating neuralgic pain. Major side effects: nausea, vomiting, dizziness, ataxia, lethargy. May cause bone marrow suppression.
	Clonazepam	Found to be most effective in comparative studies. Causes the most drowsiness of all the anticonvulsants.
	Phenytoin	Least toxic but also the least effective for neuropathic pain.
	Valproate	More GI side effects than other anticonvulsants.
Local anesthetics	Mexiletine (PO) Flecainide (PO) Lidocaine (IV)	Used for neuropathic pain (not FDA-approved for this indication).
Tricyclic antidepressants	Amitriptyline Imipramine Nortriptyline	For postherpetic neuralgia, superficial dysesthesias. Dosage to produce analgesia is usually below that needed for antidepressant effect, and onset of action is usually more rapid than when used for depression (within 4–6 days). Anticholinergic side effects may be troublesome. To minimize adverse effects, start at low doses and escalate slowly. Use amitriptyline when sedation is a desired side effect.
Corticosteroids	Dexamethasone Prednisolone	Reduce bone pain of metastatic origin. Ameliorate headache due to ↑intracranial pressure. Relieve pain from epidural spinal cord compression and from tumor infiltration of a peripheral nerve or plexus. Improve overall sense of well-being.
Phenothiazines	Methotrimeprazine	The only phenothiazine with analgesic properties (15 mg IM is equianalgesic to 10 mg of IM morphine).

continued

TABLE 1.3   **Adjuvant Analgesic Drugs**   *continued*

Class	Drug	Comments
	Methotrime-prazine *cont.*	Nonopiate receptor mechanism (probably works through α-adrenergic blockade). Nonconstipating and does not cause respiratory depression. Use when sedation is a desired side effect. Also has very strong antiemetic properties.
Antihistamines	Hydroxyzine	Analgesic effect additive to that of opioids. Has additional antiemetic, antispasmodic, anxiolytic, sedative, and bronchodilator effects.
Amphetamines	Dextroamphetamine Methylphenidate Pemoline	Seem to potentiate the action of opioid analgesics. Useful when it is desirable to opioid-induced drowsiness.
Biphosphonates	Pamidronate Clodronate	May relieve malignant bone pain, especially pamidronate when given IV at 2- to 3-week intervals.

Radiation Therapy

Indications

Radiation therapy gives good to excellent relief in
- **Painful bone metastases** (55–66% experience total pain relief; 90% experience worthwhile relief).
- Pain due to acute **spinal cord compression**.
- Chest pain secondary to inoperable bronchial carcinoma.
- **Dysphagia** due to cancer of the esophagus or gastric cardia. (When combined with 5-FU/mitomycin C chemotherapy, radiation therapy provides rapid, long-duration improvement of swallowing in up to 91% of patients.)

Techniques

- **Local external beam irradiation**:
  - For palliative treatment of most localized bone metastases, a **single dose of 8 Gy** is equally effective as fractionated doses and is much easier for the patient.

- Dose fractionation may be appropriate for prevention of pathologic fracture in lytic lesions (to enhance recalcification) and for acute spinal cord compression (to minimize reactive edema).
  - **Hemibody irradiation** may be indicated for patients with widespread disease.
    - Produces overall response rates of 73% to 100%, complete response rates of 5% to 57%.
    - Most patients **respond within 48 hours.**
    - Pain relief is independent of the radiosensitivity of the tumor.
    - **Toxicity** is greater than with local external beam irradiation → patient should be premedicated with dexamethsone, antiemetics (metoclopramide), and hydration to minimize acute GI effects (nausea, diarrhea 12–24 hours after treatment).
    - Maximal tolerated doses:
      - Upper body: a single fraction of 6 Gy.
      - Lower body: a single fraction of 8 Gy.
  - **Radiopharmaceuticals**:
    - Beta-emitting radiopharmaceuticals concentrate at sites of osteoblastic activity and deliver a **localized dose of irradiation at the metastatic site**.
      - Most commonly used in cancers of the prostate and breast.
      - Response is slower than with external beam radiation (2–4 weeks).
      - Response rates range from 37% to 92%.
    - Most frequently used:
      - **Strontium 89**.
      - Phosphorus 32 (more apt to cause myelosuppression).
      - Iodine 131, for metastases from carcinoma of the thyroid.
    - Can be given as a **single outpatient injection**.
    - Very expensive.

Chemotherapy

- *In responsive tumors*, chemotherapy may provide excellent pain relief of long duration, especially when pain is due to
  - Leptomeningeal disease or intracranial metastases.
  - Multiple liver metastases.
  - Colorectal cancer.
  - Recurrent squamous cell cancers of the head and neck.
- Guidelines for the use of chemotherapy to palliate pain in advanced cancer:
  - Use **oral formulations** whenever possible.

- Choose **single-agent** rather than combination regimens.
- Choose agents with the lowest toxicity.
- Start at submaximal dosage and escalate gradually to the point of toxicity, then back down.
- Give short courses.

Hormonal Therapy

- Hormonal manipulation is used principally for cancers arising in cells that have an endocrine function (breast, endometrium, prostate).
- Some hormonal therapies *induce* pain by producing a transient (1- to 2-week) "**tumor flare**," associated with diffuse aching at sites of bone metastases. Tumor flare is most likely with
  - Breast cancer: tamoxifen, progestational agents (megestrol, medroxyprogesterone), and gonadotropin-releasing hormone analogs (goserelin, leuprorelin).
  - Prostate cancer: gonadotropin-releasing hormone analogs (goserelin, leuprorelin).
- Hormonal therapy to *relieve* pain is most likely to be effective in **carcinoma of the prostate**.
  - **Bilateral orchidectomy** brings about relief of bone pain in 60% to 80% of patients within hours of surgery; effects last up to 2 years.
  - Similar response rates can be achieved with diethylstilbestrol (1 mg PO qd), but onset of pain relief is slower.
- In carcinoma of the **breast, progestational agents** (megestrol, medroxyprogesterone) may give long-duration relief of pain from bony metastases:
  - Improvement will occur within 1 to 2 weeks in patients who are destined to respond and will be maximal in less than a month.
  - The patient should receive adequate analgesic coverage by other means during the period of tumor flare.

Surgery

- Tumor debulking by itself generally does not provide palliation of pain.
- *Indications* for palliative surgery:
  - Stabilization of a long bone with lytic metastases to prevent pathologic fracture.
  - Decompression of the spinal canal to prevent impending paralysis.
  - Relief of bowel obstruction in selected patients when conservative treatment fails (see Chapter 21).

Anesthetic Procedures

- Most helpful in treating well-localized somatic or visceral pain.
- Not very effective for deafferentation pain.

TABLE 1.4   Anesthetic Procedures Used to Control Cancer Pain

Procedure	Indications and Comments
Trigger point injection	Localized myofascial pain with an identifiable, tender trigger point.
Nitrous oxide inhalation	Generalized pain, especially when unresponsive to escalating doses of opioids. Incident pain. Patient controls the level of anesthesia. Usually is *not* sedating in the context of severe pain and may in fact increase the patient's level of alertness.
Continuous epidural infusion with opioids and/or local anesthetics	Unilateral and bilateral lumbosacral pain. Midline perineal pain. Usually allows reduction of systemic opioid dosage, but tolerance to epidural opioids develops within days to weeks.
Nerve Blocks	
Peripheral	Somatic pain in discrete dermatomes, usually in the head, chest, or abdomen (e.g., intercostal block for chest wall pain; paravertebral block for radicular pain). If successful, may proceed to neurolytic blockade with phenol for more prolonged (2- to 3-month) relief.
Epidural Intrathecal	Chest wall pain extending over several dermatomes. Unilateral lumbar or sacral pain. Midline perineal pain. Bilateral lumbosacral pain.
Autonomic	
Celiac plexus	Midabdominal pain, especially from pancreatic cancer.
Stellate ganglion	Reflex sympathetic dystrophy. Postherpetic neuralgia. Arm pain from brachial plexopathies.
Lumbar sympathetic	Reflex sympathetic dystrophy. Intractable urogenital pain.

Neurosurgical Procedures

▪ **Neuroablation:** Procedures that interrupt specific nerve tracts (e.g., rhizotomy → dorsal nerve root; cordotomy → spinothalamic tract; myelotomy → polysynaptic pain pathway that runs through the center of the spinal cord).

▪ **Neurostimulating procedures:**
   • Based on "gate theory": Electrical stimulation of large-diameter nerve fibers inhibits pain, at the level of the interneurons in the substantia gelatinosa, by "closing the gate" to impulses from the small-diameter fibers that carry noxious sensation.
   • Electrical stimulation of the dorsal columns has been used to treat deafferentation pain in the chest, midline, or lower extremities.

Physical Modalities

▪ **Local heat** (hot water bottle; electric heating pad; hot moist compresses; immersion in hot water):
   • Indications:
     - Joint stiffness.
     - Muscle spasms.
     - Pain that the patient reports is relieved by a hot shower.
   • Hot packs should be wrapped well in toweling to prevent burns.
   • Heat should not be applied to areas exposed to radiation therapy.
   • There is no conclusive evidence that the use of heat over tumor sites increases tumor growth, and there are **no contraindications to the use of heat to relieve pain in advanced cancer**.
▪ **Local cold applications** (ice packs, towels soaked in ice water):
   • May relieve burning pain or muscle spasm, when heat is ineffective.
   • Ice packs should be sealed and wrapped in toweling to prevent skin irritation.
   • Apply for no more than 15 minutes at a time.
   • Do not apply to tissue that has been damaged by radiation, in peripheral vascular disease, or in patients with allodynia (pain due to a stimulus that does not ordinarily provoke pain).
▪ **Massage:**
   • Comfort measure to ease general aches and pains.
   • Terminally ill patients generally do not tolerate deep or vigorous massage; light massage, using baby oil or alcohol-free lotion, is generally preferred.

- **Transcutaneous electrical nerve stimulation (TENS)**:
  - *Indications in palliative care*: mild to moderate pain, especially
    - Pain in the head and neck regions.
    - Pain due to nerve compression or nerve infiltration by tumor.
    - Postherpetic neuralgia.
    - Bone pain from metastases or multiple myeloma.
  - Response may be good to excellent at first but tends to decay over several weeks of use.
  - See Appendix 3 for details of TENS treatment methods.
- **Vibration therapy**:
  - Mechanism not fully understood; does not work via endogenous opioids and may involve stimulation of pacinian corpuscles.
  - Indicated primarily for pain arising in nerves or muscles.
  - Works best at frequencies around 100 Hz.
  - Apply near or distal to painful site with moderate pressure for 45 minutes.
- **Acupuncture**:
  - Very few studies have evaluated the effectiveness of acupuncture in cancer pain.
  - Acupuncture may be helpful in pain due to
    - Painful muscle spasms.
    - Bladder spasms.
    - Hyperesthesia, dysesthesia, postherpetic neuralgia.
- **Exercise**:
  - Patients should be encouraged to remain active as long as possible, to maintain muscle strength, joint mobility, coordination, and balance.
  - When patient can no longer exercise actively, gentle **passive range-of-motion exercises** should be performed to preserve muscle length and joint function (passive exercises should *not* be carried out if they increase pain).

Psychosocial Interventions

- Part of the multimodal approach to pain, in conjunction with analgesics.
- The goal of most psychosocial interventions is to help the patient **regain a sense of control** that has been undermined by illness and debility.
- Psychosocial interventions work best when introduced early in the course of the illness, when the patient still has the energy to learn and practice a given technique.

- Psychosocial interventions include
  - Patient education to provide accurate information about pain and pain control and to address fears regarding the use of opioids (e.g., fear of addiction, tolerance, side effects).
  - Relaxation techniques (e.g., focused breathing exercises, progressive muscle relaxation, meditation).
  - Guided imagery.
  - Hypnosis.
  - Cognitive and behavioral therapies.

References and Further Reading

Aaron AD. The management of cancer metastatic to bone. *JAMA* 272:1206, 1994.

Bates TD. The management of bone metastases: radiotherapy. *Palliative Med* 1:117, 1987.

Billings JA. Neuropathic pain. *J Palliative Care* 10(4):40, 1994.

Bruera E, Watanabe S. Psychostimulants as adjuvant analgesics. *J Pain Symptom Manage* 9:412, 1994.

Cherny NI, Portenoy RK. Cancer Pain: Principles of Assessment and Syndromes. In Melzack R, Wall PD (eds). *Textbook of Pain*. Edinburgh: Churchill-Livingstone, 1994, Chap. 43.

Coia LR, Soffen EM, Schultheiss TE, et al. Swallowing function in patients with esophageal cancer treated with concurrent radiation and chemotherapy. *Cancer* 71:281, 1993.

Collins TM, Ash CV, Close HJ, Thorogood J. An evaluation of the palliative role of radiotherapy in inoperable carcinoma of the bronchus. *Clin Radiol* 39:284, 1988.

Ellershaw JE, Kelly MJ. Corticosteroids and peptic ulceration. *Palliative Med* 8:313, 1994.

Fosburg MT, Crone RK. Nitrous oxide analgesia for refractory pain in the terminally ill. *JAMA* 250:511, 1983.

International Association for the Study of Pain. Subcommittee on taxonomy of pain terms: A list with definitions and notes on usage. *Pain* 6:249, 1979.

Kearsley JH. Some basic guidelines in the use of chemotherapy for patients with incurable malignancy. *Palliative Med* 8:11, 1994.

Melzack R, Wall PD. Pain mechanisms: A new theory. *Science* 150:971, 1965.

Needham PR, Hoskin PJ. Radiotherapy for painful bone metastases. *Palliative Med* 8:95, 1994.

Rakowsky E, Klein B, Marshak G, Lurie H. 5-Fluorouracil and high dose folinic acid in symptomatic advanced colorectal carcinoma: importance of symptomatic relief. *Palliative Med* 5:250, 1991.

Romond EH, Metcalfe MS, Macdonald JS. Palliative chemotherapy and hormonal therapy. *Semin Oncol* 12:384, 1985.

Saunders CM (ed). *The Management of Terminal Disease*. London: Edward Arnold, 1978.

Twycross RG, Fairfield S. Pain in far advanced cancer. *Pain* 14:303, 1982.

Vibration therapy for pain (editorial). *Lancet* 339:1513, 1992.

Watanabe S, Bruera E. Corticosteroids as adjuvant analgesics. *J Pain Symptom Manage* 9:442, 1994.

Watson CPN. Antidepressant drugs as adjuvant analgesics. *J Pain Symptom Manage* 9:392, 1994.

World Health Organization. *Revised Method for Relief of Cancer Pain and Other Symptoms Management*. Geneva: WHO, 1994.

2 Principles and Techniques of Pharmacologic Management

We must all die. But that I can save him from days of torture, that is what I feel as my great and new privilege. Pain is a more terrible lord of mankind than even death itself.

ALBERT SCHWEITZER, *ON THE EDGE OF THE PRIMEVAL FOREST*

Evaluation of the Patient with Pain

- **Believe the patient's complaint of pain**.
- **Take a careful history**:
  - Determine **extent of disease** and previous **treatments**.
  - Place the pain temporally in the patient's cancer history.
  - Define the characteristics of the pain:
    - **Site(s)**.
    - Pattern of **referral**.
    - **Timing**: constant versus intermittent versus incident (only during activity).
    - **Quality** (e.g., aching, burning, lancinating, crampy).
    - **Severity**: Use **quantitative pain scale** (e.g., visual analog, verbal numerical), and document in patient's chart (Figure 2.1).

Number each type of pain on the body diagram at
the right:

Pain #:	1	2	3	4
Severity				
Mild				
Moderate				
Severe				
Unbearable				
Duration				
1–2 weeks				
2–6 weeks				
6–12 weeks				
>12 weeks				
Timing				
Constant				
Intermittent				
Interferes with:				
Sleep				
Function or mobility				

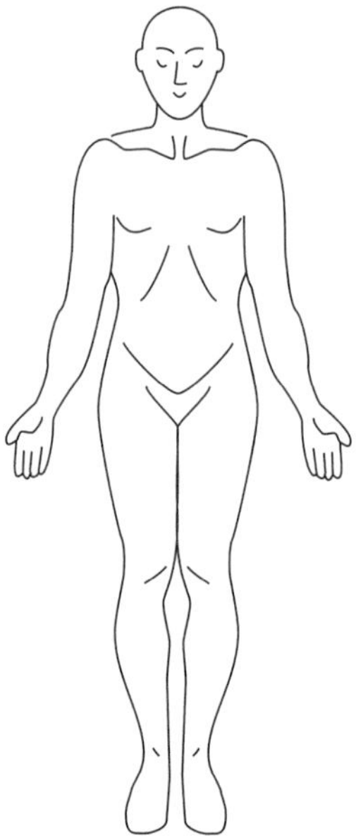

Drugs taken for pain and dosages:
1.   3.
2.   4.

Other treatment modalities:

Nerve block				
Radiation therapy				
Other:				
Effectiveness:				
No effect				
Partial pain relief				
Complete pain relief				

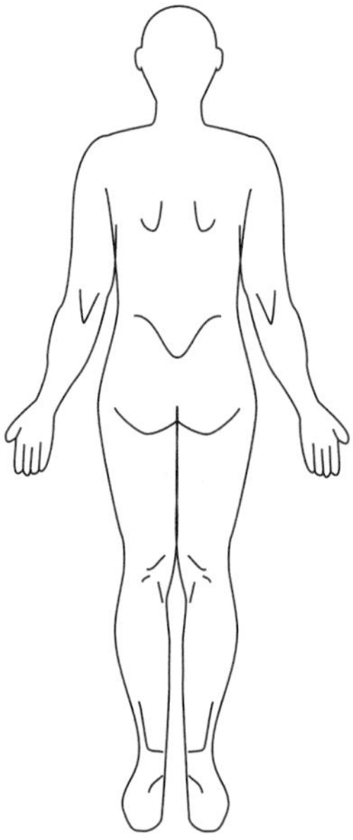

Impressions from the patient's family: _____

_____

_____

Other information: _____

_____

_____

Probable sources of the patient's pain(s):
1. _____
2. _____
3. _____
4. _____
5. _____

FIGURE 2.1   Tel Hashomer Pain Assessment Chart (based on the model from
St. Christopher's Hospice, London).

- **Aggravating/relieving factors.**
- Response to **medications.** For each medication the patient takes, find out:
  ◦ Dosage and dosing interval.
  ◦ Route of administration.
  ◦ How long the patient has taken the medication.
  ◦ To what extent the medication relieves pain and for how long.
  ◦ Whether there have been adverse effects.
- Response to other measures tried for relief (heat, cold, massage).
- **Interference** with daily activities, sleep.
- Other **medical disorders** (e.g., hypercalcemia, diabetes).
- Other **symptoms** (e.g., constipation, nausea, asthenia).
- **Functional status** (Karnofsky, ECOG).
- Characteristics of the patient:
  - Personality.
  - Psychological state (evidence of anxiety, depression).
  - Previous pain history.
- **Verify history** from a family member.
- **Careful medical/neurologic examination:**
  - Areas of skin hypo- or hypersensitivity.
  - Areas of sensory loss.
  - Trigger points.
  - Motor weakness, atrophy.
- Evaluate the patient's **extent of disease.**
- Make a specific **pain diagnosis.** → Outline the **therapeutic approach.**
- **Reassess** over and over again.

General Principles of Pain Management

The principles of managing pain in patients with cancer have been summarized as follows by the World Health Organization:

- By mouth
- By the clock
- By the ladder
- For the individual
- Use of adjuvants
- Attention to detail

- **By mouth**: The oral route is the route of administration of choice for analgesic (and other) medications whenever possible.
  - Spares patients painful injections.
  - Gives patients more control over their situation, since they are not dependent on others to receive their medication.
- **By the clock**: Analgesic medications for moderate to severe pain should be given on a fixed dose schedule around the clock and not on an "as needed" basis.
  - Patients hesitate to use medications prescribed on a "prn" basis ("I'll just wait a little longer....").
  - Scheduled dosing ensures that the next dose is given before the effect of the previous dose has worn off → more consistent and reliable pain relief.
  - When pain is allowed to reemerge before the next dose of analgesic
    - The patient experiences needless additional suffering.
    - Tolerance is more likely to occur, requiring escalating doses.
- **By the ladder**:
  - The World Health Organization (WHO) has developed a three-step analgesic ladder to guide the sequential use of drugs in treating cancer pain (Figure 2.2).
  - For patients with mild to moderate pain, the **first step** is to use a **nonopioid** drug, with the addition of an adjuvant drug as required by the situation (see discussion below).
  - If the nonopioid drug, given at the recommended dosage and frequency, does not relieve the patient's pain, the **second step** is to add a **weak opioid** (again with or without an adjuvant drug, as required).
  - If the combination of a nonopioid plus a weak opioid still does not relieve the pain, as a **third step**, a **strong opioid** should be substituted for the weak opioid.

Summary: WHO Analgesic Ladder

Step	Category	Prototype	Substitutes
1	Nonopioid	Aspirin	Acetaminophen NSAIDs
2	Weak opioid	Codeine	Propoxyphene (Darvon)
3	Strong opioid	Morphine	Hydromorphone (Dilaudid) Methadone Fentanyl Levorphanol (Levo-Dacmoran)

- **For the individual**:
  - Individual requirements for analgesics vary enormously.
    - The average patient will require the equivalent of 60 to 120 mg of oral morphine per day.
    - Some patients will require less opioid.
    - A small percentage of patients may require very high doses (e.g., > 2000 mg/day).
  - The dosage of analgesic must be titrated against the particular patient's pain.

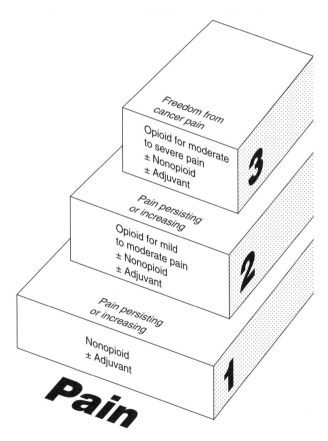

FIGURE 2.2   Three-step analgesic ladder. Redrawn, by permission from: *Cancer Pain Relief and Palliative Care: Report of a WHO Expert Committee*. Geneva: World Health Organization, 1990 (Technical Report Series, No. 804), Fig. 1.

> THE RIGHT DOSAGE OF MORPHINE IS THE
> DOSAGE THAT RELIEVES THE PATIENT'S PAIN
> WITHOUT INTOLERABLE SIDE EFFECTS.

- **Use of adjuvants:**
  - To enhance analgesic effects (e.g., corticosteroids, anticonvulsants).
  - To control adverse effects of opioids (e.g., antiemetics, laxatives).
  - To manage symptoms that are contributing to the patient's pain (anxiety, depression, insomnia).
- **Attention to detail:**
  - Take nothing for granted.
  - Be precise in history taking.
  - Explore the patient's "total pain."
  - Determine what the patient knows about the situation and what the patient believes and fears about the pain and the things that can relieve it.
  - Give the patient precise instructions, both orally and in writing, for how to take the prescribed medications.

Starting Analgesic Therapy

> - Aim for graded relief.
> - Start with a specific drug for a specific pain.
> - Choose an appropriate route of administration.
> - Titrate the dosage of opioid.
> - Provide for rescue doses.
> - Anticipate and treat side effects.

- **Aim for graded relief:**
  - The initial goal is a **pain-free night's sleep** to break the cycle of pain → insomnia → exhaustion → ↑pain (should be achievable within 24 to 48 hours).
  - The next goal is **relief of pain at rest**.
  - Finally, the aim is **relief of pain during weight bearing and movement**, if possible.
- **Start with a specific drug for a specific pain:**

Type of Pain/Quality of Pain	*Treatment (Analgesics + Adjuncts)**
Visceral ("Aches all the time")	Mild: **Acetaminophen**, 1 gm q4h, *or* **aspirin**, 650 mg qid pc, *or* **naproxen**, 500 mg bid. Moderate: **codeine**, 60 mg q4h + NSAID. Severe: **morphine** (see text for technique of dosage titration) + **dexamethasone**, 4 mg qam.
Bone ("Worse when I move")	**NSAID**: Aspirin, 650 mg q4h, *or* naproxen, 500 mg bid. Cover with misoprostol ± H$_2$ blocker, antacids. Consider **radiation therapy**: single dose of 8 Gy of radionuclide (e.g., strontium 89). Consider biphosphonates: **clodronate**, 800 mg PO bid.
Neuropathic Pain ("Burning, stabbing")	
Nerve compression	**Opioid**, as above + **dexamethasone** 2-4 mg qd.
Superficial dysesthesia	**Opioid**, as above + **amitriptyline** (Elavil), 25-100 mg hs, *or* **imipramine** (Tofranil), titrate to 100-150 mg hs.
Intermittent stabbing	**Opioid**, as above + **clonazepam** (Klonopin), 0.5 mg tid, *or* **carbamazepine** (Tegretol), 200 mg bid-tid + **mexiletine** (Mexitil), 200 mg tid. Try TENS.
Increased Intracranial Pressure	**Dexamethasone**, 16 mg qam (titrate upward if no effect).
Gastric Distention	**Metoclopramide** (Reglan), 10 mg q4h ± **activated charcoal/simethicone** (Charcoal Plus), 2 tabs qid.
Tenesmus	**Chlorpromazine** (Taroctyl), 12.5 mg q4-8h, *or* **belladonna**, 2 mg PR, *or* local application of 0.1% betamethasone cream ± 2% lidocaine gel.
Muscle Spasm	**Diazepam** (Valium), 10 mg hs, *or* **baclofen** (Baclosal), 10 mg tid. Consider trigger point injection, TENS.

continued

Type of Pain/Quality of Pain	Treatment (Analgesics + Adjuncts)*
Dysuria	**Phenazopyridine** (Pyridium), 200 mg qid. Antibiotics as indicated.
Lymphedema	**Furosemide** (Lasix), 40 mg qam + **spironolactone** (Aldactone), 100 mg qam + **dexamethasone**, 4 mg qam. Consider TENS.
Malignant Ulcer	**Metronidazole** (Flagyl), 400 mg tid, or **clindamycin** (Cleocin), 300 mg tid.

*All dosages are PO (by mouth) unless otherwise indicated.

- **Choose an appropriate route of administration:**

Route	Available Drugs	Comments
Oral (PO)	Acetaminophen All NSAIDs Codeine, propoxyphene, morphine, hydromorphone, levorphanol, methadone, oxycodone	Preferred route of administration whenever possible.
Sublingual (SL) or buccal	Buprenorphine, in some countries (not in United States)	Obviates first-pass metabolism. SL administration of an injectable formulation may be useful in patients transiently unable to swallow.
Rectal (PR)	Morphine, hydromorphone, oxymorphone	PR/PO potency of morphine = 1:1. Controlled-release morphine tablets may also be given PR. PR route contraindicated when there are lesions of the anus or rectum, diarrhea, or fecal impaction.
Transdermal	Fentanyl	Slow onset of action. Patches are applied for 48–72 hours.
Intramuscular (IM)	Morphine, hydromorphone, levorphanol, methadone, oxymorphone	IM/PO potency of morphine = 3:1. Offers no pharmacokinetic advantage over other routes.

Route	Available Drugs	Comments
Intramuscular (IM) *cont.*		Repeated IM injections are unnecessarily painful. Not recommended as a standard route for cancer pain.
Intravenous (IV)	Morphine	IV/PO potency of morphine = 6:1. May rarely be needed to give a loading dose to achieve rapid pain relief. Continuous IV infusion of opioids more likely to produce tolerance than when opioids are given by other routes.
Subcutaneous (SQ)	Morphine, hydromorphone, oxymorphone	Used for continuous infusions. Obviates the need for frequent injections. Maintains steady level of analgesia, without peaks and troughs. Preferred route when PO dosing is not possible.
Epidural and intrathecal	Morphine, hydromorphone, fentanyl and analogs	Requires specialized skills to institute treatment. Tolerance develops relatively rapidly. Significant risk of respiratory depression. Pruritus may be very troublesome.

- **Titrate the dosage of opioids**:
  - There are various methods for starting opioid therapy, and each has its merits. The method described here is the one we have found useful at the Tel Hashomer Hospice.
  - **Before starting opioids**:
    - **Find out** what the patient knows, believes, and **fears about opioids**, and address specific misconceptions and fears with specific facts (Table 2.1).
    - **Describe** anticipated **side effects** in detail, and indicate how long each might be expected to last.
    - Encourage the patient to persevere despite initial side effects.

- If the patient is *not* forewarned about side effects (such as nausea, dizziness, sleepiness), he is likely to conclude that he is "allergic to opioids," and that conviction will follow him throughout the course of his illness, depriving him of the benefits of opioids and thus causing needless misery.

TABLE 2.1   Morphine Misconceptions

Misconception	Fact
Morphine will cause addiction.	**Addiction** (i.e., psychological dependence) is exceedingly rare (4 cases/12,000) when morphine is used to relieve severe pain. **Physical dependence** (the development of a withdrawal syndrome on abrupt dosage reduction or administration of an antagonist), on the other hand, is an intrinsic property of opioid drugs but is *not important clinically* so long as patients are instructed not to discontinue their medication abruptly. If the need for opioid analgesia should decrease or cease altogether (e.g., after radiation therapy), opioids may be safely stopped by tapering the dose over several days (see text).
Tolerance to morphine's analgesic effects develops rapidly, and if it is given too early, morphine will not be effective later, when the patient really needs it.	The majority of patients can be maintained for long periods on a stable dose of morphine. If pain relief becomes inadequate at a given dosage (usually because of disease progression, not true tolerance), all that is necessary to regain a good level of analgesia is to increase the dosage. Morphine has no analgesic ceiling.
Morphine causes dangerous respiratory depression.	Clinically significant respiratory depression does not occur in cancer patients, even patients with COPD, when morphine dosage is titrated according to the patient's pain, for the pain antagonizes morphine's depressant effects. Tolerance to respiratory effects of morphine develops rapidly.
Morphine will make the patient into a "zombie."	When titrated against pain, morphine does not usually produce excess sedation, except during the first few days of treatment.

Misconception	*Fact*
Morphine hastens death.	There is no evidence that morphine given in a dosage appropriate to produce analgesia either shortens or prolongs life. The object of giving opioids is to improve the *quality* of whatever time remains to the patient, whether months or days.

- For **opioid-naive patients** (patients who have not taken opioids previously):
  - For the first day, take **immediate-release morphine** tablets, **7.5 mg** as needed to relieve pain.
  - On the second day, **add up the total** dose taken during the previous 24 hours.
  - **Divide** the total dose **by 2** to arrive at the twice-daily dosage of **controlled-release morphine.**
- For **patients already taking opioids** but whose pain is inadequately controlled:
  - Calculate the patient's current 24-hour dosage of controlled-release morphine.
  - Use ⅙ **of the current 24-hour dosage as a rescue dose** of immediate-release morphine.
  - The rescue dose may be taken as often as
    - Every hour PO, or
    - Every ½ hour IM.
  - After 1 day, **add up all the morphine** the patient has taken during the previous 24 hours (controlled-release morphine plus all the rescue doses of immediate-release morphine).
  - **Divide** the total **by 2** to arrive at the new twice-daily dosage of controlled-release morphine.

EXAMPLE: A patient taking controlled-release morphine, 90 mg bid, is having severe pain. He is instructed to take 30 mg PO (i.e., [90 × 2] × ⅙) of immediate-release morphine as needed to achieve relief of pain, as often as every hour if necessary, and to keep a record of how much he has taken. The following day, he reports that he needed four 30-mg tablets of immediate-release morphine in addition to his regular dosage of controlled-release morphine. That is, he has taken:

Controlled-release morphine: 90 mg × 2 = 180 mg
Immediate-release morphine: 30 mg × 4 = 120 mg
Total = 300 mg
Total ÷ 2 = new dosage of controlled-release morphine = 150 mg bid

- **Provide for rescue doses:**
  - Patients receiving round-the-clock opioids should also be furnished with "rescue doses" of a short-acting opioid in the event that pain breaks through the coverage with controlled-release opioid.
  - **Rescue dose = ¹⁄₆ × 24-hour dose** of controlled-release morphine.

Situation	Definition	Management
Breakthrough pain	Intermittent exacerbations of pain (occurring spontaneously or related to activity).	Supplement CR morphine with a rapid-onset, short-duration opioid at ⅙ the 24-hour morphine dosage. Patient-controlled analgesia for those receiving continuous SQ infusion.
Incident pain	Pain related to a specific activity (e.g., bathing the patient).	Give a short-acting opioid 15–20 minutes before the anticipated activity.
End-of-dose failure	Pain exacerbated predictably before the next scheduled dose of CR morphine.	Increase the dosage of CR morphine *or* decrease the dosing interval (from q12h to q8h).

- If opioid side effects are problematic and breakthrough pain is not severe, the medication prescribed for "rescue" can be a nonopioid (e.g., an NSAID).
- **Anticipate and treat side effects:**

Side Effect	Prevention or Treatment	Comments
Sedation	Discontinue other drugs that may have additive sedative effects (e.g., benzodiazepines, barbiturates). Can add: **Dextroamphetamine**, 5–10 mg PO bid, *or* **methylphenidate** (Ritalin), 10 mg PO at 0800 and 5 mg PO at 1200.	Warn patient that sedation is likely during the first 3–5 days of opioid treatment but usually improves thereafter, although drowsiness during inactivity may persist.
Respiratory depression	If severe (respiratory rate < 8–10/min) and accompanied by depressed consciousness, give **naloxone**, 0.4 mg diluted in 10 ml	Usually not clinically important. Tolerance to this side effect develops very rapidly.

Side Effect	Prevention or Treatment	Comments
Respiratory depression *cont.*	of saline *slowly* IV, titrated to the respiratory response.	
Nausea and vomiting	Prescribe an antiemetic, such as **haloperidol** (Haldol), 0.5-100 mg PO hs, *or* **fluphenazine**, 0.5-200 mg PO bid, to be taken if nausea/vomiting occurs (not as routine prophylaxis).	Occur in about 65% of patients starting morphine treatment. Tolerance develops relatively rapidly (within 5-10 days).
Constipation	Start a bowel regimen together with opioids: **bisacodyl** (Dulcolax), 5 mg PO hs + **lactulose** (Chronulac), 10-30 ml PO bid ± **docusate** (Colace), 2 tabs PO bid	Nearly universal in patients taking opioids, and can become a more intractable problem than the pain. Due to both ↓gut secretion and ↓peristalsis.
Myoclonus	**Clonazepam**, 0.5 mg PO tid or 1 mg PO hs	More likely in patients taking relatively high doses of opioids. More likely in patients taking neuroleptics, antidepressants, or NSAIDs in addition to opioids.
Sweating	**Dexamethasone**, 4 mg PO qam, *or* an NSAID	More likely in patients with primary or metastatic liver involvement.
Confusion, dizziness	Warn elderly patients that they may become confused or dizzy at times for the first few days of treatment but that the effect will wear off.	Postural hypotension may cause dizziness in the elderly.
Acute urinary retention	Urinary catheterization	
Pruritus	Try an oral antihistamine: **Diphenhydramine**, 25-50 mg PO hs, *or* **hydroxyzine**, 25 mg PO hs.	Due to morphine-induced histamine release, which may also cause bronchoconstriction.

Follow-up and Reassessment

- **Ongoing reassessment** of pain management is necessary so long as the patient is alive.
  - Pain is a dynamic process and may change from hour to hour.
    - **New pains** may arise at any time. A change in the patient's pain pattern or the development of a new pain should not be automatically attributed to preexisting causes. New pain may arise from
      - **Disease progression** with invasion of new sites.
      - **A treatable acute problem** (e.g., infection, pathologic fracture).
      - Side effects of some treatments (e.g., epigastric pain from NSAIDs).
    - **Some pains may lessen**, for example, after radiation therapy of bone metastases → decreased opioid requirements.
  - Side effects of analgesics must be monitored, as they may prevent the patient from taking pain medications.
  - **Every pain assessment should be thoroughly documented** in the patient's chart (see Figure 2.3 for one method of ongoing documentation).
- **Tolerance to opioids**:
  - Definition: The need to increase dosage of a drug over time to maintain a given level of analgesia.
  - Tolerance to most *adverse effects* of opioids (sedation, respiratory depression, nausea) develops relatively rapidly, although tolerance to the constipating and miotic effects develops slowly if at all.
  - **Tolerance to the *analgesic* effects of opioids is relatively uncommon**. In a study of 1000 patients with advanced cancer receiving regular opioids (Brescia et al., 1992):
    - Eighty-one percent were maintained on stable doses of opioids.
    - Fourteen percent were able to discontinue opioids.
    - Only 5% required an average daily dosage increase of more than 10% of the previous dose.
  - In most cancer patients, the **first indication of tolerance** is a **decrease in the *duration* of analgesia** for a given dose of opioid.
  - The **need for increasing doses** of opioids **usually signals disease progression** and not true tolerance.
  - If tolerance does develop, all that is usually needed to regain satisfactory analgesia is to increase the dosage of opioid, in the manner described earlier (i.e., add up the total opioid, including rescue doses, taken during the previous 24 hours, and recalculate the daily dosage accordingly).

Pain Severity:

DATE:																												
PAIN #:	1	2	3	4	1	2	3	4	1	2	3	4	1	2	3	4	1	2	3	4	1	2	3	4	1	2	3	4
Mild																												
Moderate																												
Severe																												
Unbearable																												

Analgesic Medication(s) and Dosage:

DATE:					
Pain #1					
Pain #2					
Pain #3					
Pain #4					

Measurements of Opioid Overdosage:

Pupillary size (mm)					
Respiratory rate					

Side Effects of Analgesics:

	0	+	0	+	0	+	0	+	0	+	0	+	0	+
Constipation														
Diarrhea														
Melena														
Epigastric pain														
Urinary retention														

0 = Absent   + = Present

SEVERITY:	0	1	2	3	0	1	2	3	0	1	2	3	0	1	2	3	0	1	2	3	0	1	2	3	0	1	2	3
Nausea																												
Vomiting																												
Sleepiness																												
Confusion																												

0 = Absent   1 = Mild   2 = Moderate   3 = Severe

Comments: _____

_____

FIGURE 2.3   Ongoing assessment of pain control and analgesic side effects.

- **Cross-tolerance** among opioids is **not complete** → if true tolerance to one opioid occurs, it is possible to switch to another opioid, starting at *half* the predicted equianalgesic dosage, then titrating the dosage upward as needed.
- **Preventing withdrawal from opioids**:
  - Patients with cancer occasionally require rapid reduction of opioid dosage or discontinuation of opioids altogether, for example:
    - When the cause of pain is neutralized by radiotherapy or other antineoplastic treatment.
    - When pain perception is altered by nerve block or neuroablative procedures.
  - In such cases, **opioid withdrawal syndrome can be avoided by tapering the opioid dosage**:
    - For the first 2 days, give half of the previous daily dosage.
    - Then reduce the daily dosage by approximately 25% every 2 days thereafter, until a daily dosage of 30 mg of morphine has been reached.
    - After 2 more days on 30 mg/day of morphine, the opioid may be stopped.

  EXAMPLE: A patient has been taking 120 mg of controlled-release morphine twice a day for many weeks. After a course of radiation therapy, he is pain free. His dosage is tapered as follows:

  Day 1 to 2: 60 mg bid.
  Day 3 to 4: 45 mg bid.
  Day 5 to 6: 30 mg bid.
  Day 7: Discontinue morphine.

- **Transdermal clonidine, 0.1 to 0.2 mg/day**, may be given if needed to reduce anxiety, tachycardia, and other autonomic symptoms that may accompany opioid withdrawal.

References and Further Reading

American Pain Society. *Principles of Analgesic Use in the Treatment of Acute Pain and Chronic Cancer Pain: A Concise Guide to Medical Practice.* Skokie, IL: American Pain Society, 1992.
Brescia FJ, Portenoy RK, Ryan M, et al. Pain, opioid use, and survival in hospitalized patients with advanced cancer. *J Clin Oncol* 10:149, 1992.
Cherny NI, Portenoy RK. The management of cancer pain. *CA* 44:262, 1994.

Coyle N, Adelhardt J, Foley KM, Portenoy RK. Character of terminal illness in the advanced cancer patient: Pain and other symptoms during last four weeks of life. *J Pain Symptom Manage* 5:83, 1990.

Coyle N, Portenoy R. Infection as a cause of rapidly increasing pain in cancer patients. *J Pain Symptom Manage* 6:266, 1991.

Foley KM. The treatment of cancer pain. *N Engl J Med* 313:84, 1985.

Jacox A, Carr DB, Payne R, et al. *Management of Cancer Pain: Clinical Practice Guideline.* No. 9. AHCPR Publication No. 94-0592. Rockville, MD: Agency for Health Care Policy and Research, U.S. Department of Health and Human Services, Public Health Service, March, 1994.

Patt RB (ed). *Cancer Pain.* Philadelphia: Lippincott, 1993.

Twycross RJ. *Pain Relief in Advanced Cancer.* Edinburgh: Churchill Livingstone, 1994.

World Health Organization. *Cancer Pain Relief.* Geneva: WHO, 1986.

Nutrition and
Hydration

3 Nutrition and Hydration

An article of food or drink which is slightly inferior, but more palatable, is to be preferred to that which is superior but less palatable.

HIPPOCRATES, *APHORISMS, II.38.*

The Impact of Cancer and Its Treatment on Nutrition

Cancer Cachexia

Cancer cachexia is the name given to a symptom complex comprising
- Anorexia.
- Early satiety.
- Weight loss.
- Anemia.
- Asthenia.
- Tissue wasting.
- Organ dysfunction.

Incidence of Cachexia in Different Cancers

Lowest Incidence	Intermediate Incidence	Highest Incidence
Breast cancer	Colon cancer	Pancreatic cancer
Sarcoma	Prostate cancer	Gastric cancer
Non-Hodgkin's lymphomas	Lung cancer	

- No correlation between tumor extent and weight loss (except in breast cancer).

Causes of Cachexia in Cancer Patients

- **Decreased nutritional intake** is probably the most important factor. It occurs as a result of
  - **Anorexia,** which is present in 80% of terminal cancer patients (see Chapter 13).
  - **Malfunction of the gastrointestinal tract:**
    - Cancer of oral cavity, pharynx, esophagus → **odynophagia/ dysphagia.**
    - Gastric cancer → **reduced gastric capacity,** partial gastric outlet obstruction → nausea and vomiting, early satiety, protein-losing enteropathy.
    - Intestinal tumors → **mechanical obstruction,** blind loop.
    - Pancreatic cancer → **malabsorption.**
  - **Psychological factors:**
    - Depression, grief, anxiety → poor appetite.
    - Fear of recurrence → fear of weight loss as a sign of tumor progression.
    - Learned food aversions.
- **Increased nutritional losses:**
  - Bleeding.
  - Protein losses through the intestine.
  - Diarrhea (carcinoid, pancreatic cancer, bowel resection, cancer-induced **lactase deficiency**).
  - **Tumor-related catabolism has little effect** (only metabolically active tumors >1.4 kg could consume more than 15% of daily caloric intake).

- **Abnormalities of substrate metabolism** that mimic insulin resistance:
  - Increased energy expenditure correlated with malignancy, unrelated to extent of disease.
  - Changes in **carbohydrate metabolism**: inefficient energy utilization.
  - Changes in **lipid metabolism**: decrease in total body fat (related to insulin deficiency) and increased oxidation of fatty acids.
  - Abnormalities in **protein metabolism**: nitrogen depletion, negative nitrogen balance, decreased muscle protein synthesis.
  - Changes in body composition:
    - Increased ECF and total body sodium.
    - Decreased ICF and total body potassium.
- **Effects of antitumor treatment** on nutrition:
  - Surgery → negative nitrogen balance.
  - Chemotherapy:
    - Nausea/vomiting (e.g., cisplatin, mustard, DTIC).
    - Mucositis/esophagitis (5-FU, MTX, Adriamycin, bleomycin, vinblastine).
  - Radiotherapy:
    - Anorexia, nausea, vomiting.
    - Dysphagia, odynophagia.
    - Xerostomia.
    - Enteritis, colitis, diarrhea.

Consequences of Malnutrition in the Cancer Patient

- Survival is shorter in patients who have experienced weight loss as a consequence of their cancer.
- **Protein depletion**:
  - Principally from peripheral rather than visceral muscle.
  - Eventually depleted enzymes, serum proteins.
  - **Impaired immunocompetence** (nutritional therapy reverses anergy).
- **Poor wound healing**.
- **Death** occurs when 30% to 50% of body protein stores are lost.

Nutritional Assessment

History

- Rate and extent of **weight loss** (weight loss >10% of body weight over 3 months = malnutrition).

- Symptoms of malabsorption.
- Special diets.
- Problems with taste, chewing, swallowing; nausea/vomiting.
- Food allergies.
- Medicine and alcohol intake.
- Learned food aversion

Physical Examination

- Dry, scaly, atrophic skin.
- Cheilosis, glossitis, or other vitamin deficiency signs.
- **Muscle wasting**, loss of muscle strength.
- Pitting **edema**.

Laboratory Tests

- Serum **albumin**:
  - Below 3.4 gm/dl associated with increased morbidity/mortality.
  - Below 3.0 gm/dl indicates significant visceral protein depletion.

Nutritional Therapy in Patients Undergoing Treatment for Cancer

General Principles

- The most effective way to improve a cancer patient's nutritional status is to **control the cancer**.
- Goals of nutritional therapy:
  - To prevent/reverse nutritional deficits → reduce morbidity from cancer treatment.
  - To increase treatment response rates and survival.
  - To improve quality of life.
  - To palliate symptoms.
- Factors to consider in choosing nutritional strategy:
  - Patient's ability to chew/swallow.
  - Patient's capacity to digest/absorb enteral nutrition.
  - Patient compliance.
  - Family support.
  - Cost.

Indications for Nutritional Therapy

- For malnourished cancer patients or those expected to become malnourished during the course of their disease:
  - Patients undergoing a major operation for upper GI malignancy.
  - Chemotherapy patient with severe GI dysfunction.
- Total parenteral nutrition (TPN) decreases operative morbidity/mortality but has *not* been demonstrated to improve survival of any group of patients with cancer and may, indeed, produce net harm (American College of Physicians, 1989; Terepka and Waterhouse, 1956).

Routes of Administration

Choice of route of administration is based primarily on functional status of the GI tract (if GI tract is normal, **enteral feeding** is always **preferred**).

- **Oral** treatment is indicated in any patient able to ingest sufficient nutrients.
  - Prescribed **diet** should take into account the pathophysiology of the patient's condition:

Condition	Dietary Prescription
Gastric resection	5-6 small meals. Separation of liquids from solids. Restrict monocarbohydrates. Restrict lactose-containing foods. Iron supplementation/parenteral B_{12}.
Short bowel	Frequent small meals. Low-fiber, low-fat diet. Restrict monocarbohydrates, lactose. Supplement with Ca, Mg, Zn (and B_{12} if terminal ileum was resected).
Pancreatic insufficiency	Low-fat diet. Pancreatic enzymes.
Chronic radiation enteritis	Low-fat, low-fiber diet. Restrict lactose-containing foods.
Esophageal strictures	Soft diet, emphasis on liquids or high-caloric nutritional supplements.
Post laryngectomy	Solids and soft foods. Avoid liquids.

- Dietitian should provide instructions regarding specific foods, size and frequency of meals, and other details.
- Diet should deal with **specific problems of oral feeding**:

Problem	Approaches to Solution
Anorexia	Small, frequent feedings. Meals high in calories and protein. Avoid fluid intake with meals to prevent early satiety. Consider **megestrol acetate** (Megace), **160 mg PO qd–tid**, if not contraindicated by disease state (also reduces nausea and vomiting).
Nausea/vomiting	Eat **salty foods**; avoid sweet, greasy, fatty foods. Clear, **cool beverages** and carbonated drinks. Popsicles, gelatin desserts. Dry foods (toast, crackers). Six small feedings. Do not lie down immediately after eating if gastric atony.
Changes in **taste sensitivity**	Acidic foods may stimulate appetite, improve taste acuity. Zinc supplements.
Mucositis	Soft foods. Avoid very hot or very cold foods. Avoid acidic, salty, spicy foods. Use a **straw** to direct nutrients away from painful areas. Smoking/alcohol strictly forbidden.
Xerostomia from radiation therapy, antihistamines, narcotics	Chewing gum, sugar-free candy to stimulate saliva. Rinse mouth with soda water or tea with lemon. Artificial saliva before meals. Gravies, sauces, or broth to moisten foods. Avoid foods likely to cause dental caries.
Constipation from narcotics, vincristine	Increase dietary fiber as tolerated. Increase **fluid** intake to 2-3 L/day, as tolerated. Increase physical activity. **Laxative** medications.

Problem	Approaches to Solution
Diarrhea	Maintain fluid intake + foods high in potassium. Water-soluble fiber. Restrict lactose.

- **Enteral** feeding:
  - Indicated in patients unable to ingest sufficient nutrients but whose GI function is adequate for digestion/absorption:
    - Anorexia.
    - Upper GI cancers.
  - Routes:
    - **Nasogastric (NG) tubes** most commonly used.
      - Suitable for short-term use in hospital.
      - Small-bore (6–8F) silicone tubes can be left in place for 4 to 6 weeks.
      - Essential to **place tip of tube in antrum** or more distally to avoid aspiration.
    - **Gastrostomy** tube:
      - Can be placed endoscopically under local anesthesia.
      - Diameter of tube is 16F to 20F (2 × NG tube) → does not clog.
      - Unlikely to be dislodged accidentally.
      - Gastric feeding allows stomach to dilute hyperosmolar solutions → less diarrhea than with jejunostomy.
      - Disadvantage (versus jejunostomy): risk of aspiration.
    - **Jejunostomy** tube:
      - Recommended when there is proximal GI obstruction or fistula.
      - Advantages: less stomal leakage, skin erosion, nausea, vomiting, bloating.
      - Disadvantage: **diarrhea** → *Start with small volumes* (25 to 30 ml/hr) of full-strength formula → gradually increase volume over 3 to 4 days. Do *not* use antidiarrheals to increase tolerance.
- **Enteral feeding solutions**:
  - Solutions requiring **full digestion**:
    - For patients with *intact GI tract.*
    - Contain whole proteins, fats as triglycerides, long-chain carbohydrates.
    - Caloric density about **1 to 2 cal/ml**.
    - Examples: Ensure, Osmolite, Sustacal.
  - Solutions requiring **partial digestion**:
    - For patients with maldigestion, malabsorption, rapid GI transit.

- ° Lower protein/fat percentages.
- ° Examples: Vivonex, Vital High Nitrogen, Criticare High Nitrogen.
- **Rate of administration**:
  - – For intact GI tract: 300- to 500-ml bolus qid.
  - – For gastrectomized: slow drip (100–200 ml/hr).
  - – For short bowel, radiation enteritis, or other malabsorption syndrome: very slow drip (<100 ml/hr).
- **Monitor** blood glucose, BUN, electrolytes, Ca^{2+}, and Mg^{2+} daily until metabolic status stable on enteral feeding → every 3 to 7 days.
- Treat **complications** of enteral hyperalimentation:

Complication	Treatment
Vomiting, bloating	Reduce flow rate.
Diarrhea and cramping	Reduce flow rate; review medications; determine stool osmolality.*
Hyperglycemia	Reduce flow rate; give insulin.
Edema	Usually no Rx; may use diuretics.
Essential fatty acid deficiency	Supplement PO or with IV Intralipid.
Congestive heart failure (CHF)	Reduce flow rate; treat for CHF.
Hypernatremia, hypercalcemia	Adjust electrolytes.
Clogged tube lumen	Flush or replace tube.
Aspiration pneumonia (rare)	D/C enteral alimentation.
Esophageal erosion (rare)	D/C NG tube.
Hyperosmolar coma (rare)	D/C enteral alimentation.

*See Edes et al., 1990.

Nutritional Support of the Terminally Ill Patient

General Principles

- There is no evidence that improving nutritional intake in advanced cancer has any beneficial effects on morbidity or mortality. → The **aim** of nutritional counseling is to **improve quality of life** by giving the patient maximum enjoyment from eating.
- Determine **whose problem it is** that the patient "is not eating enough"—the patient's or the family's.

- Listen to family's/patient's fears → explain:
  - Force-feeding a dying patient will only tire the patient.
  - Eating will not reverse the underlying pathologic process.
  - Loss of interest in food is natural near death.
  - The body takes in only what it needs.
- **Rule out reversible causes** of anorexia, such as
  - Constipation.
  - Nausea.
  - Mouth discomfort.
  - Pain.
  - Electrolyte disturbances.
  - Depression.
- **Avoid** commercial **nutritional supplements**:
  - Supplements suppress appetite and are boring and often unpalatable.
  - Supplements tend to replace foods that the patient likes and enjoys.
  - There is no evidence that nutritional supplements improve the patient's status.

Specific Strategies

Problem	Treatment Possibilities
Abnormalities of taste	**Reduce urea content** of diet (less red meat; more eggs, dairy products). If meats *are* served, marinate before cooking and season well to disguise bitter taste. Serve foods at room temperature, not hot. Try tart foods. Encourage fluids with meals.
Anorexia*	**Permission to eat less.** **Smaller, more frequent feedings.** Involve the patient in menu planning, and respect personal food preferences. Use **smaller dinner plates** for smaller helpings. Have **food available** whenever patient is hungry. **Avoid strong smells** of cooking at mealtimes. Have patient **dress for meals** and sit at the table if possible. Try appetite stimulants: ▪ The best appetite stimulant is food that the patient likes.

*See Chapter 13 for more details.

continued

Problem	Treatment Possibilities
Anorexia *cont.*	• A glass of sherry or wine may be appreciated by patients who were accustomed to a small drink before dinner. • **Dexamethasone**, 4 mg qam. • **Megestrol acetate** (Megace), 160 mg qd. • Dronabinol, 2.5 mg PO bid 1 hr pc. • Multivitamins. For small stomach or gastric atony: • Metoclopramide (Reglan), 10 mg PO ac, *or* • Domperidone (Motilium), 10 mg PO tid.
Mucositis	Soft foods. *Avoid* very hot or very cold foods. Avoid acidic, salty, spicy foods. Use a *straw* to direct nutrients away from painful areas.
Xerostomia	Chewing gum, sugar-free candy to stimulate saliva. Rinsing mouth with soda water or tea with lemon. Artificial saliva before meals. Sips of fluid before each bite of solid food. Gravies, sauces, or broth to moisten foods.
Social consequences of cachexia	Dental relining → restores chewing ability and improves facial appearance. Old and new photos of patient. New set of well-fitting clothes. Avoid routine weighing of the patient.

Hydration of the Terminally Ill Patient Near the End of Life

When patients are no longer able to take oral fluids, hydration may be provided by **hypodermoclysis** (subcutaneous fluid administration).

- Indicated for patients in good symptom control when **maintenance of cognitive status** is important.
- Volumes of **500 to 1500 ml/24 hr** can be administered by the SQ route.
- The preferred solution is **normal saline** or a 2 : 1 mixture of 5% dextrose and normal saline; 20 to 30 mEq of **potassium** may be added to each liter of fluid.
- Some centers advocate the addition of 500 to 750 U of **hyaluronidase** to each liter to promote absorption of fluid from the subcutaneous site.
- When patients are still partially mobile or are able to go home on leave for a day, hydration may be given during the night only.

- For details on initiating SQ infusions, see Appendix 2.

During the **last days of life**, patients tend to take in less and less food and fluid.

- **Reduced intake** of food and fluids preterminally is probably a **normal physiologic mechanism** that prepares the organism for death.
- **Hunger and thirst are very rare in the last days of life** and can be controlled by simple means (e.g., lubrication of the lips and mouth).

The preponderance of evidence indicates that **intravenous fluids are medically unnecessary** during the last days of life and may in fact be detrimental.

Potential Disadvantages of Intravenous Hydration at the End of Life

↑ Urine output → bed-wetting, bedpans, catheters.

↑ Respiratory tract secretions → cough, pulmonary congestion, sensations of choking and drowning.

↑ Gastrointestinal secretions → vomiting.

↑ Edema, ascites, pleural effusions.

If hydration produces ↓serum urea, ↑awareness, ↑pain.

May prolong agonal period (without prolonging life).

Interferes with family's psychological preparations for the patient's death.

Places physical barriers between the patient and family/caregivers → inhibits physical contact with patient.

Management of Terminal Dehydration

- **Explain** to the family that
  - The patient no longer needs significant amounts of food and fluids.
  - The patient does not feel hunger and thirst.
  - Parenteral fluids may increase the patient's discomfort.
- If, despite explanations, the patient or family is still uncomfortable with a decision to withhold parenteral fluid therapy, give **subcutaneous** (preferably) **or intravenous fluids at a rate not exceeding 1 to 1.5 L/day**; use furosemide as needed to control symptoms of overhydration.
- If parenteral fluids are *not* given, **prevent symptoms of thirst** by
  - Attention to oral hygiene.
  - Small sips of fluids.
  - Giving small amounts of crushed ice to suck.

References and Further Reading

Aker SN. Oral feedings in the cancer patient. *Cancer* 43:2103, 1979.

American College of Physicians. Parenteral nutrition in patients receiving cancer chemotherapy: Position paper. *Ann Intern Med* 110:734, 1989.

Bernstein IL. Physiological and psychological mechanisms of cancer anorexia. *Cancer Res* 42(suppl):715s, 1982.

Bernstein IL. Etiology of anorexia in cancer. *Cancer* 581:1881, 1986.

Bernstein IL, Sigundi RA. Tumor anorexia: A learned food aversion? *Science* 209:416, 1980.

Billings JA. Comfort measures for the terminally ill: Is dehydration painful? *J Am Geriatr Soc* 33:808, 1985.

Brennan MF. Uncomplicated starvation versus cancer cachexia. *Cancer Res* 37:2359, 1977.

Bruera E, Legris M, Kuehn N, Miller M. Hypodermoclysis for the administration of fluids and narcotic analgesics in patients with advanced cancer. *J Pain Symptom Manage* 5:218, 1990.

Burge FI. Dehydration symptoms of palliative care patients. *J Pain Symptom Manage* 8:454, 1993.

Copeland EM, Daly JM, Dudrick SJ. Nutrition as an adjunct to cancer treatment in the adult. *Cancer Res* 37:2451, 1977.

Cox SS. Is dehydration painful? *Ethics Medics* 12(9):1, 1987.

DeWys WD. Changes in taste sensation and feeding behavior in cancer patients: A review. *J Human Nutr* 32:447, 1978.

DeWys WD. Anorexia as a general effect of cancer. *Cancer* 43:2013, 1979.

DeWys W, Herbst S. Oral feeding in the nutritional management of the cancer patient. *Cancer Res* 37:2429, 1977.

Donaldson S, Lenon R. Alterations of nutritional status: Impact of chemotherapy and radiation therapy. *Cancer* 43:2036, 1979.

Edes TE, Walk BE, Austin J. Diarrhea in tube-fed patients: Feeding formula not necessarily the cause. *Am J Med* 88:91, 1990.

Ellershaw JE, Sutcliffe JM, Saunders CM. Dehydration and the dying patient. *J Pain Symptom Manage* 10:192, 1995.

Fainsinger R, Bruera E. The management of dehydration in terminally ill patients. *J Palliative Care* 10(3):55, 1994.

Fainsinger R, MacEachern T, Miller M, et al. The use of hypodermoclysis for rehydration in terminally ill cancer patients. *J Pain Symptom Manage* 9:298, 1994.

Harvey K, Bothe A, Blackburn GL, et al. Nutritional assessment and patient outcome during oncological therapy. *Cancer* 43:2065, 1979

Heber D, Byerley LO, Chi J. Pathophysiology of malnutrition in the adult cancer patient. *Cancer* 58(suppl):1867, 1986.

Holland JC, Rowland HJ, Plumb M. Psychological aspects of anorexia in cancer patients. *Cancer Res* 37:2425, 1977.

Lamerton R. Dehydration in dying patients. *Lancet* 337:981, 1991.

McCann RM, Hall WJ, Groth-Juncker A. Comfort care for terminally ill patients: The appropriate use of nutrition and hydration. *JAMA* 272:1263, 1994.

McCormick WJ. Ascorbic acid as a chemotherapeutic agent. *Arch Pediatr* 69:151, 1952.

Micetich KC, Steinecker PH, Thomasma DC. Are intravenous fluids morally required for a dying patient? *Arch Intern Med* 143:975, 1983.

Nixon DW, Heymsfield SB, Cohen AE. Protein-calorie undernutrition in hospitalized cancer patients. *Am J Med* 68:683, 1980.

Oliver D. Terminal dehydration. *Lancet* ii:631, 1984.

Padilla GV, Grant MM. Psychosocial aspects of artificial feeding. *Cancer* 55:301, 1985.

Peteet JR, Medeiros C, Slavin L, Walsh-Burke K. Psychological aspects of artificial feeding in cancer patients. *JPEN* 5:138, 1981.

Printz L. Terminal dehydration, a compassionate treatment. *Arch Intern Med* 152:697, 1992.

Rains BL. The nonhospitalized tube-fed patient. *Oncol Nurs Forum* 8(2):88, 1981.

Rapin C. Nutrition for terminally ill elderly patients. *Eur J Palliative Care* 1(2):84, 1994.

Shils M. Principles of nutritional therapy. *Cancer* 43:2093, 1979.

Shils ME. Nutritional problems induced by cancer. *Med Clin North Am* 63:1009, 1979.

Tannenbaum A, Silverstone H. Nutrition in relation to cancer. *Adv Cancer Res* 1:451, 1953.

Terepka AR, Waterhouse C. Metabolic observations during the forced feeding of patients with cancer. *Am J Med*, February 1956, p. 225.

Terminal dehydration (editorial). *Lancet* i:301, 1986.

Theoglides A. Is vitamin therapy helpful for advanced cancer patients? *JAMA* 235:956, 1976.

Waller A, Hershkowitz M, Adunsky A. The effect of intravenous fluid infusion on blood and urine parameters of hydration and on state of consciousness in terminal cancer patients. *Am J Hospice Palliative Care* 11(6):22, 1994.

Yan E, Bruera E. Parenteral hydration of terminally ill cancer patients. *J Palliative Care* 7(3):40, 1991.

Zerwekh JV. Should fluid and nutritional support be withheld from terminally ill patients? Another opinion. *Am J Hospice Care* 4:37, 1987.

Weakness

4 Weakness

Spontaneous weariness indicates disease.

HIPPOCRATES, *APHORISMS* ii, 5.

Incidence

Weakness is one of the most common symptoms in advanced cancer and is **nearly universal in the terminal stages** of illness.

- In one prospective study of 54 patients with advanced breast cancer (Bruera and MacDonald, 1988), there was a 72% prevalence of asthenia (i.e., fatigue, easy tiring, weakness).
- In other studies of cancer patients in various stages of their disease, the prevalence of weakness is reported to be from 36% to 78%.

Causes of Weakness in Advanced Cancer

- Weakness in any given patient with advanced cancer usually has **multiple causes**.
- Some **causes** are **related to the tumor** itself:
  - Tumor burden.
  - Altered metabolism.
  - Cancer cachexia (wasting affects both skeletal and cardiac muscle).
  - Paraneoplastic syndromes (e.g., Eaton-Lambert and other myopathies).
  - Spinal cord compression.

- **Look for reversible causes** that may be contributing to weakness:
  - Insufficient sleep.
  - Depression.
  - Anemia.
  - Bed rest.
  - Drugs (opioids, antidepressants, phenothiazines).
  - Metabolic disturbances, especially
    - Hypercalcemia.
    - Hypokalemia.
  - Endocrine imbalances, especially
    - Hypothyroid.
    - Hypoadrenalism (most often due to too rapid withdrawal of corticosteroid medication).
  - Occult sepsis.

Evaluation of the Patient with Weakness

Taking the History

- **Find out what the patient means** by weakness:
  - Evaluate for symptoms of depression (feelings of worthlessness, excessive guilt).
  - Determine what the *patient* thinks is causing the weakness (e.g., does the patient see it as a sign that the disease is worsening?)
- **Characterize** the weakness:
  - **Onset**: sudden or gradual?
  - **Location**: localized or generalized?
  - **Quantitation**: Use an objective scale, such as the **performance status** scale of the Eastern Cooperative Oncology Group (ECOG):

Performance Status Scale

ECOG Score	Description
0	Carries on all normal activities.
1	Has symptoms, but is ambulatory and able to carry out normal activities.
2	Symptomatic, but out of bed >50% of the time.
3	Symptomatic and in bed >50% of the time.
4	Bedridden.

- Is the patient having problems with **sleep**? How much sleep does the patient get in 24 hours, and what is the sleep pattern (naps during the day? insomnia at night?).
- Are there problems with **appetite**? How much **weight** has the patient **lost** in the past month?
- What **medications** does the patient take regularly (including over-the-counter medications)?

Physical Examination

Look especially for the following:

Region	Look for:	Suggests:
Head	Coarse hair	Hypothyroid
	Lid lag	Hypothyroid
	Thinning of lateral third of eyebrows	Hypothyroid
Eyes	Miosis	Opioid overdose
	Conjunctival pallor	Anemia
Mouth	Cheilosis, reddened shiny tongue	Vitamin deficiencies
Abdomen	Palpable bladder	Cord compression
Extremities	Asterixis	Hepatic or renal insufficiency
		Hypokalemia
Back	Tenderness to percussion over vertebrae	Spinal cord involvement
Neurologic	Proximal myopathy	Eaton-Lambert or other myopathic syndrome
	Absent deep tendon reflexes (DTRs) that reappear after 10 seconds of maximal voluntary contraction	Eaton-Lambert syndrome
	Prolonged relaxation time of DTRs	Hypothyroid
	Hyperactive DTRs	Acute cord compression
	Spasticity, sensory loss, extensor plantar	Acute cord compression

Laboratory Studies

- Hemoglobin, WBC count.
- Serum sodium, potassium, calcium, magnesium.

- Blood glucose.
- Serum urea, creatinine, liver enzymes.
- Triiodothyronine (T_3), thyroxine (T_4).
- Drug levels where relevant (phenytoin, digoxin).

Management of Weakness in the Patient with Advanced Cancer

Although weakness is the most common and often most vexing symptom in patients with advanced cancer, it is the symptom for which we have the least satisfactory solutions.

- **Address treatable contributing causes**:

Contributing Cause	Treatment
Anemia	Transfuse with whole blood for Hb < 9.0 if patient so wishes.
Hypokalemia	If patient is taking a loop diuretic, substitute a potassium-sparing diuretic (spironolactone, 100 mg qam) for a few days, then recheck serum potassium. For severe hypokalemia (K^+ < 2.8 mEq/L), give potassium supplementation via potassium-rich foods (citrus juice, tomatoes, bananas) or potassium chloride tabs (Slow-K), 600 mg bid–tid pc.
Hypercalcemia	Hydration. For serum Ca^{2+} > 12, **pamidronate**, 60 mg in 250 ml of normal saline infused over at least 4 hours (see Chapter 42).
Medications	Try to reduce dosage of drugs such as antidepressants or benzodiazepines, or switch to an alternative drug. Drugs with sedative effects are best given in the evening when possible. For oversedation produced by narcotic analgesics, a trial of **methylphenidate**, 10 mg at 0800 and 5 mg at 1200, may enable increased activity levels.
Insomnia	Determine cause (anxiety? bad dreams?). Sedative/hypnotic medication, e.g., **flunitrazepam**, 1–2 mg PO hs.
Anorexia/cachexia	**Dexamethasone**, 4 mg PO qam. Multivitamins. For patients with life expectancy > 1 month, **megestrol acetate**, 160 mg PO qd.

Contributing Cause	Treatment
Suspected sepsis	Antibiotics where appropriate.
Depression	Start antidepressive medications (see Chapter 37).
Prolonged immobilization	Physiotherapy.
Endocrine imbalance	Replacement therapy (thyroid hormone, restart corticosteroids if recently withdrawn).
Eaton-Lambert syndrome	**Guanidine HCl**, 125–500 mg PO tid.
Cord compression	**Dexamethasone**, 100 mg IV stat + radiation therapy (see Chapter 35).

- Help patient to **establish priorities**.
  - Explain to the patient that his or her strength will fluctuate.
  - Help patient **plan periods of rest and periods of activity** to maximize the energy the patient has available for things that are really important to him (e.g., for a particular project or for spending time with friends and family).
  - Help the patient to delegate tasks that he or she is no longer able to perform (e.g., housework), and arrange for assistance where necessary.
- **Before important events** (e.g., wedding of a son or daughter), help the patient to achieve the maximum possible strength and sense of well-being:
  - Ensure **adequate rest** during the days preceding.
  - Start **corticosteroids**, or increase the dosage of corticosteroids already prescribed.
  - **Transfuse** with whole blood for hemoglobin <9.0, especially if accompanied by tachycardia and dyspnea.
  - Pay meticulous attention to **control of other symptoms** (e.g., pain, nausea, cough).
  - For the event itself, give **dextroamphetamine, 2.5 mg bid,** *or* **methylphenidate, 10 mg bid,** *or* **pemoline, 18.75 to 37.5 mg PO** a few hours before.

References and Further Reading

Bruera E, Chadwick S, Brenneis C. Methylphenidate associated with narcotics for the treatment of cancer pain. *Cancer Treat Rep* 71:120, 1987.

Bruera E, MacDonald RN. Asthenia in patients with advanced cancer. *J Pain Symptom Manage* 3:9, 1988.

Erlington G. The Lambert-Eaton myasthenic syndrome. *Palliative Med* 6(2):9, 1992.

Grant R. Nonmetastatic manifestation of malignancy: neurological. *Palliative Med* 3:181, 1989.

Josh J, DeJongh C, Schnapper N, et al. Amphetamine therapy for enhancing the comfort of terminally ill patients with cancer. *Proc Am Soc Clin Oncol*, C-213, 1982.

Lichter I. Weakness in terminal illness. *Palliative Med* 4(2):73, 1990.

Regnard CFB, Mannix KA. Weakness and fatigue in advanced cancer: a flow diagram. *Palliative Med* 6(2):253, 1992.

Theoglides A. Asthenia in cancer. *Am J Med* 73:1, 1982.

Dermatologic
and Related
Problems

5 Smelly Tumors

Few complications can cause so much misery as the infiltration of the skin by primary or metastatic tumor and the subsequent development of ulcerating or fungating wounds.

- Unsightly and bad-smelling lesions are a severe blow to self-image.
- Malodorous wounds lead to social isolation.
- Ulcerated cutaneous metastases often cause severe pain.

Incidence and Pathology

- Metastases to skin may occur in various primary malignancies:

Site of Primary Cancer	Incidence of Skin Metastases	Usual Site(s) of Skin Metastases
Breast	25%	Chest wall, scalp
Lung	7%	Chest wall, scalp
Kidney	5%	Lower abdominal wall, genitalia, scalp
Colon	3%	Abdominal wall, often periumbilical
Other solid tumors	1–2%	

- Average survival from the time of detection of skin metastasis is 3 months.
- Malignant ulceration occurs in about 8% of all patients with advanced cancer.

Principles of Management of Fungating and Malodorous Wounds

- Palliative **oncologic treatment** may provide excellent temporary control of malignant ulceration.
  - Chemotherapy may bring about regression of cutaneous lesions of breast cancer.
  - Radiation therapy will control bleeding from widespread malignant ulceration and will achieve healing of fungating lesions (especially in breast cancer).
  - Toilet mastectomy may be indicated for massive breast lesions.
- Aspects of **symptomatic treatment**:

Cleansing the wound	▪ When wound is draining profuse or purulent exudate, cleanse thoroughly by **irrigation with sterile saline**. Unless the wound has a very bad odor, do *not* use antiseptic cleansing solutions or hypochlorites, which may be toxic to granulation tissue.
Debridement	▪ For debridement of encrusted, purulent materials, use **wet-to-dry dressings**. ▪ For purulent slough, use xerogel dressing, such as Debrisan. ▪ For black, necrotic tissue, carry out enzymatic debridement by applying streptokinase to the necrotic area.
Controlling odor	▪ Regular cleansing with **disinfectant** solution such as povidone-iodine, freshly prepared Dakin's solution (sodium hypochlorite), or 1% chlorhexidine solution may be sufficient in some cases to control bad odor. ▪ The bad odor of malignant ulceration is due to anaerobic organisms, primarily *Bacteroides*. Therefore the treatment of choice for malodorous cutaneous lesions is **metronidazole**, 0.8% gel applied topically with or without systemic treatment (200–400 mg PO tid). ▪ **Charcoal dressings** are very effective in adsorbing odors from smelly wounds (see under "Dressing the wound," below). ▪ Where metronidazole gel is not available or is not tolerated, a suspension of aluminum hydroxide/magnesium hydroxide (**Maalox**) may be applied to the skin after thorough cleansing and drying.

Controlling odor *cont.*	▪ Another alternative to metronidazole gel is **yogurt**, applied to the skin after it has been cleansed and dried. ▪ Application of **honey** has also been successful in controlling odor from malignant ulceration and has been reported to enhance wound healing.
Controlling bleeding	▪ Apply **pressure** to visible bleeding vessels. If pressure alone is ineffective, hold a piece of gauze that has been soaked in 1:1000 epinephrine over the bleeding point. ▪ For widespread oozing, apply **sucralfate paste** (crush a 1-gm sucralfate tablet in 2–3 ml of water-soluble gel). ▪ Alternatively, apply a topical absorbable hemostatic sponge such as Gelfoam. ▪ Small bleeding points can be controlled with silver nitrate sticks. ▪ Consider **radiotherapy**.
Dressing the wound	▪ Requirements for type of dressing vary with the amount of exudate from the wound. Dressings for exudative wounds should incorporate three layers: 1. Layer next to wound: sterile, nonadherent, permeable to exudate. 2. Middle layer: absorbent; protects outer layer from becoming wet. 3. Outer layer: charcoal, to adsorb odor. ▪ Change dressing only as required by volume of exudate. ▪ To remove dressings, *soak them off* with normal saline. ▪ Cleanse wound surface with saline irrigation before applying fresh dressing.
Controlling pain	▪ Aluminum hydroxide/magnesium hydroxide suspension (**Maalox**) or **yogurt** applied to the ulcerated area will often relieve burning sensations. ▪ Consider **NSAIDs**.

References and Further Reading

Ashford RFU, Plant G, Maher J, Teare L. Double-blind trial of metronidazole in malodorous ulcerating tumours. *Lancet* i:1232, 1984.

Ashford RFU, Plant GT, Maher J, et al. Metronidazole in smelly tumours. *Lancet* i:874, 1980.

Beckett R, Coombes TH, Frost MR, et al. Charcoal cloth and malodorous wounds. *Lancet* ii:594, 1980.

Cherife J, Scarmato G, Herzsage L. Scientific basis for use of granulated sugar in treatment of infected wounds. *Lancet* i:560, 1982.

Doll DC, Doll KJ. Malodorous tumors and metronidazole. *Ann Intern Med* 94:139, 1981.

Foltz AT. Nursing care of ulcerating metastatic lesions. *Oncol Nurs Forum* 7:8, 1980.

Jacob M, Markstein C, Liesse M, Deckers C. What about odor in terminal care? *J Palliative Care* 7(4):31, 1991.

Keast-Butler J. Honey for necrotic malignant breast ulcers. *Lancet* ii:909, 1980.

Management of smelly tumours (editorial). *Lancet* 335:141, 1990.

Mossel DAA. Honey for necrotic malignant breast ulcers. *Lancet* ii:1091, 1980.

Newman V, Allwood M, Oakes RA. The use of metronidazole gel to control the smell of malodorous lesions. *Palliative Med* 3:303, 1989.

Thomlinson RH. Kitchen remedy for necrotic malignant breast ulcers. *Lancet* ii:707, 1980.

Wood DK. The draining malignant ulceration: Palliative management in advanced cancer. *JAMA* 244:820, 1980.

6 Pressure Sores

Definition

- Damage to the skin as the result of extrinsic pressure and shearing forces.
- Affect 20% of terminally ill patients.
- The word *decubitus* comes from the Latin *decub*, meaning "lying down." Since many of these lesions develop while the patient is sitting, *pressure sore* is a more accurate term than *decubitus ulcer*.

Pathophysiology

Multiple factors contribute to the development of pressure sores. The **most important contributing factors** are as follows:

Major Factors in the Development of Pressure Sores
Pressure
Shearing forces
Moisture
Fiction

▪ **Pressure** is the immediate cause of pressure sores.
  • Decreased blood flow → tissue anoxia → increased capillary permeability → edema → cell death (starting at epidermis).
  • Inverse relation between pressure and time in producing damage.
    - High pressure exerted over brief periods is less damaging than **low pressures applied over prolonged periods**.
    - Initial skin breakdown can occur in 6 to 12 hours, even in a healthy person—more quickly in the debilitated (< 2 hours).
▪ **Shearing forces** occur when adjacent surfaces slide with respect to one another (e.g., bone moves but skin sticks to the sheet), as when the head of the bed is raised and the patient's body slides downward → pressure transmitted to sacrum and deep fascia.
▪ **Friction** occurs when two surfaces move across one another (e.g., when a patient is dragged across bedsheets) → removes protective outer skin layer (stratum corneum).
▪ **Moisture**, especially that due to fecal incontinence, encourages maceration and infection of skin. Notably, excessively *dry* skin is also a significant risk factor for pressure sores.

Other Contributing Factors

▪ **Immobility** of all or part of the body (from pain, paralysis, sedation, coma, massive ascites/edema).
▪ **General malnutrition** and specific deficiencies:
  • **Vitamin C** deficiency → impaired wound healing.
  • **Zinc** deficiency → impaired wound healing.
  • **Hypoproteinemia** → interstitial edema.
▪ **Cachexia**.
▪ **Anemia**.
▪ **Immunosuppression** from any source (chemotherapy, debility) → damaged skin becomes portal of infection.
▪ **Chronic corticosteroid therapy** → opportunistic infection, poor wound healing.
▪ Neurologic: **sensory loss** and/or **motor deficit**.
▪ Peripheral **vascular disease**.
▪ **Obesity** or contractures, which make it difficult to turn the patient.
▪ Maceration of the skin.
▪ Conditions causing tissue edema or devitalization.
▪ Old **age**.
▪ Medical/nursing deficiencies:
  • Improperly applied casts, bandages.

- Folds in **bed linens** or **hard mattresses** under immobilized patients.
- Restraints, bed rails.

Sites of Pressure Sores in Terminally Ill Patients

- Occur over bony prominences and weight-bearing areas.
- Most commonly **sacrum**, **hips**, and **heels**.

Posture	Site of Pressure Sore
Supine	Rim of ear
	Inner knee
	Heel
Lateral	Trochanter
	Lateral condyle of knee
	Malleolus
Sitting	Sacrum
Semirecumbent	Outer ankle

Prevention of Pressure Sores

Pressure Redistribution

- Appropriate **mattress**—options:
  - Egg-crate mattress.
  - Water bed or water-filled camping mattress.
  - Air bed.
  - Clinitron bed (flotation support system that distributes the patient's weight evenly): reduces skin pressure to < 25 mm Hg/cm^2.
- **Reposition patient** by turning as often as necessary to prevent erythema (usually at least every 2–3 hours). Use **pillows** or wedge cushions at strategic locations.
- **Wheelchair cushion**: Shift weight every 15 minutes if able.
- **Elbow** and **heel pads**; baby sponge taped to sacrum.
- **Raise heels/ankles** off sheets with wedge-shaped foam pads placed under the calves.
- Bed cradles.
- *Avoid* ring cushions ("donuts") because they are apt to compromise circulation.

Skin Care

- **Inspect** skin at each change of position.
- **Keep the patient dry** (change soiled linens; if necessary, urinary and fecal diversions).
- Keep the **skin moisturized**: Apply silicone-based cream gently over bony prominences.
- *Avoid trauma* to the skin:
  - To minimize forward sliding/shear, **do not elevate** the patient > 30 **degrees**.
  - To minimize friction, **lift** patients, don't drag.
  - **No restraints.**
  - **No bed rails.**
  - Avoid overheating → sweating.
  - Micropore tape for IVs, dressings.
  - Avoid vigorous massage.
  - Avoid alcohol or astringents on areas under pressure.

Nutrition

- Try to keep plasma **albumin above 3 gm/dl, hemoglobin above 10 gm/dl**.
- Supplements:
  - **Vitamin C**, 500 mg qd PO or IV.
  - **Zinc**, 50 mg PO hs.

General Measures

- Try to get the patient **out of bed** as much as possible, but
- Do not seat patient in chair/wheelchair longer than 1 hour if obese or 2 hours if thin.
- Increase circulation to extremities with **active/passive range of motion** exercises.

Treatment of Pressure Sores

Objectives of Treatment

The objectives of treatment in terminally ill patients are **different** from those in other patients. Cure of pressure sores is difficult if not impossible during the last months and weeks of life; overzealous attempts to achieve complete cure can simply add to the patient's discomfort and misery.

- To **improve the physical, mental, and spiritual condition of the patient** to the degree feasible.
- To **reduce the pain** of pressure sores by local and systemic therapy.
- To **prevent exudation and bad odors** from the pressure sore.
- Via interdisciplinary intervention (including a psychologist when necessary), to **help the patient cope** with the blow to body image that decaying tissue represents.

General Principles

- **Relief of pressure**: Healing cannot occur without good blood supply.
- **Cleanliness** and **dryness**.
- Effective, **prompt removal of debris**, pus, and necrotic material from wound surface.
- **Protect** granulation tissue **from reinfection** and from **cytotoxic agents** (e.g., silver nitrate solutions, acidifiers, hypotonic solutions).
- Administer appropriate **antibiotics**.

Treatment of Pressure Sores by Stage

Stage	Appearance of the Sore	Treatment Measures
1	**1A**: Blanching erythema; skin not broken **1B**: Nonblanching erythema; skin not broken	**Pressure relief**: No pressure until erythema has resolved • Stage 1A: 4 hours or less. • Stage 1B: 48 hours. **Semipermeable membrane** dressing (Omiderm, Tegaderm) especially for elbows, hips, insides of knees; apply after wound cleansing; place over entire wound and leave in place for 3–4 days (change only when necessary).
2	Superficial skin loss	**Pressure relief**. Cover with **Omiderm** dressing after wound cleansing.
3	Blister and eschar formation	**Pressure relief**. Do *not* open blisters; cover with Omiderm. Eschar: • If prognosis < 4 weeks, leave intact. • If prognosis > 4 weeks, debride piecemeal with scalpel.

continued

Stage	Appearance of the Sore	Treatment Measures
4	Clean ulcer with red granulomatous base	**Pressure relief.** Clean with **povidone-iodine 10%** (avoid hypochlorite antiseptics). Hydrocolloid dressings, for low exudate (e.g., Duoderm, Granuflex), *or* Calcium alginate dressings, for high exudate (covered with semiocclusive dressing), *or* Honey or sugar-povidone-iodine packing.
5	Infected ulcer or gray slough in base	**Pressure relief.** **Wet-to-dry dressings** or alginate dressings or Debrisan until debridement is complete. **Enzymatic debridement** (e.g., streptokinase) → irrigate with warm saline to remove exudate; if unsuccessful: **Surgical debridement** for thick eschar or extensive necrosis. If the patient is not a candidate for surgical debridement, try: • Sugar-povidone-iodine packing. • **Charcoal** dressings for malodorous wounds. Systemic **antibiotic** for surrounding *cellulitis* (metronidazole ± clindamycin).

Properties of Different Types of Dressings for Pressure Sores

Type of Dressing	Indications and Uses
Semipermeable film (Omiderm, Bioclusive, Tegaderm)	Protects very early damage from shear forces. Prevents bacterial contamination. Maintains humidity in shallow ulcers, producing ideal conditions for granulation and healing. Provides immediate pain relief. Best applied when there isn't exudation from the sore.
Hydrocolloids (Granuflex, Duoderm)	For low-exudate wounds. Maintains moist environment. Fluidizes to produce a gel useful for debridement. Provides environment for granulation.
Alginates (Kaltostat, Kaltocarb)	For heavy exudates: controls secretion and bacterial contamination by absorption and formation of hydrophilic gel.

Type of Dressing	Indications and Uses
Hydrogels/xerogels	For debridement in the presence of slough and infection: rehydrates eschar and makes it easier to remove.
Enzymatic (Elase, Travase)	For eschar and necrotic tissue: Loosens necrotic tissue by liquefaction, thereby aiding in its removal. (Protect edges of wound with zinc paste, and apply to eschar under an occlusive dressing.)
Polysaccharide dextra- nomer (Debrisan)	For exudative, infected wounds: On contact with wound exudate, the beads absorb fluid and swell, forming a gel; bacteria and dead cells are drawn away from the wound. Applied q24h until wound is clean and granulation tissue is developing.
Charcoal (Actisorb)	Malodorous infected pressure sores: adsorbs bacteria, cellular debris, toxins, and odors.

References and Further Reading

Allman RM, Goode PS, Patrick MM, et al. Pressure ulcer risk factors among hospitalized patients with activity limitation. *JAMA* 273:865, 1995.

Alper JC, et al. Moist wound healing under a vapor permeable membrane. *J Am Acad Dermatol* 8:347, 1983.

Andersen KE, Jensen O, Kvorning SA, Bach A. Prevention of pressure sores by identifying patients at risk. *Br Med J* 284:1370, 1982.

Bromfield R. Honey for decubitus ulcers. *JAMA* 224:905, 1973.

Cherife J, Scarmato G, Herzsage L. Scientific basis for use of granulated sugar in treatment of infected wounds. *Lancet* i:560, 1982.

DeConno F, Ventafridda V, Saita L. Skin problems in advanced and terminal cancer patients. *J Pain Symptom Manage* 6:247, 1991.

Dolinger RD. Pressure sores and optimum skin care. *J Palliative Care* 6:50, 1990.

Efem SEE. Clinical observations on the wound healing properties of honey. *Br J Surg* 75:679, 1988.

Goren D. Use of Omiderm in treatment of low-degree pressure sores in terminally ill cancer patients. *Cancer Nurs* 12:165, 1989.

Guggisberg E, Terumalai K, Carron J, Rapin C. New perspectives in the treatment of decubitus ulcers. *J Palliative Care* 8(2):5, 1992.

Jepson BA. Relieving the pain of pressure sores (letter). *Lancet* 339:503, 1992.

Knutson RA, Merbitz LA, Creekmore MA, Snipes HG. Use of sugar and povidone-iodine to enhance wound healing: Five years' experience. *South Med J* 74: 1329, 1981.

Rao DB, Sane PG, Giorgiev EL. Collagenase in the treatment of dermal and decubitus ulcers. *J Am Geriatr Soc* 23:22, 1975.

Reuler JB, Cooney TG. The pressure sore: Pathophysiology and principles of management. *Ann Intern Med* 94:661, 1981.

Seiler W, Stahelin H. Decubitus ulcers: Treatment through five therapeutic principles. *Geriatrics* 9:30, 1985.

7 Stomas and Fistulas

Definitions

- **Stoma**: A surgically created opening to divert feces or urine out of the body through an artificial conduit in the abdominal wall.
- **Fistula**: An abnormal passage between two internal organs or from an internal organ to the surface of the body.

Bowel Stomas

Location of the Stoma

- Depends on the level of obstruction or the amount of bowel that had to be removed.
- Determines the character and volume of the fecal effluent.

Type of Stoma	Area of Bowel Bypassed	Special Considerations
Ileostomy	Entire colon and rectum	Continuous, liquid, high-volume fecal output. Contains digestive enzymes → extra skin protection required.
Ascending or transverse colostomy	Colon and rectum distal to the stoma	Large-volume, semiliquid fecal output.

continued

Type of Stoma	Area of Bowel Bypassed	Special Considerations
Descending or sigmoid colostomy	Rectum and part of distal colon	Formed stool.

Stoma Care: General Principles

- Respect the patient's established regimen for stoma care. The patient will feel more secure doing things his or her own way.
- Be sure the patient's skin is clean and dry before applying a fresh ostomy bag over the stoma.
  - Use only mild soaps to clean the skin around the stoma.
  - Rinse the skin thoroughly to remove all soap.
  - Pat the skin dry *gently* with a soft towel; do not rub.
- Use a specially formulated powder or ointment around the stoma to protect the skin from contact with fecal effluent.
- Replace a full ostomy bag promptly.
- Make sure the patient's appliance fits properly (the appropriate size may change as the patient's stoma shrinks or his weight changes).

Stoma Care: Special Considerations

- **Inflammation of the skin** around the stoma is very common.

Cause of Inflammation	Symptoms & Signs	Management
Allergic dermatitis	Itching Erythema corresponding to area of contact between the skin and the appliance	Change to another type of appliance (made from a different material).
Effluent dermatitis (due to prolonged contact with fecal effluent)	Desquamation Signs of infection	Protect inflamed skin (Stomahesive paste). Steroid creams for inflammation. Antifungal/antibacterial creams for infection. Do not allow ostomy bag to overfill; change promptly.

Cause of Inflammation	Symptoms & Signs	Management
Mechanical trauma	Persistent erythema → denudation and erosions	Change pouching system every 4–7 days or when leakage occurs.

- **Gas and odors**:
  - Dietary modifications: Avoid onions, cabbage, beans, lentils, and carbonated beverages.
  - Give an **activated charcoal** preparation (Charcoal Plus, 2 tabs PO pc and hs).
  - Activated charcoal can also be added to the ostomy bag.
  - Avoid changing ostomy bags around mealtime, since odor may disturb the patient's appetite.
- **Diarrhea**:
  - Try to increase stool bulk (Metamucil, bananas, rice, pasta).
  - Use a drainable ostomy bag to permit removal of fecal effluent without frequent ostomy bag changes.
  - In severe cases, give an antidiarrheal (tincture of opium or loperamide).
- **Constipation**:
  - Constipation should be *prevented* by prescribing appropriate laxatives at the same time that opioid treatment is started.
  - When the patient has not passed stool via the stoma for more than 2 days, examine the stoma to determine whether there is stool within range of the examining finger:
    - If so, give an oil retention **enema** (using a Foley catheter with inflated balloon to facilitate retention of the oil for 10 minutes).
    - If stool is beyond the reach of the examining finger, give an **osmotic laxative** (lactulose) with or without a bowel stimulant (bisacodyl) and wetting agent (docusate).
    - If those measures fail to produce results, give Fleet enema.
    - *Note*: A stoma cannot retain suppositories.
- **Bleeding from the stoma** occurs commonly and usually is not serious.
  - Most stomal bleeding can be stopped by applying firm pressure with a gauze pad for a few minutes.
  - When bleeding persists or recurs, it may be due to tumor infiltration → consider local radiation or cryosurgery.

Ileal Conduits

- An ileal conduit is created surgically by
  - Isolating a segment of ileum with its mesentery;
  - Reanastomosing the remaining bowel;
  - Implanting the distal ureters into the isolated segment of ileum;
  - Sealing one end of the ileal segment, and bringing the other end to the abdominal wall as a cutaneous stoma.
- Urine is collected in an ostomy bag placed over the stoma. **Pouching systems** resemble those for ostomies:
  - A skin barrier of some sort (paste or solid) is always required to protect the peristomal skin.
    - Assess peristomal skin daily for signs of chemical or mechanical irritation.
    - Make sure the skin barrier opening is an appropriate size.
  - The pouch should be odor-proof and have a drainage valve at the bottom to allow the pouch to be emptied into a toilet (or connected to gravity drainage at night).
  - The patient may be bathed with the pouch on or off.
- Alkaline urine may cause formation of **crystals** and predispose to stone formation. If crystals form:
  - Swab the skin around the pouch with a solution made from **1 part vinegar : 1 part water**.
  - Instill 1 to 2 ounces (30–60 ml) of the same solution into a fresh ostomy pouch, and have the patient lie supine for half an hour to allow the inside of the stoma to be flushed; then empty the pouch and rinse with cool water.
- Routine stoma care is similar to that for bowel stomas (see Bowel Stomas).

Nephrostomy

- Definition: A surgically created fistula from the renal pelvis to the outside of the body, to permit drainage of urine when there is ureteral obstruction.

Routine Care

- Change the bandage every 2 days or as needed, preferably after the patient showers.

- Remove the old bandage.
- Cleanse the skin with bactericidal soap, then paint with povidone-iodine solution.
- Apply slit gauze pads around the nephrostomy tube → loop the tubing to prevent inadvertent dislodgment → place a large gauze pad over the looped tubing.
- Secure with an elastic bandage over the large gauze pad. (If elastic bandaging produces an allergic reaction, use hypoallergenic tape).
- Connect the tubing to a standard urine collection bag or (in the ambulatory patient) a leg bag.

Possible Problems

- **Purulent discharge around the nephrostomy tube**:
  - If there is only a small amount of discharge, cleanse the skin with povidone-iodine and bandage as usual.
  - If there is a lot of discharge (enough to soak the previous dressing), cleanse the skin; protect the skin with Stomahesive; bandage.
- **Blockage**: If there is no urine output from the nephrostomy for more than 2 to 3 hours, seek urologic consultation. Do not attempt to flush the nephrostomy tube unless there is backup available to reintroduce it should it become dislodged.
- **Dislodgment** of the nephrostomy tube: Apply a pressure dressing to the cutaneous fistula and seek urologic consultation.

Cutaneous Fistulas

Incidence

- Occur in approximately 1% of patients with advanced malignancy.
- Patients at highest risk are those with GI cancers and those who received irradiation to pelvic organs.

Management

- Wherever anatomically possible, apply an **ostomy bag** over the fistula to collect its effluent and reduce odor.
  - Clean the skin surrounding the fistula with warm water (without soap or antiseptics).
  - Use fillers to create a flat surface to which to attach the bag.

- Apply Stomahesive paste to the skin edges around the fistula.
- Pediatric colostomy bags have a softer, more flexible flange and may be easier to fit onto anatomically difficult areas. Making several cuts in the flange of the Stomahesive wafer may also help it to conform better to an irregular skin surface.
- Fill crevices between the skin and the wafer with carmellose paste.
- Empty the bag frequently (use drainable bags for high-output fistulas).
▪ *For high-output fistulas*, consider giving **octreotide, 300 μg/24 hr SQ**.
▪ **Protect the surrounding skin** with barrier creams.
▪ **Control odor**:
  - For odors due to anaerobic infection, give metronidazole, 400 mg PO tid.
  - Carry out changes of ostomy bag in a well-ventilated room.
▪ Special problems:
  - Fistulas that are particularly difficult to manage include
    - Fistulas in anatomically awkward areas, where it is not possible to cover the opening with an ostomy bag.
    - Multiple fistulas.
  - Approaches:
    - For fistulas in anatomically difficult areas, one source recommends using self-polymerizing silicone rubber as a plug (Walls et al., 1994). We have not had success with this technique, but it may be worth trying in difficult cases.
    - For multiple fistulas or fistulas in difficult areas, there may be no option but to use absorbent pads with a charcoal layer to reduce odor.

References and Further Reading

Mercadante S. Treatment of diarrhea due to enterocolic fistula with octreotide in a terminal cancer patient. *Palliative Med* 6:257, 1992.

Walls AWG, Regnard CFB, Mannix KA. The closure of an abdominal fistula using self-polymerizing silicone rubbers. *Palliative Med* 8:59, 1994.

Watt R. Nursing management of a patient with a urinary diversion. *Semin Oncol Nurs* 2:265, 1986.

8 Peripheral Edema

Definition

Accumulation of excess, low-protein fluid in the subcutaneous tissues.

Incidence

The incidence of peripheral edema has been reported to be between 20% and 80% of patients in the terminal stages of cancer.

Causes of Edema in Patients with Advanced Cancer

Usually multifactorial, with several causes acting together:
- **Immobility** →
  - Gravitational effect on dependent limbs.
  - Lack of normal muscle activity that ordinarily facilitates venous and lymphatic return to the central circulation.
- **Hypoalbuminemia**, resulting from
  - Malnutrition.
  - Metabolic effects of tumor.
  - Hepatic dysfunction.
  - Drainage of protein-rich exudates from third-space collections (ascites, pleural effusions).

- **Salt and fluid retention** due to
  - Drugs: corticosteroids, NSAIDs, some antibiotics.
  - Cardiac, renal, or hepatic failure.
- Increased **intra-abdominal pressure** (ascites, hepatomegaly).
- **Peripheral venous disease.**

Consequences of Edema in the Cancer Patient

- Decreased mobility (legs feel heavy; shoes no longer fit) → worsening of edema.
- Skin breakdown and cellulitis.

Clinical Findings

- Swollen extremity with pale, cold skin that pits easily (if skin is warm and dusky, suspect venous obstruction).
- Differentiate low-protein edema from lymphedema:

	Low-Protein Edema	*Lymphedema*
Response to external pressure	Pitting	Usually nonpitting
Response to elevation	Alleviates edema	Little or no response
Response to diuretics	Alleviate edema	Little or no response
Appearance of skin	Taut, smooth	Brawny, hyperkeratotic
Limbs affected	Usually lower limbs before upper limbs; usually bilateral	Often unilateral; may involve one upper limb

- Laboratory studies useful in elucidating the source(s) of edema:
  - Serum electrolytes, urea, creatinine, osmolality.
  - Hepatic enzymes.
  - Serum albumin.
  - Urine electrolytes and osmolality.

Management of Edema in Patients with Advanced Cancer

▪ **Encourage exercise.**
  • **Walking** is the best exercise to counteract lower-extremity edema (massaging effect of calf muscles).
  • If the patient is unable to walk, encourage isometric exercises in bed.
▪ **Elevate edematous extremities to the level of the heart** or above.
  • Simply raising the legs on a footstool is not effective.
  • The patient should, instead, be at **bed rest** with his legs raised on pillows for 30 to 60 minutes every few hours.
▪ For active patients, apply full-length **compression stockings** first thing in the morning.
  • Use low-pressure garments (10–30 mm Hg at the ankle).
  • Stockings should be worn all day and removed at night.
  • Bedridden patients do not benefit from stockings.
▪ Review patient's medications, and when possible, **stop medications that predispose to fluid retention**:
  • Corticosteroids.
  • NSAIDs.
▪ Provide **skin care**:
  • Use lanolin cream on taut skin to improve elasticity.
  • Assess skin several times daily for signs of breakdown, infection, or pressure injury.
▪ **Diuretics** are indicated when edema produces significant discomfort or limitation of mobility.
  • The patient should be capable of reaching toilet facilities easily or should be catheterized.
  • Use diuretics with caution in uncatheterized male patients who give a history of prostatism (hesitancy, frequency, decreased force and caliber of urinary stream).
  • Give diuretics to uncatheterized patients as a **single morning dose**, to reduce nocturia.
  • Usual starting regimen:
    - **Furosemide, 20 to 40 mg PO qam**.
    - **Spironolactone, 100 mg PO qam**.
    - If there is no response in 3 to 4 days, the morning dosage of each drug may be doubled. (In catheterized patients, a second dose may be added in the evening.)

- If there is still no response, a second dose (half of the morning dose) may be added at noon.
- Rigid fluid and salt restriction for the treatment of edema have no place in palliative care, since such restrictions decrease quality of life.

References and Further Reading

Badger C, Regnard CFB. Oedema in advanced disease: a flow diagram. *Palliative Med* 3:213, 1989.
Flombaum C, Isaacs M, Scheiner E, et al. Management of fluid retention in patients with advanced cancer. *JAMA* 245:611, 1981.

9 Lymphedema

Definition

Accumulation of lymph in the soft tissues as a result of disturbed lymph drainage.

Incidence

- Among patients with cancer, lymphedema is seen most commonly in women with breast cancer after **axillary lymph node dissection** (especially when combined with **radiotherapy**) →
  - Lymphedema of the ipsilateral *upper extremity*.
  - Can develop at any time after surgery (immediately or many years later).
  - Incidence of lymphedema following axillary node dissection + radiation is about 40%.
- Lymphedema of the *lower extremity* is most likely in patients who have undergone inguinal node dissection or patients with **intrapelvic tumors** (transitional cell carcinoma [TCC] of the bladder, prostate cancer, ovarian cancer).

Pathophysiology

- Damage to regional lymph nodes by surgery ± radiation (most commonly) or by tumor invasion →
- ↓Removal of fluid and protein from the distal limb →

- Accumulation of protein-rich fluid in the tissues of the limb →
- ↑Fibroblast activity → ↑fibrogenesis → tissues become fibrotic ("brawny") → further closure of lymphatics → ↓lymph clearance →
- Remaining lymphatics engorged → lymphatic valves become nonfunctional → further ↓lymph clearance → further fibrosis, etc.

Clinical Findings

Symptoms

- Limb feels **heavy, clumsy, tight, and/or bursting**.
- **Pain** caused by tissue pressure is generally **deep** and **aching**.
  - Exacerbated by exercise and hot weather.
  - Increasing in severity as the day goes on.
- Severe pain is *not* a feature of lymphedema. If the patient complains of severe pain in the lymphedematous limb, suspect infection, bone metastases, or recurrence of tumor.

Signs

Any of the following may be present:
- **Persistent swelling** of a limb or part of a limb.
  - Early, the edema may indent to external pressure ("pitting").
  - When interstitial fibrosis has developed, lymphedema is *usually* nonpitting.

	Simple Edema	Lymphedema
Response to external pressure	Pitting	Usually nonpitting
Response to elevation	Alleviates edema	Little or no response
Response to diuretics	Alleviates edema	Little or no response
Appearance of skin	Taut, smooth	Brawny, hyperkeratotic
Limbs affected	Usually lower limbs before upper limbs; usually bilateral	Often unilateral; may involve one upper limb

- Deepening of skin creases.
- **Stemmer's sign**: Skin at the base of the digits is thickened and cannot be easily pinched between two fingers.
- **Cutaneous changes**: Depending on the stage of lymphedema, the skin may be
  - Taut and shiny when edema develops rapidly.
  - Weeping (lymphorrhea).
  - Dotted with small lymphangiomas ("lymph blisters").
  - Hyperkeratotic, with papillomas (elephantiasis).
  - Ecchymotic (especially lower extremities).

Management of Lymphedema in the Patient with Advanced Cancer

Drug Treatment

Drug treatment is mostly disappointing but should be tried:
- Trial of **diuretics** (to treat secondary venous component of lymphedema):
  - Furosemide, 40 mg PO qam +
  - Spironolactone, 100 mg PO qam.
- If diuretics do not produce results within 2 to 3 days, a trial of high-dose **corticosteroids** is warranted, particularly for lymphedema involving the face, trunk, or lower extremities (to reduce tumor mass compressing lymphatic drainage channels):
  - Dexamethasone, 8 mg PO qam (taper dose by ¼ every 3 days).
- Benzopyrones have been quite effective in the long-term treatment of lymphedema but are not useful in palliative care because they take too long (8 months or more) to exert their effects.

Complex Physical Therapy

Complex physical therapy consists of
- **Skin care**, to improve skin condition and prevent infection:
  - Keep the lymphadematous limb as **clean** as possible.
    - A soapless cleanser (such as Alpha Keri Oil) is preferred.
    - Dry the limb *gently* with a soft cloth, making sure to dry all skin creases and between digits.
  - **Protect** the lymphadematous limb **from trauma**.
    - Avoid sunburn.
    - Use insect repellent to prevent bites.

- Use protective gloves for gardening.
- Be careful cutting nails.
- Do not use the lymphadematous limb for measuring blood pressure, taking blood, giving injections, or intravenous or subcutaneous infusions.
- Apply **lanolin** or similar unscented oil to keep the skin moist and supple.
- **Erythema** on a lymphadematous limb means **cellulitus** and must be treated *immediately* when noticed (within the hour): phenoxymethyl **penicillin, 500 mg PO q6h** (or, if allergic to penicillin, erythromycin, 500 mg q6h) for 2 weeks. (If recurrent infection, continue maintenance penicillin, 500 mg qam for 6 months.)
- Lymphatic **massage**, to remove excess fluid and protein:
  - The patient should be recumbent, and the area to be massaged should be bared.
  - Do not apply oil or lotion to the area to be massaged.
  - Massage is performed in the direction of normal lymph flow, starting on the trunk and working toward the distal extremity.
  - Massage of the trunk and one limb takes at least 20 minutes.
- **Compression bandaging** and compression garments to prevent reaccumulation of fluid in the massaged limb:
  - The compression garment or bandage must be worn at all times, including at night.
  - The limb should be washed and dried thoroughly when compression bandages are changed.
  - Compression garments and undergarments must be kept clean and dry.
  - The bandage or garment should be removed and reapplied just before bedtime.
  - Compression pumps ("pressure sleeve") may be useful in some cases, but only after massage has cleared the area; otherwise pressure sleeves may lead to accumulation of excess fluid and protein proximal to the sleeve.
- Special **exercises** to encourage lymphatic outflow (best performed while wearing compression garment or compression bandage to provide counterpressure).
  - **Avoid immobilizing** a lymphadematous limb (e.g., in a sling).
  - Involved joints should be put through **full range of motion** (passive range of motion exercises at least twice daily for patients too weak to move by themselves).

- The lymphadematous limb need not be elevated, but in bedridden patients the limb should be supported on a pillow in a position of comfort.

Transcutaneous Electrical Nerve Stimulation (TENS)

▪ Experience gained at the Tel Hashomer Hospice suggests that TENS can rapidly and dramatically reduce even long-standing lymphedema, at least in the short term.
- This use of TENS is still investigational.
- Studies are now under way to determine the optimal TENS settings and schedule of treatments for lymphedema.
▪ Current **protocol** of the Tel Hashomer Hospice for TENS treatment of lymphedema:
  - Apply one electrode of the electrode pair to the distal lymphedematous extremity.
  - Apply the second electrode to the same extremity, proximal to the margin of lymphedema if possible. (If using a dual channel TENS, electrode pairs may be crossed on the same limb, or one pair may be placed distally and the other pair proximally.)
  - Settings:
    - Rate: **130 Hz**.
    - Pulse width: < **130 μsec**.
    - Amplitude: Start from zero and increase until the patient reports a comfortable level of paresthesias.
    - Mode: Start with **C** (conventional) mode → switch to **M** (modulated) mode after 5 minutes.
  - Frequency of treatments: Start with **1 hour tid**.

References and Further Reading

Badger C, Regnard CFB. Oedema in advanced disease: a flow diagram. *Palliative Med* 3:213, 1989.

Brennan M. Lymphedema following the surgical treatment of breast cancer: A review of pathophysiology and treatment. *J Pain Symptom Manage* 7:110, 1992.

Casley-Smith JR. Modern treatment of lymphoedema. *Mod Med Aust* 35(5):70, 1992.

Casley-Smith JR. Modern treatment of lymphoedema. I. Complex physical therapy: the first 200 Australian limbs. *Australas J Dermatol* 33(2):61, 1992.

Casley-Smith JR, Morgan RG, Piller NB. Treatment of lymphedema of the arms and legs with 5,6-benzo[α]pyrone. *N Engl J Med* 329:1158, 1994.

Farncombe M, Daniels, G, Cross L. Lymphedema: The seemingly forgotten complication. *J Pain Symptom Manage* 9:269, 1994.

Foldi E, Foldi M, Clodius L. The lymphedema chaos: A lancet. *Ann Plast Surg* 22:505, 1989.

Kissin MW, Querci della Rovere G, Easton D, Westbury G. Risk of lymphoedema following the treatment of breast cancer. *Br J Surg* 73:580, 1986.

10 Pruritus

Definition

An irritating sensation in the skin that produces a desire to scratch.

Incidence

Pruritus occurs in 5% to 12% of cancer patients at some time during their illness.

Pathophysiology of Pruritus

- Itch and pain share common neuroanatomic pathways.
- There are a variety of *itch mediators*:
  - Histamine, proteases, bile salts, and trypsin all cause itch.
  - Prostaglandin E lowers threshold to itching.
  - Opiate receptors are involved:
    - Naloxone *decreases* itch.
    - Opiates relieve pain but exacerbate itch.
- The perception of itch is increased by
  - Dehydration, heat.
  - Anxiety.
  - Boredom.

Causes of Pruritus in Terminally Ill Patients

Primary Skin Problems

Most common source of pruritus in cancer patients:
- **Xerosis** (dry, flaky skin), especially in the elderly.
- Wet, **macerated skin.**
- **Contact dermatitis:**
  - Antihistamine creams.
  - Neomycin ointments.
  - Local anesthetic creams.
- Dermatitis herpetiformis.
- **Infestations:**
  - Scabies.
  - Pediculosis.
  - Fleas, mites (inquire about pets).

Drugs

- Drugs that commonly produce *allergic reactions:*
  - Penicillins, sulfonamides, streptomycin, nitrofurantoin.
  - Allopurinol.
  - Carbamazepine.
- Drugs that *cause histamine release* from mast cells:
  - Morphine, codeine, meperidine (*not* dose-dependent; more common after epidural administration).
  - Aspirin.
  - Vancomycin.
  - Radiocontrast agents.
- Drugs that produce itch by *hepatic cholestasis:*
  - Anabolic steroids, oral contraceptives.
  - Captopril.
  - Chlorpropamide.
  - Phenothiazines (chlorpromazine).
  - Tolbutamide.
  - Trimethoprim-sulfamethoxazole.

Systemic Disease

- Chronic **renal failure:**
  - Pruritus occurs in up to 90% of dialysis patients.
  - Itch worsens during hemodialysis; worse in summer.

- **Obstructive hepatobiliary disease**:
  - Bile salts cause hepatocytes to release itch mediator.
  - The incidence and severity of the pruritus are not dose-related to the bilirubin level.
- **Hodgkin's disease** → B symptoms (fever, night sweats, weight loss) and pruritus.
- **Cutaneous infiltration** of malignancy.
- Hyperthyroidism.
- Polycythemia vera.
- Iron deficiency.

Diagnostic Workup of Pruritus

History Taking

- *Location*: Localized or generalized.
- *Onset*: Pruritus of acute onset less suggestive of underlying systemic disease as the cause.
- *Duration*.
- *Nature* of the itch:
  - Scabies: severe unremitting itching worse in the evening.
  - Dermatitis herpetiformis: "burning."
  - Polycythemia vera: "prickling."
- *Severity*: Pruritus that wakes patient from sleep likely to have systemic cause.
- *Bathing habits* (overbathing, harsh soaps).
- Use of *topical medications*, lotions, creams, alcohol.

Physical Examination

- Thorough examination of the *skin*:
  - Look for primary skin lesions.
  - Long linear excoriations along the back → pediculosis.
  - Inflammatory papules on legs with small central vesicle → flea bites.
  - Butterfly sign on middle upper back → hepatobiliary disease.
  - Excoriations in web spaces of fingers, in groin → scabies.
  - Uremic "frost."
- Icterus.
- Lymphadenopathy.
- Hepatomegaly.

Laboratory Examinations

- CBC with differential.
- BUN, creatinine.
- Liver function tests.
- Thyroxine (T4) and thyroid-stimulating hormone (TSH).

Management of Pruritus

General Measures

- *Avoid* traumatizing the skin by
  - Alcohol rubs.
  - Woolen clothing.
  - Frequent bathing, especially with strong soaps, hot water.
- Add medicinal oils to bath.
- Dry skin by patting with a soft towel; **don't rub.**
- **Apply oil** to the skin immediately after bathing and at night (lanolin, bland creams, emollient creams, olive oil, or petrolatum).
- Avoid overheating and sweating.
- Keep patient's fingernails cut short.

Nonspecific Local Measures

- Bland cool compresses.
- An ice pack will often relieve severe episodic local itching.
- Topical lotions:
  - **Menthol-containing lotions** (see appendix to this chapter).
  - **Lubricating ointment** to which menthol 0.25% to 0.5% is added.
  - For worst affected areas:
    - **Calamine lotion** (can add menthol).
    - **Crotamiton** (Eurax) cream, bid to tid.

Nonspecific Pharmacologic Treatment

- A **sedating antihistamine** can be prescribed for use 1 hour before bedtime (can switch to twice-daily dosing if the effect does not last throughout the day). Possibly useful drugs include
  - Hydroxyzine (Atarax, Vistaril), 25 mg PO hs.
  - Doxepin (Sinequan, Adapin), 25 mg PO hs.
  - Promethazine (Phenergan), 25 mg PO hs.
  - Chlorpheniramine maleate, 2 to 4 mg PO hs.

- Diphenhydramine (Benadryl), 50 mg PO q6h.
- Where available, dimetindenum (Fenestil), 1 mg PO qd plus 0.1% gel applied locally tid will take care of the majority of difficult pruritus cases (not currently available in the United States).
  - Nonsedating antihistamines have *not* been effective.
  - *Avoid* topical corticosteroids, especially fluorinated steroids.

Specific Management Measures for Pruritus of Known Etiology

Cause of Pruritus	Treatment Measures
Xerosis	Stop using soap. Bathe in lukewarm, not hot, water. Oil skin after bathing and hs. Cover dry, itchy area with wet cloth × 15-20 minutes → apply ointment to area.
Wet skin	Protect skin with barrier (zinc oxide paste). Do *not* use petroleum jelly under breasts, in groin. Wet → dry dressings (Burow's solution) to dry skin.
Uremia	Treat underlying problem to the extent possible.

Cholestasis	**Ondansetron**, 8 mg IV, then 8 mg PO bid.
	Methyltestosterone, 25 mg SL bid.
	  • 7-10 days for maximum effect.
	  • Contraindicated in prostate or male breast cancer.
	Aluminum hydroxide (Maalox), 15 ml q6h.
	Cholestyramine (Questran), 4 gm qid, is theoretically of benefit, but it is difficult for ill patients to take and causes constipation as well as malabsorption of oral medications.
	May require **stent** for biliary drainage.
	Radiotherapy to nodes at porta hepatis.

Skin infiltration by breast cancer	Aspirin or another NSAID (naproxen, 250-500 mg bid).
Cutaneous lymphoma	Electron beam radiotherapy.
Candidiasis	**Miconazole** nitrate 2% (Monistat) lotion, qd-bid.

- When specific measures fail to control pruritus, try **dimetindenum** (Fenestil)—where available—orally and applied topically, as described above.

References and Further Reading

Goldman BD, Koh HK. Pruritus and Malignancy. In Bernard JD (ed). *Mechanisms and Management of Pruritus*. New York: McGraw Hill, 1994, Chap. 21.

Raderer M, Müller C, Scheithauer W. Ondansetron for pruritus due to cholestasis (letter). *N Engl J Med* 330:1540, 1994.

Savin JA. Do systemic antipruritic agents work? *Br J Dermatol* 102:113, 1980.

Schworer H, Ramadori G. Improvement of cholestatic pruritus by ondansetron. *Lancet* 341:1277, 1993.

Appendix: Antipruritic Agents—Formulations

Commonly used components:

- **Camphor**: applied in 1% to 3% concentration; anesthetic effect.
- **Menthol** (0.25-0.5%) substitutes cool sensation for itch.
- **Phenol** (0.5-2%) anesthetizes cutaneous nerve endings.
- **Salicylic acid** (1-2%) and **tars** (3-10%): mode of action unknown.

Calamine lotion USP (drying)

calamine (zinc oxide with 0.5% ferric oxide for coloring)	8 gm
zinc oxide	8 gm
glycerin	2 ml
bentonite magma (suspending agent)	25 ml
calcium hydroxide solution qs	100 ml

Phenolated calamine USP
1% phenol added to the above

Calamine liniment (less drying)

calamine	15 gm
peanut oil	50 gm
calcium hydroxide qs	100 ml

Menthol lotion with phenol (Schamberg's)

menthol	0.5 gm
phenol	1 gm
zinc oxide	20 gm
calcium hydroxide solution	40 ml
peanut oil qs	100 ml

Antipruritic lotion

menthol	0.5-1 gm
phenol	0.5-1 gm
benzyl alcohol	5-10 gm
olive oil	5 ml
propylene glycol	5 ml
camphor water qs	100 ml

Antipruritic ointment

phenol	1 gm
menthol	0.25 gm
salicylic acid	1 gm
coal tar	2 gm
hydrophilic ointment qs	100 gm

11 Other Skin Problems

Dry Skin (Xerosis)

Incidence

Dry skin is very common among all elderly, especially during cold months of the year.

- Represents dehydration of the stratum corneum.
- **Skin becomes dry because it lacks *water*,** not skin oils → therapy is directed at replacing water in the skin.
- Xerosis is a common source of **itching** (pruritus) in patients with cancer.
- When xerosis is associated with inflammation and itch → asteatotic eczema.

Clinical Findings

- Dry skin covered with fine scale, particularly over anterior tibias, dorsa of the hands, forearms.
- In more severe cases, skin becomes fissured and takes on the appearance of cracked porcelain.
- Itching → scratching → inflammation → more itching, etc.

Prevention of Xerosis

- Keep room temperature as low as possible consistent with the patient's comfort.

- Use a portable humidifier to increase the ambient moisture in the patient's surroundings.
- Avoid mechanical trauma from rough clothing or bedding.
- Avoid excessive use of soap and water.
- Rub the skin surface with emollient oil immediately after bath and in the evening before sleep.

Management of Xerosis

- Rationale: First add water to the skin; then take measures to keep it there.
  - *Add water to the skin* by soaking affected part (or by **bathing**) for 5 to 10 minutes in warm (not hot) water.
    - For patients who cannot bathe, place a wet cloth over the area of xerosis for 15 to 20 minutes.
    - Do not use soaps; bath emollients (Alpha Keri, Aveeno) preferred.
  - Immediately after bathing, *while skin is still moist,* apply fatty hydrophobic **ointment** to skin to keep the moisture in (**petrolatum** excellent in the elderly; otherwise protective ointment such as Aquaphor).
- For *inflamed, eczematous skin,* use a **topical corticosteroid ointment** with occlusive dressings for 24 to 48 hours.

Sweating

Incidence

Sweating, with or without fever, occurs in approximately 5% of cancer patients.
- *Night sweats* are particularly common in lymphomas and small cell lung cancer.
- Sweating in patients with advanced cancer may be caused by
  - Morphine.
  - Other drugs that cause autonomic hyperactivity.
  - Liver metastases.
  - Tumor pyrogens.
  - Occult infection (fever often masked by corticosteroids, dehydration, debility).

Management of Sweating

- Frequent sponge baths with tepid water.
- Lightweight pajamas and bedding.

- Change bedding frequently.
- In hot weather, use an electric fan to promote evaporation of sweat from the skin and air conditioning to cool ambient temperature.
- If the patient is *febrile* and uncomfortable from fever, give an **antipyretic** such as acetaminophen, 500 mg qid, or aspirin, 325 mg qid.
- If there is reason to suspect occult *infection* (with or without fever) and sweating is distressing to the patient, give a trial of antibiotic therapy with a broad-spectrum agent.
- For *morphine-induced sweating*, or sweating in the context of *liver metastases*, try **dexamethasone**, 2 to 4 mg PO qam, or **indomethacin**, 25 mg PO qam.
- For *wet, macerated skin* in *intertriginous areas*, protect skin with **zinc oxide paste**.

Radiation Damage to the Skin

Newer megavoltage machines cause much less skin damage at the entry site, but orthovoltage x-ray, which is particularly useful for palliation of bone pain, may produce **skin changes**:
- Erythema →
- Dry desquamation (heals 2-4 weeks after treatment) →
- Moist desquamation (heals 4-8 weeks after treatment) →
- Pigmentation (usually disappears in 3-4 months).

Preventing Skin Damage During Radiation Treatment

- Do not apply antiperspirants, lotions containing alcohol, or other irritating substances to the skin.
- Avoid physical irritants against irradiated skin.
- Avoid direct sunlight on the irradiated field (during treatment and forever after).
- Do not use tape on the skin that lies within the radiation port.

Management of Acute Radiation Damage to the Skin

- For severe erythema or moist desquamation: cool compresses × 10 minutes → air dry.
- For dry desquamation: unscented lubricating ointment.

Herpes Infections

Herpes Simplex ("Cold Sores")

Herpes labialis is caused by type 1 herpesvirus.
- After primary infection, the virus remains latent in sensory ganglia.
- Can be reactivated by stress, fever, infection, and anything that depresses immunity (lymphoma).
- Most common sites: perioral, cheeks, nose, and neck (but can occur anywhere on the skin).

Clinical Findings

- Primary infection:
  - Appearance of lesions preceded by local tenderness for 1 to 2 days.
  - With the appearance of the lesions, there is *severe pain* and tender submandibular lymphadenopathy.
  - Pain may be severe enough to prevent eating and drinking.
  - Buccal mucosa shows vesicles and erosion; gingiva is red and edematous.
- Recurrent infection:
  - Lesions are preceded by burning or tingling sensations for several hours.
  - Less painful than primary infection.
  - Clusters of clear vesicles then appear at the site of earlier burning sensations → vesicles become cloudy → prurulent → dry and crust.
  - Tender lymphadenopathy.
  - Healing occurs within 7 to 10 days if bacterial superinfection does not occur.

Management of Herpes Simplex Infections

- Primary infections:
  - Adequate **analgesia** may require opioids during the first week or so.
  - **Topical anesthetics** may provide relief of mouth pain (Benadryl Elixir or viscous lidocaine).
  - **Benzalkonium chloride mouthwash** (Zephiran) helps soothe mucous membranes and prevent secondary infection.
- Recurrent infection:
  - **Topical** ethyl **ether**:
    - Soak a small cotton pledget in ethyl ether, and place it over the entire lesion for 5 minutes (lesion and surrounding skin will blanch).

- Repeat in 12 or 24 hours and again in 48 hours.
- Slight burning on application is quickly followed by relief of pain and itching.
- When lesions are in the healing stage, **topical bacitracin** ointment will help prevent superinfection.

Herpes Zoster ("Shingles")

Primary infection usually occurs in childhood (varicella).

▪ Herpes zoster results from *reactivation* of virus that lies latent in the dorsal root or cranial nerve ganglion.
▪ Tends to follow a **dermatomal distribution**. The location of the dermatome may be affected by
  • Previous radiation therapy.
  • Malignant lesions involving the spinal cord.
  • Peripheral metastatic deposits.

Clinical Findings

▪ Eruption of zoster lesions often *preceded for 3 to 10 days by itch, tenderness, or pain.*
  • There may be dysesthesia, hypesthesia, or hyperesthesia in the affected dermatome.
  • Pain of zoster sometimes taken for myocardial infarct, cholecystitis, or ureteral colic, depending on location.
  • Pain may persist for several months.
▪ Lesions start posteriorly (most commonly in thoracic or cervical segments) → anterior and peripheral distribution of the affected nerve.
  • Red macules, papules, plaques → clusters of vesicles → crusting and shedding within 1 to 2 weeks.
  • In more severe cases, lesions may become hemorrhagic or infarcted.

Management of Herpes Zoster Infections

Problem	Treatment Measures
Pain during acute attack	Analgesia as required (opioids).
Vesicular rash	Cool compresses (1 : 20 Burow's solution). Paint lesions with tincture of benzoin/collodion. Drying shake lotion (alcohol/menthol). Splinting, as for rib fracture: Cover lesions with cotton, then wrap with elastic bandage.

continued

Problem	Treatment Measures
Crusted or infected lesions	Topical antibiotic cream (e.g., bacitracin).
Prevention of postherpetic neuralgia	Acyclovir (Zovirax) ointment, tid × 1 week. Dexamethasone, 10 mg PO qam × 1 week → 5 mg PO qam × 1 week → 2 mg PO qam × 1 week, starting within the first week of the eruption.
Treatment of postherpetic neuralgia	Start standard analgesic regimen according to the WHO ladder (nonopioid → weak opioid → strong opioid). If no improvement is noted within the first 3-4 days of treatment, add: **Amitriptyline**, 10-25 mg PO hs; increase dosage by 25 mg q3 days thereafter until maximum dosage of 75-100 mg has been reached. If results are not satisfactory, add **carbamazepine**, starting at 200 mg PO hs, and gradually escalating the dosage (by 200 mg q3-5 days) up to about 800 mg, as tolerated. Try **TENS** (transcutaneous electrical nerve stimulation) to the affected dermatome (electrodes placed on either side of the herpetic lesions).

References and Further Reading

DeConno F, Ventafridda V, Saita L. Skin problems in advanced and terminal cancer patients. *J Pain Symptom Manage* 6:247, 1991.

Eaglestein WH, Katz R, Brown JA. The effects of early corticosteroid therapy on the skin eruption and pain of herpes zoster. *JAMA* 211:1681, 1970.

Farrell RG, Nesland RS. Topical ethyl ether therapy of herpes simplex lesions. *JACEP* 6:372, 1977.

Levine N. State of the art: Topical corticosteroids. *Ariz Med* 361:904, 1979.

Sabin AB. Misery of recurrent herpes: What to do? *N Engl J Med* 293:986, 1975.

Schimpff S, Serpick A, Stoler B, et al. Varicella-zoster infections in patients with cancer. *Ann Intern Med* 76:241, 1972.

Taub A. Relief of postherpetic neuralgia with psychotropic drugs. *J Neurosurg* 39:235, 1973.

Gastrointestinal
and Abdominal

12 Oral Complications and Mouth Care

Clinical Findings Relevant to Oral Hygiene

History

In taking the history, ask about
- Dryness of the mouth.
- Sores in the mouth.
- Oral pain.
- Bleeding from the mouth.
- Changes in taste.
- Dysphagia.
- Recent chemotherapy.
- Previous radiation therapy.
- Current medications.
- Previous dental/periodontal disease.
- Dentures.

Physical Examination

In performing the physical examination of the mouth, pay particular attention to
- Odor of the breath.
- Lips: cracking, cheilosis, herpetic lesions.
- Tongue: papillae, coating, moisture.

- State of the gingiva and teeth.
- Buccal membranes: ulcers, candidal pseudomembrane.
- Oropharynx: erythema, lesions.
- Lesions of the hard or soft palate.
- Dentures: Do they fit properly? In what condition are they?

Dry Mouth (Xerostomia)

Incidence in Patients with Advanced Cancer

- Xerostomia is mentioned as a specific complaint by 40% of patients admitted to a hospice.
- Xerostomia probably affects all cancer patients to some degree during the terminal stages of their illness.

Causes of Xerostomia in Cancer Patients

- **Candidiasis**.
- **Drugs**: anticholinergics, antihistamines, phenothiazines, antidepressants, morphine, β-blockers, diuretics, anticonvulsants, antipsychotics.
- **Radiation** therapy to the head and neck.
- **Dehydration**.
- **Mucositis** secondary to chemotherapy.
- **Mouth breathing**.

Management of Dry Mouth in Patients with Advanced Cancer

Objective	Possible Means
Treat empirically for candidiasis	Antifungal agents (see section on candidiasis, below).
Stimulate salivary flow	Crushed ice. Sugar-free lemon drops or gum. Pineapple chunks. Pilocarpine, 5–7.5 mg tid or qid, especially for postradiation xerostomia.
Replace lost secretions	Saliva substitutes: ▪ Carboxymethylcellulose preparations (Glandosane). ▪ Mucin-based preparations.

Objective	Possible Means
Protect the teeth	Avoid dietary sugar. Scrupulous oral hygiene and fluoride rinses. Toothbrushing with fluoride gel toothpaste, soft brush. Regular dental flossing. Fluoride applications: Elmex Gelee A297, 25 gm q2 weeks.
Treat dehydration with local measures	Sips of water. Spray bottle to lubricate mouth with water. Swab the patient's mouth periodically with a moistened gauze sponge.
Prevent complications of xerostomia	Mouth care every 2 hours (teach family members).

Sore Mouth

Most common **causes** in patients with advanced cancer:
- Candidiasis.
- Herpes simplex, especially in patients receiving chemotherapy.
- Mucositis.
- Aphthous stomatitis.

Oral Candidiasis

Incidence

- In ambulatory patients, 16% of patients with leukemia, 7% of patients with solid tumors.
- Occurs in 10% of hospitalized, debilitated elderly patients regardless of underlying diagnosis.
- Incidence probably approaches 90% as the patient with cancer nears death.

Risk Factors in Cancer Patients

- Recent chemotherapy or radiation therapy.
- Antibiotic treatment.
- Corticosteroids.
- Smoking.

Clinical Findings

▪ Most common oral form of candidiasis is **thrush** (acute pseudo-membranous candidiasis):
 • Painless white strands, flecks, or patches resembling milk curds that adhere firmly to underlying mucosa (bleeds if scraped off).
 • Lesions may develop in any part of the mouth, but most often the sides/dorsum of the tongue, buccal mucosa, gums, and oropharynx.
▪ **Acute atrophic candidiasis**:
 • Usually follows antibiotic therapy.
 • Patchy loss of papillae on the tongue with painful erosions of the oral mucosa.
▪ **Chronic atrophic candidiasis**:
 • Occurs in as many as 65% of denture wearers.
 • Chronic erythema and edema of the palate where it comes in contact with the dentures; cheilosis.

Treatment of Oral Candidiasis

Antifungal Agent	Dosage	Comments
Clotrimazole troches (Mycelex)	10 mg × 5/day (q4h while awake) × 2 weeks	Agent of choice because of low cost, high patient acceptability, and absence of adverse side effects. Excellent prophylactic agent in high-risk patients.
Fluconazole (Diflucan)	150 mg PO × 1	Effective in a single dose. Useful in patients with short prognosis.
Nystatin oral suspension	3–6 ml q6h (100,000 U/ml)	No prophylactic activity. Must be held in the mouth for 5 minutes, then swallowed. Unpleasant, bitter taste. May be more soothing if diluted with flavored water and frozen (nystatin popsicle).
Amphotericin B lozenges	10-mg lozenge PO qid	Many patients respond slowly or not at all. Not currently available in the United States.
Miconazole 3% gel (Monistat)	2.5 ml applied to oral mucosa qid	Extremely unpleasant taste.

Antifungal Agent	Dosage	Comments
Ketoconazole (Nizoral)	200 mg PO qd	High incidence of adverse reactions: ▪ Especially nausea/vomiting (dose-related). ▪ Gynecomastia. ▪ Elevation of serum transaminase. For resistant cases only.

Herpes Simplex

Incidence

▪ Incidence in patients receiving chemotherapy reported anywhere from 11% to 65%; incidence higher in patients with lymphoma.

Clinical Findings

▪ Start as vesicles that rupture to form ulcers 4 to 6 mm in diameter with irregular borders, gray center, and swollen erythematous margin.
▪ Swollen, bleeding, very painful gingiva.
▪ If lips affected, they are swollen and encrusted.

Treatment of Oral Herpes Infections

Acyclovir (Zovirax) suspension, **200 mg (5 ml) × 5/day for 5 days.**

Mucositis

Causes of Mucositis in Cancer Patients

▪ **Radiation therapy:**
  • Mucositis usually appears by second week of radiation therapy (at dose of 2000 rad) →
  • Mucositis intensifies → may persist 2 to 3 weeks after completion of radiation.
▪ **Chemotherapy:**
  • Most commonly occurs after treatment with 5-fluorouracil, methotrexate, bleomycin, or doxorubicin.
  • Begins as early as 3 days after starting treatment, peaks 1 week after completing treatment, then slowly recedes (unless complicated by infection).
  • Early symptoms: increased sensitivity to hot/cold foods; intolerance to citrus fruits.
  • Oral mucositis may indicate ulceration of entire GI tract.

- Grading system for mucositis:

Stage	Signs and Symptoms
0	None
I	Pain
II	Ulcers, but able to eat
III	Ulcers; can take liquids only

Management of Mucositis

- **General measures**:
  - Serve **food at room temperature**, not hot.
  - Avoid heavily seasoned or acid foods (or any foods that trigger pain).
  - Avoid alcohol and tobacco.
  - Moisten foods with sauces; dry foods may be difficult for patient to swallow.
  - Chilled or frozen yogurt soothes oral mucosa and provides a high-protein snack.
  - Institute **infection prevention** measures:
    - Clotrimazole troches 10 mg × 5/day. If clotrimazole is not locally available, use nystatin oral suspension, 300,000 U tid to qid (3 ml can be frozen in sweetened, flavored water as a popsicle).
    - Remove and clean dentures before each dose; at night, soak dentures in water containing 5 ml of nystatin suspension.
- **Mouth care** every 4 hours around the clock:
  - Remove patient's dentures, if present.
  - Use a soft toothbrush to apply dilute hydrogen peroxide solution (1 part H_2O_2 to 4 parts saline) to the teeth, gums, and tongue.
  - Rinse mouth with the same peroxide solution until the mouth is free of debris.
  - Final rinse with tap water.
  - Cleanse the patient's dentures, and replace them gently if tolerated.
- **Pharmacologic treatment possibilities**:
  - **Xylocaine viscous 2%** solution: Swish 15 ml for 30 seconds, then spit out (q3h maximum).

- **Analgesic cocktail:** 1 to 2 tbsp 15 minutes ac and hs; hold for 2 minutes in mouth, then spit out. (To prepare: Maalox, 345 ml; xylocaine viscous, 79 ml; Benadryl Elixir, 47 ml.)
- **Choline salicylate** (Teejel) or **benzydamine HCl 5%** applied to affected area (benzydamine is not currently available in the United States).
- **Orabase** applied prn pc and hs to ulcerated areas.
- **Sucralfate 1-gm tabs:** Crush and spread through mouth.
- **Sucralfate suspension:** Swish for 2 minutes and swallow, pc and hs. (To prepare: Dissolve eight 1-gm sucralfate tabs in 40 ml of sterile water; add 40 ml of 70% sorbitol and shake; in a separate container, dissolve 3 Ensure flavor packs in 10 ml of water; add to drug mixture; water qs to 120 ml.)
- **Vitamin E:** Puncture capsule and apply directly on lesion.

Aphthous Stomatitis

Clinical Findings

- Well-circumscribed, 1- to 15-mm discrete, painful lesions (no vesicular stage).
- Most often found in the soft oral mucosa (i.e., not on the gingiva or hard palate).

Management of Aphthous Stomatitis

Treatment possibilities:
- Triamcinolone oral rinses, 5 ml qid after meals and hs. (To prepare the rinse fluid, add 60 ml of Kenalog-40 to 200 ml of normal saline), *or*
- Tetracycline suspension, 250 mg swished in the mouth for 2 minutes, then swallowed, qid, *or*
- Levamisole, 50 mg PO tid × 2 days/week.

Halitosis (Offensive or Unpleasant Breath)

Halitosis may be a serious problem in the care of the terminally ill because it creates a barrier between the patient and those around him (family, friends, caregivers) and may worsen social isolation at the end of life.

Most Common Causes of Halitosis in Patients with Advanced Cancer

- Problems in the oral cavity account for the majority of cases:
  - Poor oral hygiene ± xerostomia → periodontal and gingival disease.
  - Infection (herpetic, candidal).
  - Necrotic tumor in the oral cavity.
  - Bleeding within the mouth, from infection, tumor, or chemotherapy.
- Respiratory tract disease:
  - Chronic sinusitis.
  - Necrotic tumors involving the pharynx, larynx, or bronchi.
- Gastrointestinal problems, primary gastric stasis.
- Renal or hepatic failure.
- The nature of the bad odor may provide a clue to the diagnosis:

Odor of the Breath	Possible Source
Sewer breath	Anaerobic organisms anywhere in the mouth, respiratory tract, or GI tract, especially: • Necrotic tumor in mouth or throat. • Pulmonary abscess or bronchiectasis. • Intestinal obstruction.
Sickly, sweet breath	*Pseudomonas* pneumonia.
Fishy or uriniferous breath	Renal failure.
Fetor hepaticus: musty, ammoniac odor	Hepatic failure.

Management of Halitosis in the Terminally Ill

General Measures

- Good mouth care every 4 hours (see next section).
- Disinfection of dentures every night.
- Avoid foods that contribute to bad breath odor (garlic, onions).

Specific Measures

Contributing Cause of Halitosis	Treatment Measures
Poor oral hygiene	Mouth care (see below).
Necrotic tumor in oropharynx	Metronidazole, 250 mg PO tid–qid or applied topically to visible lesion. 1% Hydrogen peroxide mouthwash: Gargle qid (pc and hs).

Contributing Cause of Halitosis	Treatment Measures
Bleeding in the mouth	Apply topical thrombin to the bleeding area. Consider tranexamic acid, 500 mg PO tid.
Suppurative process in the lungs (copious, foul-smelling sputum)	Metronidazole, 250 mg PO tid-qid ± amoxicillin, 250-500 mg PO tid while awaiting results of sputum culture.
Gastric stasis	Metoclopramide, 10 mg PO qid ac and hs, *or* Cisapride, 5 mg PO qid, ac and hs.

Routine Mouth Care for Terminally Ill Cancer Patients

General Principles

- Regular mouth care can prevent the majority of oral problems in patients with advanced cancer.
- Routine mouth care should be given at least **every 4 hours**.
- Mouth care is especially important **before each meal**, to stimulate appetite and flow of saliva.
- Cleansing of the mouth should also follow each meal and snack, to avoid accumulation of debris.
- The **family should be involved** in the patient's oral care when the patient is no longer able to carry out oral hygiene measures for himself.

Oral Care Protocol (Every 4 Hours)

- **Remove** patient's **dentures**, if present, and brush thoroughly with a denture brush and appropriate solution (if patient has candidiasis, dentures should be soaked each night in nystatin suspension).
- With a **soft** (baby) **toothbrush**, brush the patient's teeth by placing the brush at the gingival margin and making a sweeping motion toward the crowns of the teeth. If use of a brush causes bleeding, use a disposable foam stick soaked in sterile saline to clean the dental surfaces and gingival margins.
- **Clean** the patient's **tongue**:
  - Gauze pad dipped in dilute peroxide solution.
  - Some authorities recommend giving fresh pineapple.

- Have patient **rinse** mouth:
  - **Normal saline rinse** for normal mucosa.
  - If there is thick mucus, use **sodium bicarbonate mouthwash** (2 tsp of sodium bicarbonate to 1 L of water or saline).
  - If there is hardened debris in the mouth, use **hydrogen peroxide mouthwash** (1 part 3% hydrogen peroxide to 4 parts water, prepared just before use).
  - Final rinse with saline or tap water.
- Apply water-soluble jelly to **lips**.

References and Further Reading

Bodey GP. Candidiasis in cancer patients. *Am J Med* 77D:13, 1984.

Bodey GP, Samonis G, Rolston K. Prophylaxis of candidiasis in cancer patients. *Semin Oncol* 17(3, Suppl 6):24, 1990.

Cottone JA, Langlais RP. Recurrent aphthous stomatitis—literature review. *J Oral Med* 32:21, 1977.

Daeffler R. Oral hygiene measures for patients with cancer. *Cancer Nurs*, Part I: 3(5):347, 1980; Part II: 3(6):427, 1980; Part III: 4(1):29, 1981.

DeConno F, Ripamonti C, Sbanotto A, Ventafridda V. Oral complications in patients with advanced cancer. *J Palliative Care* 5:7, 1989.

Degregorio MW, Lee WMF, Ries CA. *Candida* infections in patients with acute leukemia: Ineffectiveness of nystatin prophylaxis and relationship between oropharyngeal and systemic candidiasis. *Cancer* 50:2780, 1982.

Dreizen S. Oral candidiasis. *Am J Med* 77D:28, 1984.

Finlay I. Oral fungal infections. *Eur J Palliative Care* 2(Suppl):4, 1995.

Graykowski EA, Kingman A. Double blind trial of tetracycline in recurrent aphthous ulceration. *J Oral Pathol* 7:376, 1978.

Johnston JT, Ferreti GA, Nethery WJ, et al. Oral pilocarpine for post-irradiation xerostomia in patients with head and neck cancer. *N Engl J Med* 329:390, 1993.

Krishnasamy M. The nurse's role in oral care. *Eur J Palliative Care* 2(Suppl):8, 1995.

Meyer JD, Degraeve M, Claryss J, et al. Levamisole in aphthous stomatitis. *Br Med J* 1:671, 1977.

Quintiliani R, Owens NJ, Quercia RA, et al. Treatment and prevention of oropharyngeal candidiasis. *Am J Med* 77D:44, 1984.

Scully C. Other causes of oral soreness. *Eur J Palliative Care* 2(Suppl):13, 1995.

Walls A. Dental causes of sore mouth. *Eur J Palliative Care* 2(Suppl):10, 1995.

Yeo E, Alvarado T, Fainstein V, Bodey GP. Prophylaxis of oropharyngeal candidiasis with clotrimazole. *J Clin Oncol* 3:1668, 1985.

13 Anorexia

Definition

Loss of appetite.

Incidence

- Anorexia is the **second most common symptom** in patients with advanced cancer (after weakness and fatigability) and is present in 65% to 85% of cases.
- Studies have shown that appetite and the ability to eat were the **most important** physical **aspects of** patients' **quality of life** (Padilla, 1986)—more important to the patient than physical strength or the ability to work.

Causes of Anorexia in Patients with Advanced Cancer

- Impaired gastric emptying.
- Constipation.
- Pain.
- Squashed stomach syndrome.
- Medications (e.g., opioids, antibiotics).
- Oral candidiasis.
- Peptides produced in response to tumor (e.g., tumor necrosis factor, interleukin-1).

- Changed tastes and new food aversions (e.g., to red meat).
- Low morale.

Clinical Assessment

History

In taking the history, ask:
- What **foods does the patient like** and **dislike?**
- Are there problems with **taste** or **smell?**
- Does the patient have sores or dryness in his **mouth?**
- Are there **problems with chewing** and **swallowing?**
- Does the patient suffer from **nausea** and vomiting?
- How often does the patient move his bowels? When was the last bowel movement?
- Are there symptoms of **malabsorption** (diarrhea, bulky or fatty stools)?
- What **medications** is the patient currently taking?
- Does the patient enjoy an occasional **alcoholic drink?**

Physical Examination

On physical examination, look particularly for:
- Signs of nutritional deficiency (e.g., atrophic skin, angular stomatitis, red tongue, bleeding gums).
- Oral candidiasis.
- Decreased bowel sounds.
- Fecal impaction.

Laboratory Studies

- Blood sugar.
- Serum electrolytes.
- Serum calcium.
- Total protein and serum albumin.

Management of Anorexia in Advanced Cancer

Objective

To improve the patient's quality of life:

- Patients find anorexia depressing, a reminder that they are "wasting away" from their disease → improvement in appetite boosts morale.
- It is usually not realistic to try to achieve significant improvement in the patient's nutritional state. (For nutritional therapy while the patient is still undergoing active treatment, see Chapter 3.)

General Measures

- Give the patient **permission to eat less** than previously.
- Find out what the patient likes to eat, and prepare **foods that the patient chooses**.
- Use **smaller dinner plates**, and give smaller portions.
- **Make food attractive** to the eye and to the palate.
- **Avoid strong cooking smells** at mealtime.
- The patient's hands and face should be washed for mealtimes, and his mouth cleaned.
- When possible, have the patient **dress for meals** and sit at the table, preferably with others; eating is a social as well as a nutritional occasion.
- Have **food available** whenever the patient is hungry.
- Treat conditions that may be contributing to anorexia (e.g., hypercalcemia, constipation).

Pharmacologic Interventions

Class of Drug	Example(s)	Comments
Gastrokinetic agents	**Metoclopramide**, 10 mg PO tid **Domperidone**,* 10 mg PO tid	Useful in patients complaining of nausea or early satiety.
Corticosteroids	**Dexamethasone**, 4 mg PO qam, then taper gradually to the minimum effective dosage	Highly effective in improving appetite in the short term, with few side effects at the dosage recommended; may lose efficacy after a few weeks.

*Not currently available in the United States.

continued

Class of Drug	*Example(s)*	*Comments*
Progesterone analogs	**Megestrol acetate**, 40 mg PO qid **Medroxyprogesterone acetate**, 100 mg PO tid	80% of patients will show marked improvement in appetite; significant decreases in nausea and vomiting occur in more than 50%; abnormalities of taste are often reduced, and weight gain (of fat and lean body mass) is often seen in nearly all patients except those in the most terminal stages. Treatment with recommended dosage costs $2/day (more expensive than steroids).
Cannabinoids	**Dronabinol**, 2.5 mg PO bid 1 hour pc	An effective appetite stimulant at low doses, without the usual side effects of drowsiness and muddled thinking.
Alcohol	1 glass of **beer** or **sherry** before meals	May improve appetite and morale in patients who enjoyed a drink before dinner when they were well.
Vitamins	Multivitamins Vitamin C, 500 mg qid	Anecdotal evidence of improved appetite (may be due to placebo effect).

In the Last Days of Life

- Anorexia is normal in the last days of life → feeding should be for comfort only.
- It is often necessary to help the patient's family to accept the situation and to desist from their attempts to force food on the patient.

References and Further Reading

Billings JA. Anorexia. *J Palliative Care* 10(1):51, 1994.

Bruera E, MacMillan K, Kuehn N, et al. A controlled trial of megestrol acetate on appetite, caloric intake, nutritional status and other symptoms in patients with advanced cancer. *Cancer* 66:1279, 1990.

Bruera E, Roca E, Cedaro L, et al. Action of oral methylprednisolone in terminal cancer patients: A prospective randomized double-blind study. *Cancer Treat Rep* 69:751, 1985.

Della Cuna GR, Pellegrini A, Piazzi M. Effect of methylprednisolone sodium succinate on quality of life in preterminal cancer patients: A placebo-controlled multicenter study. *Eur J Cancer Clin Oncol* 25:1817, 1989.

Kerr D. Alcohol and palliative care. *Palliative Med* 6:185, 1991.

Loprinzi CL, Eillison NM, Schaid DJ, et al. Controlled trial of megestrol acetate for the treatment of cancer anorexia and cachexia. *JNCI* 82:1127, 1990.

Moertel CG, Schutt AJ, Reitmeier RJ, Hahn RJ. Corticosteroid therapy of preterminal gastrointestinal cancer. *Cancer* 33:1607, 1974.

Nelson K, Walsh D, Deeter P, Sheehan F. A phase II study of delta-9-tetrahydrocannabinol for appetite stimulation in cancer-associated anorexia. *J Palliative Care* 10(1):14, 1994.

Padilla GV. Psychological aspects of nutrition and cancer. *Surg Clin North Am* 66(6), 1986.

Popiela T, Lucchi R, Giongo F. Methylprednisolone as palliative therapy for female terminal cancer patients. *Eur J Cancer Clin Oncol* 25:1823, 1989.

Reitmeier M, Volkl S, Hartenstein R. Determination of Body Compartments Using Bioelectrical Impedance Analysis in Cachectic Cancer Patients on Megestrol Acetate Therapy. In *Hormones in Cancer Cachexia: Megestrol Acetate*. Munich: Zuckschwerdt Verlag, 1991, pp. 49–58.

Taylor MB, Moran BJ, Jackson AA. Nutritional problems and care of patients with far-advanced disease. *Palliative Med* 3:31, 1989.

Wadleigh RM, Spaulding M, Lembersky B, et al. Dronabinol enhancement of appetite in cancer patients (abstract). *Proc Am Soc Clin Oncol* 9:331, 1990.

Willox JC, Corr J, Shaw J, et al. Prednisolone as an appetite stimulant in patients with cancer. *Br Med J* 228:27, 1984.

14 Dysphagia

Definitions

- *Dysphagia*: Difficulty in swallowing.
- *Odynophagia*: Pain on swallowing.

Incidence

- Twelve to 23% of patients dying of cancer experience dysphagia.
- Incidence is highest among patients with
  - Cancer of the **head and neck** (40-80%).
  - **Esophageal** cancer.
  - **Gastric** cancer.
  - Cancers involving mediastinal or pharyngeal lymph nodes (bronchogenic cancer, lymphoma).

Pathophysiology and Etiology

Swallowing proceeds through **three phases**, any or all of which may be disturbed by the malignant process.

Phase	Normal Action	Signs of Disturbance
Buccal	Food or fluid passes into the oropharynx via voluntary action of tongue and palate.	Drooling; leakage of food from mouth. Retention of food in mouth.
Pharyngeal	Swallowing reflex is initiated with closure of the epiglottis.	Choking, coughing. Food sticking in *throat*. Nasal regurgitation.
Esophageal	Peristaltic waves propel food to the stomach.	Sensation of food sticking in retrosternal area. Pain: retrosternal, throat, intrascapular.

Causes of Dysphagia in Advanced Cancer

- **Mechanical obstruction** (→ dysphagia for solids early, later for liquids as well):
  - Intraluminal tumor mass within the esophagus.
  - External compression by circumferential tumor, mediastinal mass.
  - Tumor in the mouth or pharynx.
  - Esophageal stricture secondary to radiation therapy.
- **Neuromuscular defects** (→ dysphagia for solids *and* liquids):
  - Perineural invasion into vagal trunk or sometimes sympathetic chain.
  - Damage to intramural esophageal nerve plexus by tumor invasion.
  - Cranial nerve palsies (V, VII, IX, X, XII) due to spread of tumor to base of skull.
  - Cerebral metastases → bulbar palsies.
- **Odynophagia**:
  - Candidiasis.
  - Mucositis secondary to chemotherapy or radiation therapy.
  - Reflux esophagitis.
- **Dystonic reactions** to drugs (metoclopramide, haloperidol, phenothiazines).
- Severe **weakness** and general debility.

Clinical Findings

Taking the History—Relevant Questions

Relevant Question	Implications of Answer
Does it hurt to swallow? Where?	Pharyngeal pain on swallowing suggests an inflammatory process, such as candidiasis. Severe retrosternal pain suggests esophageal spasm.
Do you have more trouble swallowing solids than swallowing liquids?	In mechanical obstruction, dysphagia for solids usually precedes dysphagia for liquids; in neuromuscular disorders, liquids are more difficult to swallow.
Do you feel as if the food is sticking on the way down? If so, point to where it seems to be getting stuck.	Usually indicates mechanical obstruction; two thirds of patients can accurately localize the site of obstruction.

Physical Examination

- Examine the **mouth and throat** carefully for signs of
  - Candidiasis.
  - Mucositis.
  - Pharyngeal inflammation.
  - Obstructing masses.
- Pay special attention to **cranial nerves** V, VII, IX, X, and XII.
- Give the patient sips of water to **observe him swallowing**:

Problem Observed in Swallowing	Suggests
Drooling	Bulbar or other neuromuscular deficit
Nasal regurgitation	Bulbar palsy
Coughing after liquids	Esophagotracheal fistula
Larynx does not elevate on swallowing	Tenth cranial nerve lesion

Management of Dysphagia

Specific Measures

- Conservative treatment alone will ameliorate dysphagia in 60% of patients.

Contributing Cause	Management Measures
Dystonic reaction to drugs	Switch to another medication. Give diphenhydramine, 25–50 mg PO/IM, *or* benztropine, 2 mg PO/IM.
Candidiasis	**Analgesia** + **Ketoconazole**, 200 mg PO qd × 5 days, *or* fluconazole, 150 mg PO × 1, *or* nystatin, 3–6 ml PO tid.
Mucositis after chemotherapy	Soft diet. Avoid hot food and beverages. Mucositis analgesic cocktail (see Chapter 12).
Radiation mucositis	**Indomethacin**, 25 mg PO bid–tid.
Suspected perineural infiltration by tumor	Trial of **dexamethasone**, 8 mg PO qam.
Mechanical obstruction of esophagus by tumor	Trial of **dexamethasone**, 8–12 mg PO qam. Expansile metal stent (preferred procedure: lowest morbidity; 90% experience improvement), *or* high-dose (60 Gy) radiation and concurrent chemotherapy (5-FU/mitomycin C), *or* intracavitary laser therapy (80% experience improvement), *or* intracavitary irradiation (65% experience improvement) or external beam irradiation.
Total obstruction	Reduce secretions to reduce drooling: **scopolamine patch**, 1.5 mg applied every 3 days.

Measures to Optimize Swallowing

- Patient sitting up to eat, with head stabilized as necessary.
- Patient should wear dentures to eat.
- Give small amounts of food, slowly.
- Remind patient to chew carefully.
- Give fluids from a nearly full cup so that patient need not tilt head back to drink.

Special Diets for Patients with Dysphagia

Type of Patient	Dietary Advice
Patient who can still swallow some solids	Frequent, small feedings. Moisten food with sauces; avoid dry food. Cut food into small pieces. Avoid sticky foods, soft bread, etc.
Patients who cannot swallow solids	Experiment with different consistencies to find food consistency that is optimal for the particular patient (paste, puree, liquid).
Patients with esophageal stent	Sit upright to eat. Increase fluid intake. Sip carbonated beverages during and after each meal. Avoid soft bread and rolls (eat bread toasted). Avoid fish, hard-boiled eggs, stringy foods. Avoid pithy fruits (e.g., oranges). Chew carefully; swallow slowly. Take medications in crushed or liquid form.

References and Further Reading

Ahlquist DA, Gostout CG, Viggiano TR, et al. Endoscopic laser palliation of malignant dysphagia: A prospective study. *Mayo Clin Proc* 62:867, 1987.

Barr H, Krasner N. Prospective quality of life analysis after palliative photoablation for the treatment of malignant dysphagia. *Cancer* 68:1660, 1991.

Bown SG. Palliation of malignant dysphagia: surgery, radiotherapy, laser, intubation alone or in combination? *Gut* 32:841, 1991.

Carter RL, Pittam MR, Tanner NSB. Pain and dysphagia in patients with squamous carcinomas of the head and neck: the role of perineural spread. *J R Soc Med* 75:598, 1982.

Coia LR, Soffen EM, Schultheis TE, et al. Swallowing function in patients with cancer treated with concurrent radiation and chemotherapy. *Cancer* 71:281, 1993.

Herskovic A, Martz K, Al-Sarraf M, et al. Combined chemotherapy and radiotherapy compared with radiotherapy alone in patients with cancer of the esophagus. *N Engl J Med* 326:1593, 1992.

Knyrim K, Wagner H-J, Bethge N, et al. A controlled trial of an expansile metal stent for palliation of esophageal obstruction due to inoperable cancer. *N Engl J Med* 329:1302, 1994.

Regnard C. Managing dysphagia in advanced cancer—a flow diagram. *Palliative Med* 4:215, 1990.

Rowland CG, Pagliero KM. Intracavitary irradiation in palliation of carcinoma of oesophagus and cardia. *Lancet* ii:981, 1985.

Sykes NP, Baines M, Carter RL. Clinical and pathological study of dysphagia conservatively managed in patients with advanced malignant disease. *Lancet* ii:726, 1988.

15 Hiccups

In the case of a person afflicted with hiccough, sneezing coming on removes the hiccough.

HIPPOCRATES, *APHORISMS*, VI, 13.

Definitions

- *Singultus* from the Latin *singul*: the act of attempting to catch one's breath while sobbing.
- *Hiccup* or *singultus:* Intermittent, reflex clonic spasm of the diaphragm and accessory inspiratory muscles associated with closure of the glottis.
- Duration:
  - *Bout:* an episode of hiccups.
  - *Persistent* or *protracted* hiccups: an episode of hiccups lasting > 48 hours.
  - *Intractable* hiccups: an episode of hiccups lasting > 1 month.

Anatomy and Physiology of Hiccups

Components of the Hiccup Reflex

Afferent Arm	Supraspinal Hiccup Center	Efferent Arm
Phrenic and vagus nerves.	Anatomic location unknown.	Phrenic and vagus nerves →

continued

135

Afferent Arm	Supraspinal Hiccup Center	Efferent Arm
Pharyngeal plexus. Sympathetic chain arising from T6–T12.	Probably involves interaction among brainstem and midbrain → respiratory center → phrenic nerve nuclei → medullary reticular formation → hypothalamus.	recurrent laryngeal nerve → hemidiaphragms and laryngeal muscles. Nerves to anterior scalene and intercostal muscles.

Characteristics of Hiccups

- Hiccups are most often **unilateral**; usually the *left* diaphragm is involved.
- If more than several hiccups occur sequentially, they become "established."
- Hiccup *frequency* is usually **4 to 60 per minute**, usually consistent for each individual.
  - ↑PCO_2 → ↓frequency of hiccups (rationale for rebreathing from paper bag).
  - ↓PCO_2 → ↑frequency of hiccups.
- Hiccups have only a minimal effect on ventilation; may be more gastrointestinal than respiratory in nature.
- Function of hiccups unknown; may serve to dislodge food caught in the esophagus.

Pathophysiology

- **Benign, self-limited hiccups** in the general population are usually due to excessive food or alcohol, aerophagia, or gastric distention.
- **Persistent or intractable hiccups** in terminally ill patients are more likely to be caused by the following:

Cause of Hiccups	Examples
Gastric distention (most common cause)	Impaired gastric motility Squashed stomach syndrome
CNS disturbance → release of higher center inhibition of hiccup reflex	Tumor Stroke
Irritation of **vagus nerve** anywhere along its course	Tumors of the neck, lung, mediastinum Esophagitis or esophageal obstruction Chest surgery

Cause of Hiccups	Examples
Irritation of the **phrenic nerve**	Tumors of the neck, mediastinum
Metabolic derangements	Uremia Hypocalcemia, hyponatremia Sepsis
Pharmacologic agents	IV corticosteroids Barbiturates Benzodiazepines

Complications of Intractable Hiccups

- Most common: **dehydration** and **weight loss.**
- Occasionally **insomnia** and **exhaustion.**
- Rarely, ventricular dysrhythmias.
- Hyponatremia (caused by polydipsia in an attempt to relieve the hiccups).
- **Esophagitis,** from recurrent gastroesophageal reflux (may also be a *cause* of hiccups).

Workup of the Patient with Persistent or Intractable Hiccups

History

- *Severity* and *duration* of current episode (severity does not always imply a serious organic cause; benign hiccups may also be intractable).
- *Relationship* of hiccups *to sleep* (hiccups that stop during sleep → psychogenic cause).
- Associated signs and symptoms.
- Recent *trauma, surgery,* or *acute illness.*
- *Medication* history.
- Previous episodes of hiccups.

Physical Examination

To detect potentially treatable causes of the episode.
- General appearance: toxic?
- Head: tenderness of temporal artery.
- Ears: foreign body irritating tympanic membrane.

- Throat: pharyngitis.
- Neck: goiter, cyst, cervical lymphadenopathy; rigidity.
- Chest: signs of pneumonia, pericarditis.
- Abdomen: distention, bowel sounds, tenderness.
- Neurologic: signs of stroke; delirium suggesting toxic/metabolic cause.

Laboratory Studies

- Chest x-ray: to rule out pulmonary, mediastinal, or cardiac sources of phrenic/vagal nerve irritation.
- CBC with differential (→ infectious causes).
- Electrolytes, especially sodium (→ hyponatremia).
- Other chemistries as suggested by history and physical examination: calcium, BUN, blood sugar, LFTs, CSF, toxicology screen.

Treatment of Intractable Hiccups

> ...[T]he amount of knowledge on any subject such as this can be considered as being in inverse proportion to the number of different treatments suggested and tried for it.
>
> MAYO (1932)

Nonpharmacologic Management

- Methods that involve **nasopharyngeal stimulation**:
  - Swallowing **granulated sugar** (1 tsp swallowed dry).
  - Stimulating the nasopharynx with a **nasogastric tube** (7.5–10 cm from tip of nares, so that tip is opposite C2; rapid, oscillating motion for 30 seconds) .
  - **Lifting the uvula** with a spoon or cotton-tip applicator.
  - Swallowing dry bread.
  - Rapid ingestion of 2 glasses of liqueur.
  - Forcible traction of the tongue to produce a gag reflex.
  - Gargling with water.
  - Sipping ice water or swallowing crushed ice.
  - Biting on a lemon.
  - Inhaling noxious agents (e.g., ammonia).
  - Drinking from the far side of a glass.
- **Stimulation of dermatome C5** (?interrupts hiccup reflex arc):
  - Tapping or rubbing the back of the neck.

- Cold key dropped inside the back collar.
- Vapocoolant spray or acupuncture to dermatomal area on the neck.
- Methods of **vagal afferent stimulation** (besides those already mentioned):
  - Nasogastric suction.
  - Iced lavage.
  - **Valsalva**, carotid massage, ocular globe pressure, digital rectal massage (!!).
- Interference with normal respiratory function:
  - Induction of sneezing or coughing.
  - **Breath holding**; hyperventilating, "gasping."
  - Rebreathing into a paper bag.
- Behavioral conditioning and hypnosis.
- Invasive techniques:
  - Pacing electrodes for direct phrenic nerve or diaphragmatic stimulation.
  - Phrenic nerve blockage with bupivacaine.
  - Surgical phrenic nerve interruption.

Pharmacologic Management

- In our experience, because a large proportion of cancer patients with hiccups suffer from gastric distention, the first line of approach, after trying simple mechanical remedies, is to give **metoclopramide** plus a simethicone or **simethicone/charcoal** preparation.
- First-line therapeutic agents:

Drug	Dosage	Comments
Metoclopramide (Reglan)	10 mg IV push over 2 minutes or IM; may repeat q4h. Maintenance: 10–20 mg PO qid	Increases gastric emptying *and* has central antidopaminergic activity.
Antacids containing **simethicone**	Charcoal Plus, 2 tabs PO qid (pc & hs) Silain-Gel, 2 tsp PO ½ hour pc & hs	Useful when gastric distention contributes to etiology.
Peppermint water		Relaxes lower esophageal sphincter → useful for hiccups from esophageal causes.

continued

Drug	Dosage	Comments
Peppermint water *cont.*		Do not use together with metoclopramide (has opposing action).
Haloperidol (Haldol)	2-5 mg IM Maintenance: 1-4 mg PO tid	Lower potential for hypotension, especially in the elderly. High efficacy rates.
Methotrimeprazine	25 mg PO tid	Strong sedative effect.
Chlorpromazine (Thorazine)	25-50 mg IM Maintenance: 25-50 mg tid	Postural hypotension a frequent complication. "Permanent" cure in 80%.

▪ Second-line therapeutic agents (reported effective in small, uncontrolled series):

Drug	Dosage	Comments
Phenytoin (Dilantin)	200 mg by slow IV push (< 50 mg/min) Maintenance: 300 mg/day	May be most effective for hiccups of central neurologic etiology. Monitor for bradycardia, heart block, hypotension.
Carbamazepine (Tegretol)	200 mg PO tid	Used successfully in hiccups due to multiple sclerosis.
Valproic acid (Depakene)	15 mg/kg/day titrated upward by 250 mg/day q2 weeks until hiccups stop or adverse side effects occur	May be associated with prolonged PT and PTT.
Methylphenidate (Ritalin)	10-20 mg IV	
Amitriptyline (Elavil)	10 mg PO tid	
Lidocaine	Loading dose of 1 mg/kg IV, followed by infusion of 2 mg/min	Second-line drug, when others fail.

Drug	Dosage	Comments
Baclofen (Atrofen, Lioresal)	5-10 mg PO bid	
Nifedipine (Adalat)	10-20 mg PO tid	

References and Further Reading

Pathophysiology

Baethge B, Lidsky M. Intractable hiccups associated with high dose intravenous methylprednisolone therapy. *Ann Intern Med* 104:58, 1986.

Davis J. An experimental study of hiccup. *Brain* 93:851, 1970.

Fisher C. Protracted hiccup: A male malady. *Trans Am Neurol Assoc* 1:128, 1967.

Jones J, Lloyd T, Cannon L. Persistent hiccups as an unusual manifestation of hyponatremia. *J Emerg Med* 5:283, 1987.

Kolodzik PW, Eilers MA. Hiccups (singultus): Review and approach to management. *Ann Emerg Med* 20:565, 1991.

Mayo C. Hiccup. *Surg Gynecol Obstet* 55:700, 1932.

Nathan MD, Leshner RT, Keller PA. Intractable hiccups. *Laryngoscope* 90:1612, 1980.

Samuels L. Hiccup: A ten-year review of anatomy, etiology, and treatment. *Can Med Assoc J* 67:315, 1952.

Shay S, Myers R, Johnston L. Hiccups associated with reflux esophagitis. *Gastroenterology* 87:204, 1984.

Souadjian JV, Cain JC. Intractable hiccups: Etiologic factors in 220 cases. *Postgrad Med* 43:72, 1968.

Stromberg BV. The hiccup. *Ear Nose Throat J* 58:354, 1979.

Travell J. A trigger point for hiccup. *J Am Osteopath Assoc* 77:308, 1977.

Wagner MS, Stapczynski JS. Persistent hiccups. *Ann Emerg Med* 11:24, 1982.

Treatment

Bellingham-Smith E. The significance and treatment of obstinate hiccough. *Practitioner* 150:1273, 1943.

Bendersky G, Baren M. Hypnosis in the termination of hiccups unresponsive to conventional treatment. *Arch Intern Med* 104:417, 1959.

Burke A, White A, Brill N. Baclofen for intractable hiccups (letter). *N Engl J Med* 319:1354, 1988.

Davignon A, Laureieux G, Genest J. Chlorpromazine in the treatment of persistent hiccough. *Union Med Can* 84:282, 1955.

Davis J. Diphenylhydantoin for hiccups (letter). *Lancet* 1:997, 1974.

Dorcus R, Kirkner F. The control of hiccoughs by hypnotic therapy. *J Clin Exp Hypnosis* 3:104, 1955.

Dunst M, Margolin K, Horak D. Lidocaine for severe hiccups (letter). *N Engl J Med* 329:890, 1993.

Engleman EG, Lankton J, Lankton B. Granulated sugar as treatment for hiccups in conscious patients (letter). *N Engl J Med* 285:1489, 1971.

Friedgood C, Ripstein C. Chlorpromazine (Thorazine) in the treatment of intractable hiccups. *JAMA* 157:309, 1955.

Fry E. Management of intractable hiccup. *Br Med J* 2:704, 1977.

Gigot AF, Flynn PD. Treatment of hiccups. *JAMA* 150:760, 1952.

Ives T, Fleming M, Weart C. Treatment of intractable hiccups with intramuscular haloperidol. *Am J Psychiatry* 142:1368, 1985.

Jacobson P, Messeneimer J, Farmer T. Treatment of intractable hiccups with valproic acid. *Neurology* 31:1458, 1981.

Lamphier T. Methods of management of persistent hiccups. *Md State Med J* 26:80, 1977.

Lewis J. Hiccups: Causes and cures. *J Clin Gastroenterol* 7:539, 1985.

Macris SG, et al. Intravenous methylphenidate for the treatment of singultus. *Anesth Analg* 42:440, 1963.

Madanagopolan N. Metoclopramide in hiccup. *Curr Med Res Opin* 3:371, 1975.

McFarling J, Susac J. Carbamazepine for hiccoughs (letter). *JAMA* 230:962, 1974.

Mukhopadhyay P, Osman M, Wajima T, et al. Nifedipine for intractable hiccups (letter). *N Engl J Med* 314:1256, 1986.

Petrosky D, Patel A. Diphenylhydantoin for intractable hiccups (letter). *Lancet* 1:997, 1974.

Salem MR, Baraka A, Rattenborg CC, Holiday DA. Treatment of hiccups by pharyngeal stimulation in anesthetized and conscious subjects. *JAMA* 202:126, 1967.

Stalnikowicz R, Fich A, Troudart T. Amitriptyline for intractable hiccups (letter). *N Engl J Med* 315:64, 1986.

Vasiloff N, Cohen D, Dillon J. Effective treatment of hiccup with intravenous methylphenidate. *Can Anaesth Soc J* 12:306, 1965.

Williamson BWA, MacIntyre IMC. Management of intractable hiccup. *Br Med J* 2:501, 1977.

16 Dyspepsia

Definitions

- *Dyspepsia:* Upper abdominal or retrosternal pain, discomfort, heartburn, nausea, vomiting, or other symptom considered to be referable to the proximal alimentary tract (Colin-Jones, 1988).
- *Nonulcer dyspepsia:* Dyspepsia (as defined above) lasting more than 4 weeks, unrelated to exercise, and for which no focal lesion or systemic disease can be found responsible (Colin-Jones, 1988).
- *Organic dyspepsia:* Dyspepsia due to specific lesions—peptic ulcer, reflux esophagitis, gastric carcinoma, and cholelithiasis—that could be readily identified on routine investigation (Colin-Jones, 1988).

Principal Causes of Dyspepsia in Cancer Patients

- **Tumor** producing obstruction or extrinsic compression on stomach or esophagus.
- Gastric **surgery** → small stomach; esophageal reflux.
- **Delayed gastric emptying** (due to autonomic damage, drugs).
- **Irradiation** damage to alimentary tract.
- **Peptic ulcer** disease (stress, NSAIDs, corticosteroids).
- Anxiety → aerophagia.

Dyspepsia Syndromes

In this chapter, we shall consider the most common clinical presentations of dyspepsia:

- Reflux esophagitis.
- Gastric hypomotility.
- Squashed stomach syndrome.
- Peptic ulcer disease.
- Aerophagia.

In terminally ill patients, it is not generally worthwhile to attempt to distinguish organic from "nonorganic" (or preorganic) dyspepsia, since initial treatment is in any event empirical, dictated by the clinical presentation, and diagnostic procedures, such as endoscopy, usually merely subject the patient to unnecessary discomfort.

Reflux Esophagitis

Pathophysiology

- Inappropriate *relaxation* of the *lower esophageal sphincter* (LES).
  - LES tone can be decreased by
    - Foods: fatty foods, chocolate, mints.
    - Drugs: theophylline, calcium channel blockers.
  - ↑Intra-abdominal pressure (from hepatomegaly, ascites, tumor) may also compromise LES.
- Composition of *gastric contents* influences degree of mucosal damage: acid/pepsin + bile + pancreatic juice (e.g., after gastrectomy) more injurious than acid alone.
- *Delayed esophageal clearance* due to motility disorders and gravity (recumbency during sleep) → prolonged mucosal contact with gastric acid.
- *Delayed gastric emptying* and increased gastric acid secretion → ↑tendency to reflux.

Symptoms

- **Heartburn**: burning epigastric or substernal sensation radiating into the throat, often occurring after meals, worse on lying down or bending over. Sometimes described as a sensation of hot water in the back of the throat.
- **Regurgitation** of acid, occasionally of food.

- **Belching.**
- **Dysphagia.**
- Can produce **chest pain** that mimics angina pectoris.
- Atypical presentations include **hoarseness** or nocturnal **cough** and **wheezing.**

Management of Esophageal Reflux-like Dyspepsia

- **Elevation of the head of the patient's bed** on 4- to 6-inch blocks to accelerate esophageal clearance gives results approaching those of therapy with H_2 receptor antagonists.
- **Dietary** advice:
  - *Avoid* foods that decrease LES tone: fatty foods, chocolate, mint, coffee, onions.
  - *Avoid* foods that irritate the esophageal mucosa: tomatoes, alcohol.
  - Do not take snacks at bedtime.
- Encourage cessation of **smoking.**
- Try not to prescribe **medications** that decrease LES tone (theophylline, calcium channel blockers, progesterone, anticholinergics, benzodiazepines, meperidine) or that irritate esophageal mucosa (NSAIDs). If the patient *must* take such medications, he should do so with plenty of water, to ensure rapid passage into the stomach.
- If the above measures are not sufficient, prescribe an **antacid** liquid, 15 to 30 ml PO ½ hour pc and hs, or **sucralfate, 1 gm PO qid.**
- If symptoms still persist, give an H_2 **receptor antagonist,** such as **famotidine, 40 mg PO hs,** *or* **ranitidine, 150 mg PO bid,** along with a prokinetic agent such as **cisapride, 10 mg tid to qid.**
- If symptoms still persist despite all the above measures, substitute the proton pump inhibitor **omeprazole, 20 mg qd,** for the H_2 receptor antagonist. (Dosage may be increased to 20 mg bid if the lower dosage is not effective.)

Gastric Hypomotility Disorders

Pathophysiology and Etiology

- Pain.
- Drugs: opioids, anticholinergics.
- Autonomic dysfunction: gastroparesis, perineural spread of cancer.
- General weakness and debility.
- Stress.

Symptoms and Signs

- Epigastric heaviness or fullness; feelings of **bloating**.
- **Early satiety.**
- **Nausea**, especially in the early morning, sometimes with retching.
- Diffuse abdominal **pain**.
- Abdominal **distention.**

Management of Dysmotility-like Dyspepsia

- Give a prokinetic agent, such as **metoclopramide (10 mg PO)**, or **cisapride (10 mg PO) ½ hour ac and hs.**

Squashed Stomach Syndrome

Pathophysiology

Stomach cannot distend normally to accommodate food, because of
- Extrinsic pressure from **hepatomegaly, ascites**, or intra-abdominal **tumor.**
- Stiffening of the gastric wall (**linitus plastica**).
- Reduction in gastric mass (**gastrectomy** → small stomach syndrome).

Symptoms

- Usually worse after eating.
- May be similar to those of hypomotility syndromes (epigastric fullness, early satiety, nausea).
- **Vomiting.**
- **Hiccups.**
- **Flatulence.**
- Heartburn.

Management of Squashed Stomach Syndrome

- Frequent, small feedings.
- Prokinetic agent, such as **metoclopramide (10 mg PO)** or **cisapride (10 mg PO) ½ hour ac and hs.**
- Give **activated charcoal–simethicone** combination, such as Charcoal Plus, 2 tabs qid (pc and hs) as a deflatulent.

Peptic Ulcer

Pathophysiology

- Occurs when there is an imbalance between intraluminal acid and pepsin and the epithelial protective mechanisms of the stomach and duodenum.
  - Factors that increase acid/pepsin secretion: high-protein diet.
  - Factors that decrease mucosal resistance: drugs (NSAIDs), alcohol, smoking.
- The bacterium *Helicobacter pylori* is a primary causative factor in peptic ulcer disease.

Symptoms

Gnawing, localized **epigastric pain**:
- Usually relieved by food or antacids.
- May wake the patient from sleep at night.
- Worse on waking in the morning.
- May be perceived as a sensation of hunger.

Management of Peptic Ulcer-like Symptoms

- Start an H₂ receptor antagonist: **Famotidine, 20 mg PO bid × 4 to 8 weeks**, then 20 mg PO hs, is the drug of choice because of (1) its higher potency and longer duration of action than ranitidine and (2) its ease of administration—the tablet is smaller than ranitidine. (*Note:* Cimetidine is not used for oncology patients because of its adverse interactions with many drugs used in palliative care.)
- Additional relief may be provided by an ulcer-coating agent such as **sucralfate, 1 gm PO qid**. (Rates of ulcer healing with sucralfate are equivalent to those with H₂ receptor antagonists, and relapse rates are lower.)
- If the patient's life expectancy is > 3 to 6 months, definitive **triple therapy** of *H. pylori* infection (with or without endoscopic or serologic confirmation of infection) should be considered:
  - Bismuth subsalicylate (Pepto-Bismol), 1 tsp qid (or 2 tabs qid) × 4 weeks +
  - Metronidazole, 250 mg PO tid × 10 to 14 days +
  - Tetracycline, 500 mg PO qid × 2 weeks.

Prevention of Gastric Ulcer in Patients Taking NSAIDS

- The drug of choice for this purpose is the synthetic prostaglandin E_1 analog, **misoprostol, 100 to 200 μg PO qid** with meals and hs.
- Concurrent administration of misoprostol may permit continuation of analgesic treatment in patients who require NSAIDs for management of bone pain but suffer epigastric distress when NSAIDs are administered.

Aerophagia

Pathophysiology

- May result from exaggeration of normal swallowing or abnormal swallowing mechanism.

Symptoms and Signs

- Bloating and belching, especially after meals.
- Frequent swallowing.
- Forward movement of the neck when swallowing.

Management

- Diversion of attention after meals.
- Sucking sweets or sipping drinks.
- Trial of an antiflatulent, such as activated charcoal/simethicone (Charcoal Plus, 2 tabs tid pc).

Summary: Dyspepsia Syndromes and Their Management

Syndrome	Symptoms	Management
Reflux esophagitis	Heartburn Regurgitation Belching Dysphagia and/or chest pain	Elevate head of patient's bed. Avoid foods/drugs that decrease LES tone. Sucralfate, 1 gm PO qid, or antacids, 15–30 ml qid (1 hour pc & hs). If insufficient response, give famotidine, 40 mg hs + cisapride, 10 mg tid. If still inadequate response, give omeprazole, 20 mg qd.
Gastric hypomotility	Bloating and distention Early satiety Nausea Diffuse abdominal pain	Prokinetic agent: metoclopramide, 10 mg PO qid (½ hour ac & hs), or cisapride, 10 mg PO qid (½ hour ac & hs).
Squashed stomach syndrome	Nausea and vomiting Hiccups Epigastric fullness Flatulence	Frequent, small feedings. Prokinetic agent: metoclopramide, 10 mg PO qid (½ hour ac & hs), or cisapride, 10–20 mg PO qid (½ hour ac & hs). Activated charcoal–simethicone combination, such as Charcoal Plus, 2 tabs qid (pc & hs).
Peptic ulcer	Gnawing, aching epigastric pain that Is worse on waking Is relieved by food/antacids May waken patient from sleep	Famotidine, 20 mg PO bid ± sucralfate, 1 gm PO qid. For patients with extended life expectancy, consider triple therapy against H. pylori: Pepto-Bismol, 2 tabs qid + Metronidazole, 250 mg tid + Tetracycline, 500 mg qid.
Aerophagia	Bloating Repetitive belching	Distraction after meals. Slow sips of fluids. Trial of activated charcoal/simethicone combination.

References and Further Reading

Bardham K, Bjamason I, Scott D, et al. The prevention and healing of acute non-steroidal anti-inflammatory drug-associated gastroduodenal mucosal damage by misoprostol. *Br J Rheumatol* 32:990, 1993.

Colin-Jones DG. Management of dyspepsia: Report of a working party. *Lancet* i:576, 1988.

Graham DY, Agrawal NM, Roth S. Prevention of NSAID-induced gastric ulcer with misoprostol: Multicentre, double-blind, placebo-controlled trial. *Lancet* ii:1277, 1988.

Hosking SW, Ling TK, Chung SC, et al. Duodenal ulcer healing by eradication of *Helicobacter pylori* without anti-acid treatment: Randomised controlled trial. *Lancet* 343:508, 1994.

Morrisey JF, Barreras RF. Antacid therapy. *N Engl J Med* 290:550, 1974.

NIH Consensus Development Panel. *Helicobacter pylori* in peptic ulcer disease. *JAMA* 272:65, 1994.

Pope CE. Acid-reflux disorders. *N Engl J Med* 331:656, 1994.

Richter JE, Long JF. Cisapride for gastroesophageal reflux disease. *Am J Gastroenterol* 90:423, 1995.

Robinson M. Gastroesophageal reflux disease. *Postgrad Med* 95(2):88, 1994.

Spiro HM. Pharmacology, clinical efficacy, and adverse side effects of sucralfate, a nonsystemic agent for peptic ulcer. *Pharmacotherapy* 2(2):67, 1982.

Tasman-Jones C. Initial and long-term management of peptic ulcer. *Patient Management* 16(3):43, 1987.

17 Gastrointestinal Bleeding

Definitions

- *Hematemesis*: The vomiting of (fresh) blood.
- *Melenemesis*: Black or coffee-ground vomitus (also referred to as "melena" in some texts).
- *Hematochezia*: The passage of bloody stools.
- *Melena*: The passage of black, tarry stools.

Sources of Gastrointestinal Bleeding in Terminally Ill Cancer Patients

- Gastrointestinal bleeding in patients with cancer is usually (80% of cases) caused by benign disease (e.g., gastritis, peptic ulcer).
  Bleeding from benign ulcers ceases spontaneously in > 80% of cases.
- Most primary cancers of the GI tract produce slow blood loss, not massive hemorrhage (but see exceptions below).
- Bleeding from ostomy stoma usually signifies recurrent malignant disease.

Anatomic Source	Pathology
Esophagus	Varices[a] secondary to hepatic tumors or liver metastases. Prolonged vomiting in a patient with reflux esophagitis.
Stomach	Gastritis (common in malignancy), caused or worsened by NSAIDs, other drugs, uremia. Benign gastric ulcer.[b] Gastric adenocarcinoma or lymphoma. Leiomyosarcoma of the stomach.[a] Melanoma involving the stomach.[a]
Small intestine	Duodenal ulcer.[b] Intestinal fistulas from tumor growth.
Colorectum	Major bleeding is rare (primary tumors usually bleed insidiously). Rectal carcinoma.

[a]Bleeding may be massive.
[b]Bleeding may be massive but usually self-limited.

Management of Gastrointestinal Bleeding in Terminally Ill Cancer Patients

- For patients with *life expectancy > 1 to 2 months*, treat as for patients without cancer, consistent with the wishes of the patient regarding endoscopy, transfusions, surgery, and so on.
  - Avoid surgery in patients whose life expectancy is less than 2 months.
  - For persistent GI bleeding from unresectable *tumor*, treat with **radiation therapy**.
- For patients in *terminal phase* of cancer for whom resuscitation is not appropriate:

Problem	Management
Melenemesis or melena	Stop NSAIDs. **Sucralfate**, 1 gm PO qid. **Ranitidine**, 150 mg PO bid.

Problem	Management
Hematemesis or hematochezia, with signs of shock (cold, clammy skin; tachycardia, restlessness)	Use green sheets/towels to soak up blood. **Keep the patient warm** (electric blanket, warm room). Sedation: **midazolam**, 5-10 mg IM.
Bleeding from rectal carcinoma	Apply **sucralfate paste** (1 gm sucralfate tab in 2-3 ml of K-Y Jelly) topically. Give **tranexamic acid**, 500 mg PO bid-tid, *or* **tranexamic acid enema** (5 gm in 50 ml of warm water) bid.

- Measures that have *not* proved beneficial in the management of GI hemorrhage:
  - Gastric lavage with any fluid at any temperature.
  - Vasoconstrictors.
  - Antacids.
  - Antipepsin agents (pepstatin).
  - Intravenous H_2 receptor antagonists.
  - Tranexamic acid (except perhaps in bleeding from rectal carcinoma).

References and Further Reading

Berstad A. Antacids, pepsin inhibitors, and gastric cooling in the management of massive upper gastrointestinal haemorrhage. *Scand J Gastroenterol* 22(Suppl 137): 33, 1987.

Henry DA, O'Connell DL. Effects of fibrinolytic inhibitors on mortality from upper gastrointestinal hemorrhage. *Br Med J* 298:1142, 1989.

Hollander D, Tamawski A. The protective and therapeutic mechanisms of sucralfate. *Scand J Gastroenterol* 25(Suppl 173):1, 1990.

Lane L, Peterson WL. Bleeding peptic ulcer. *N Engl J Med* 331:7171, 1994.

McElligot E, Quigley C, Hanks GW. Tranexamic acid and rectal bleeding (letter). *Lancet* 337:431, 1991.

Ponsky JL, Joffman M, Swayngim DS. Saline irrigation in gastric hemorrhage: The effect of temperature. *J Surg Res* 28:204, 1980.

Regnard C. Control of bleeding in advanced cancer (letter). *Lancet* 337:94, 1991.

Regnard C, Markin W. Management of bleeding in advanced cancer—a flow diagram. *Palliative Med* 6:74, 1992.

18 Nausea and Vomiting

Incidence

- Nausea and vomiting occur in 60% of terminally ill cancer patients at some stage (usually intermittent).
- The *prevalence* of nausea and vomiting is 40% in patients during the last week of life.
- Nausea and vomiting are particularly prevalent in patients with breast, stomach, or gynecologic cancers.
- Nausea and vomiting occur in up to **60% of patients receiving opioids**, especially at the initiation of opioid treatment; tolerance to this side effect usually develops within a few days to weeks.

Pathophysiology

- Vomiting reflex begins with nausea (salivation, cold sweat, gastric relaxation, tachycardia, diarrhea, swallowing).

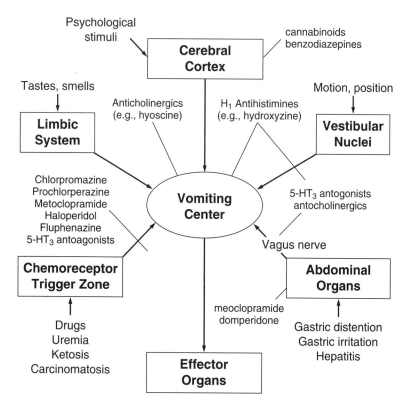

FIGURE 18.1   Pathophysiology of vomiting.

- **Vomiting center** located in dorsolateral reticular formation of the medulla coordinates the act of vomiting (see Figure 18.1). Afferents from
- Chemoreceptor trigger zone (CTZ) in the area postrema in floor of fourth ventricle. Stimulated by
  - Metabolic products (uremia, diabetic acidosis).
  - Chemotherapeutic agents.
  - Irradiation.
  May involve dopaminergic pathways → use of *dopamine antagonists* (chlorpromazine, prochlorperazine, metoclopramide, haloperidol).
- **Viscera:** Upper GI tract sends afferents to CNS via *sympathetic* and *vagal* stimulation:

- Myocardial infarction.
- Drugs, bacterial toxins, irritation.
- Chemotherapy (especially cisplatin).
- Metastatic disease to GI tract.
- **Cerebral:**
  - Cortical: psychological mechanisms (e.g., anticipatory vomiting).
  - Limbic: tastes, smells.
  - Increased intracranial pressure.
- **Vestibular nuclei**, as in motion sickness.

Etiology of Nausea and Vomiting in the Cancer Patient

Cause	Example
Physiologic	Small stomach syndrome Constipation Gastric hypomotility or stasis Intestinal obstruction Oral thrush Brain metastases Hepatomegaly Blood in stomach Cough Pain High fever
Treatment related	Chemotherapy Radiotherapy Other drugs: antibiotics, aspirin, carbamazepine, iron, steroids, digoxin, estrogens, expectorants, NSAIDs, opioids, theophylline
Metabolic	Uremia Electrolyte imbalance Endocrine (e.g., Addison's) Hypercalcemia Hyponatremia
Psychophysiologic	Anxiety Anticipatory nausea and vomiting

- The cause of nausea in any given patient is usually multifactorial (e.g., side effect of a drug + anxiety + constipation).

Diagnostic Workup of Nausea and Vomiting
History

Ask about the presence of	Suggests
Epigastric pain	Gastritis, PUD
History of peptic ulcer	PUD (pain may be masked)
Pain on swallowing	Oral thrush
Pain on standing	Mesenteric traction
Excessive thirst	Hypercalcemia
Hiccups	Uremia
Heartburn	Small stomach syndrome; esophageal reflux
Dysuria	UTI
Constipation	Nausea due to constipation
Large volume of vomitus	Reduced gastric emptying
Vomiting without nausea	↑Intracranial pressure

- Determine **pattern** of nausea: postprandial, with motion, certain smells.

Physical Examination

Examine	For Signs of
Mouth	Oral thrush
Abdomen	Hepatomegaly, abnormal bowel sounds, rigidity, tenderness
Rectum	Impaction
Neurologic	Brain metastases

Laboratory Studies

- Electrolytes.
- Urea.
- Calcium.
- Liver function tests.
- Urine for urinalysis and culture.
- Drug levels, where appropriate (e.g., digoxin or aminophylline level).

Pharmacologic Treatment
of Nausea/Vomiting

▪ General principles:
  • **Drug therapy is most likely to succeed if given prophylactically.**
  • The **oral route** is best for prophylaxis.
  • If the patient is already nauseated, oral drugs will not be reliably absorbed (duodenal reflux) → use rectal or parenteral route for at least 24 hours before trying oral antiemetics again.
▪ **Combination regimens** may be required in intractable vomiting.
  • Use each agent at optimal dosage/route.
  • Combine agents that have *different mechanisms of action* (e.g., acting at CTZ + acting directly on stomach).
  • Combine agents that *do not have overlapping toxicities*.

Cause of Vomiting	Antiemetic Regimen of Choice
Delayed gastric emptying	Metoclopramide, 10–20 mg tid–qid. Add simethicone/charcoal preparation when gas is prominent.
Initiation of opioid therapy	Metoclopramide, 10–20 mg tid–qid. In ambulatory patients, a transdermal scopolamine patch may also be effective.
Bowel obstruction	Meclizine, 25 mg bid, *or* octreotide, 150 μg IM bid or 300 μg/24 hr by continuous SQ infusion.
Vagal stimulation (e.g., oral candidiasis, stretched hepatic capsule)	Meclizine, 25 mg bid.
Increased ICP	Dexamethasone, 16–36 mg qd; increase as needed up to 100 mg.
Uremia Hypercalcemia	Haloperidol, 0.5 mg tid, *or* fluphenazine, 2 mg bid-tid.
Radiotherapy	Dexamethasone, 16 mg qam, + Prochlorperazine, 5–10 mg PO tid or 25 mg PR bid. Haloperidol, 1.5 mg hs, *or* ondansetron, 8 mg 2 hours before RT, then q8h, *or* ibuprofen, 400 mg q4h prn.

continued

Cause of Vomiting	Antiemetic Regimen of Choice
Chemotherapy	
Cisplatin	Metoclopramide, 1–3 mg/kg IV 30 minutes before and 90 minutes after chemotherapy + Dexamethasone, 20 mg IV 40 minutes before chemotherapy + Lorazepam, 1.5 mg/m^2 IV 35 minutes before chemotherapy OR Ondansetron, 8 mg slowly IV before chemotherapy, then 8 mg PO tid + Dexamethasone, 20 mg IV 40 minutes before chemotherapy
Cyclophosphamide/ Adriamycin	Metoclopramide, 2 mg/kg IV q2h × 3, then 40 mg PO q3h × 3 + Dexamethasone, 20 mg 40 minutes before chemotherapy + Diphenhydramine, 50 mg IV or PO with first metoclopramide dose, then with every other dose.

Characteristics of Commonly Used Antiemetic Drugs

See Table 18.1.

Pharmacology of the Antiemetics

Metoclopramide (Reglan)

- Gastrointestinal cholinergic effects:
  - Increases tone of lower esophageal sphincter.
  - Promotes gastric emptying.
  - Stimulates motility of upper GI tract.
- Has some blocking effect on receptors in the CTZ of the medulla.
- Drug of choice for **chemotherapy-induced vomiting** and vomiting due to **gastric stasis**.
  - For vomiting due to chemotherapy, give 2 mg/kg IV q2h starting 30 minutes before chemotherapy for 2 to 5 doses.
  - In terminal illness, doses of 10 mg PO/PR/IM tid are usually sufficient.
  - Often combined with steroid + benzodiazepine or antihistamine.

TABLE 18.1 Characteristics of Commonly Used Antiemetic Drugs

Class	Drug	Principal Action	Route	Dose Range	Frequency
Dopamine antagonist	Chlorpromazine (Thorazine)	CTZ/vomiting center	PO	6.25 mg	q8h
			IM/IV	6.25 mg	q8h
	Prochlorperazine (Compazine, Stemetil)	CTZ	PO	5–10 mg	q4–6h
			Rectal	25 mg	q4–6h
			IM/IV	10–20 mg	q3–6h
	Metoclopramide (Reglan)	CTZ/GI cholinergic	IV	10–20 mg	q2h
			PO	10–20 mg	q2–4h
	Haloperidol (Haldol)	CTZ	IV	0.5–1 mg	q8h
			PO	0.5–1 mg	q8h
	Fluphenazine (Prolixin)	CTZ	PO	2 mg	q8–12h
Anticholinergic	Scopolamine (Transderm Scōp)	Vestibular; vomiting center	Trans-dermal	0.5 mg	q3 days
	Hydroxyzine (Atarax, Vistaril)	Periphery; GI tract	PO	6.25 mg	q8h
H₁ antihistamine	Diphenhydramine (Benadryl)	Vomiting center; vestibular	PO	50–75 mg	q4–6h
	Dimenhydrinate (Dramamine, Gravol)		IM/IV	25–50 mg	q4–6h
	Promethazine (Phenergan) Hydroxyzine (Atarax, Vistaril)	UGI tract; vomiting center	PO/IM	6.25 mg	q8h
5-HT₃ antagonist	Ondansetron (Zofran)	UGI tract/ ?CNS	PO/IV	8 mg	q12h
	Granisetron (Kytril)		IV	10 µg/kg	
Steroids	Dexamethasone (Decadron)	Not known	PO/IV	4–24 mg	qam
	Methylprednisolone (Solu-Medrol)	Not known	IV	200–500 mg	q6h
Cannibinoids	Dronabinol (Marinol)	Vomiting center	PO	7.5–15 mg	q3–4h
	Nabilone (Cesamet)	Vomiting center	PO	1–2 mg	1–3 hours before, *then* q8–12h after chemo-therapy
Benzodiazepines	Lorazepam (Ativan)	Adjunctive	IV	1–2 mg/m²	q4h

- Side effects:
  - Mild **sedation**.
  - **Dystonic reactions**:
    - More common in patients < 30 years old.
    - More likely when given in combination with haloperidol.
    - Can be **controlled with diphenhydramine** (50 mg with the first dose of metoclopramide and with every other dose thereafter).
  - **Akathisia** (restlessness); anxiety, pacing, agitation.
  - **Muscle rigidity**; tardive dyskinesias.
  - **Diarrhea** (reduced by dexamethasone).

Phenothiazines

- Examples: prochlorperazine (Compazine, Stemetil); chlorpromazine (Thorazine); methotrimeprazine (Levoprome, Nozinan), the strongest but most sedating of the antiemetics.
- Work by partial inhibition of the CTZ (antidopaminergic).
- *Drugs of choice for radiation-induced nausea and vomiting.*
- Have *not* been useful in emesis induced by highly emetic chemotherapeutic agents like cisplatin (requires high dosage → extrapyramidal effects).
- *Oral* route preferred.
- Side effects:
  - **Extrapyramidal reactions**: muscle rigidity, acute dystonia, akathisia, cogwheeling, akinesia.
  - **Hypotension**.

Butyrophenones

- Haloperidol (Haldol).
- Among the most potent inhibitors of the CTZ.
- Fewer cardiovascular side effects than phenothiazines.
- Side effects: extrapyramidal reactions.

Benzodiazepines

- Lorazepam (Ativan).
- Indications:
  - Cisplatin-induced vomiting.

- Refractory anticipatory vomiting.
- Amnesic effects are helpful.

Antihistamines

- Act on the vomiting center, vestibular apparatus, and cholinergic receptors peripherally.
- Diphenydramine (Benadryl); hydroxyzine (Atarax, Vistaril); dimenhydrinate (Dramamine, Gravol); meclizine (Antivert).
- Used for motion sickness.
- In cancer patients, for control of metabolically related nausea and (diphenhydramine in particular) to combat extrapyramidal effects of phenothiazines, metoclopramide, and haloperidol.
- Relative safety in seriously ill patients.
- Side effects: *anticholinergic crisis*—usually in elderly patient or cancer patient who is receiving other medications with anticholinergic properties.

Anticholinergics

- Hydroxyzine (Atarax, Vistaril); scopolamine.
- Decrease activation of vomiting center.
- Peripherally increase gastroesophageal sphincter tone.
- Decrease retrograde GI tract motility.
- Inferior to phenothiazines in combating nausea/vomiting.

Corticosteroids

- Mechanism of antiemetic action unclear (?prostaglandin synthesis).
- Useful in ameliorating diarrhea due to metoclopramide.
- Other indications—vomiting caused by
  - Raised intracranial pressure.
  - Hypercalcemia.
  - Malignant pyloric stenosis.
- Side effects: agitation, mood changes.

Cannabinoids

- Dronabinol, nabilone.

- Equivalent or superior to prochlorperazine in chemotherapy-induced nausea and vomiting.
- Side effects frequent but usually manageable:
  - Sedation.
  - Dry mouth.
  - Orthostatic hypotension; dizziness.
  - Ataxia.
  - Euphoria/dysphoria.
- Caution in the *elderly*; best used in young patients.
- *Contraindicated*: cardiovascular or psychiatric illness.

Serotonin Antagonists

- Ondansetron (Zofran); granisetron (Kytril); tropisetron (Navoban).
- Most effective drugs against cisplatin-induced vomiting.

Factors Affecting the Choice of Antiemetic Drugs

Choose the **drug, dosage**, and **dosage schedule** according to the **desired outcome**:

- For example, if the objective is to achieve *evening sedation* but to maintain *alertness during the day*, give the whole 24-hour dose at bedtime (e.g., haloperidol, 1.5 mg hs instead of 0.5 mg tid).
- Prefer **portmanteau drugs** (drugs that can achieve more than one objective). For example, *diphenhydramine* can provide antiemetic action, antiparkinsonian action, and mild sedation (if sedation is desired).
- **Exploit the side effects of antiemetics.** For example, chlorpromazine is more sedating than haloperidol; therefore, choose the former when sedation is a desired objective in a patient requiring a drug acting on the CTZ.

Strategy for Treatment of Nausea and Vomiting in Terminally Ill Patients

---

Control of Nausea and Vomiting in the Terminally Ill

1. **Start** with **metoclopramide, 10–20 mg q6–8h** for dual effect (on gastric stasis and CTZ). As with opioids, dosing should be around the clock.
2. If metoclopramide by itself is not sufficient to control nausea and vomiting, choose a **second drug** according to the suspected mechanism causing the vomiting:
   - If secondary to *opioids, uremia, liver metastases* → give **haloperidol, 0.5 mg tid**, *or* **chlorpromazine, 6.25 mg tid**.
   - If secondary to *brain metastases*, give **dexamethasone, 16–36 mg qam**.
3. If therapy with two drugs still does not adequately control the problem, add a **third drug**: an **antihistamine** such as **hydroxyzine, 6.25 mg tid**, *or* **diphenhydramine, 25 mg tid–qid** (the addition of diphenhydramine is also useful in preventing the dystonic reactions that are more likely to occur when metoclopramide and haloperidol are given together).
4. If treatment with three drugs still does not entirely solve the problem, and if corticosteroids have not already been given for suspected brain metastases, add **dexamethasone, 4 mg qam**.
5. When vomiting persists despite the above measures, try a serotonin receptor antagonist, such as **ondansetron, 8 mg q12h PO/IV**.

Giving Medications by Syringe Driver to Control Nausea and Vomiting

- **Indication**: patient with nausea and vomiting unable to take oral medications.
- Sometimes it will be possible to bring symptoms under control with parenteral medications and thereafter switch to oral dosing.
- See suggested **starting mixture** on the next page:

Metoclopramide, 30 mg + haloperidol, 1.5 mg
+ promethazine, 6.25 mg/24 hr

▪ See Appendix 2 for details of how to use a syringe driver.

Nonpharmacologic Measures

▪ **Discontinue** as many of the patient's **drugs** as possible.
▪ Change or reduce opioid drug.
▪ Frequent small feedings.
▪ Removal from the sight/smell of food.
▪ **Acupuncture**: P6 point 10 Hz × 5 minutes.
▪ **Behavioral** therapies:
  • **Hypnosis** with imagery.
  • Progressive muscle relaxation training.
  • **Systematic desensitization**.

References and Further Reading

Aapro MS. Present role of corticosteroids as antiemetics: Recent results. *Cancer Res* 21:91, 1992.

Baines M. Nausea and vomiting in the patient with advanced cancer. *J Pain Symptom Manage* 3:81, 1988.

Bruera E, MacDonald RN, Brenneis C, et al. Metoclopramide infusion with a portable disposable pump. *Ann Intern Med* 104:896, 1986.

Campora E, Merlini L, Pace M, et al. The incidence of narcotic-induced emesis. *J Pain Symptom Manage* 6:428, 1991.

Cole R, Robinson F, Harvey L, et al. Successful control of intractable nausea and vomiting requiring combined ondansetron and haloperidol in a patient with advanced cancer. *J Pain Symptom Manage* 9:48, 1994.

Dundee JW, Ghaly KM, Bill KM, et al. Effect of stimulation of the P6 antiemetic point on postoperative nausea and vomiting. *Br J Anaesth* 63:612, 1989.

Ferris F, Kerr I, Sone M, Marcuzzi M. Transdermal scopolamine use in the control of narcotic-induced nausea. *J Pain Symptom Manage* 6:389, 1991.

Kris MG, Yeh DJ, Gralla RJ, Young CW. Symptomatic gastroparesis in cancer patients: A possible cause of cancer-associated anorexia that can be improved with oral metoclopramide (abstract). *Proc Am Soc Clin Oncol* 4:267, 1985.

Lichter I. Results of anti-emetic management in terminal illness. *J Palliative Care* 9(2): 19, 1993.

Morrow G, Morrell C. Behavioral treatment for the anticipatory nausea and vomiting induced by cancer chemotherapy. *N Engl J Med* 307:1476, 1982.

Reuben DV, Mor V. Nausea and vomiting in terminal cancer patients. *Arch Intern Med* 146:2021, 1983.

Watson M, Marvell C. Anticipatory nausea and vomiting among cancer patients: A review. *Psychology Health* 6:97, 1992.

Chemotherapy-Induced Nausea/Vomiting

Allan SG, Farqhuar DL, Harris D, Leonard RCF. Antiemetic efficacy of dexamethasone in outpatient chemotherapy. *Cancer Chemother Pharmacol* 18:86, 1986.

Dundee JW, Ghaly RG, Fitzpatrick KTJ, et al. Acupuncture prophylaxis of cancer chemotherapy-induced sickness. *J R Soc Med* 82:268, 1989.

Herrstedt J, Sigsgaard T, Boesgaard M, et al. Ondansetron plus metopimazine compared with ondansetron alone in patients receiving moderately emetogenic chemotherapy. *N Engl J Med* 328:1076, 1993.

Jones AL, Hill AS, Soucop M, et al. Comparison of dexamethasone and ondansetron in the prophylaxis of emesis induced by moderately emetogenic chemotherapy. *Lancet* 338:483, 1991.

Levitt M, Warr D, Yelle L, et al. Ondansetron compared with dexamethasone and metoclopramide as antiemetics in the chemotherapy of breast cancer with cyclophosphamide, methotrexate, and fluorouracil. *N Engl J Med* 328:1081, 1993.

Malone JM, Christianson CW, Yashinsky D, et al. Prochlorperazine and transdermal scopolamine added to a metoclopramide antiemetic regimen: A controlled comparison. *J Reprod Med* 35:932, 1990.

Smith DB, Newland ES, Rustin GJ, et al. Comparison of ondansetron and ondansetron plus dexamethasone as antiemetic prophylaxis during cisplatin-containing chemotherapy. *Lancet* 338:487, 1991.

19 Constipation

*Anyone who lives a sedentary [life] and does not exercise
or he who postpones his excretions or he whose intestines
are constipated, even if he eats good foods and takes care
of himself according to medical principles—all his days
will be painful ones and his strength will wane.*

MOSES MAIMONIDES, *MISHNEH TORAH, HILCHOTH DEOTH,*
CHAP. 4, NO. 15 (TRANSLATED BY FRED ROSNER)

Constipation is a very common and potentially debilitating problem in patients with far-advanced cancer. In one study (Curtis et al., 1991), constipation was present in 40% of patients referred to a palliative care unit; its prevalence in patients receiving opioids approaches 90%. The aim of management is to *prevent* constipation and, if it should occur, to treat it *promptly.*

Definition

The difficult passage of hard or infrequent stools (less often than every 3 days), or the passage of stool less frequently than is usual for the patient.

Causes of Constipation in Patients with Advanced Cancer

- Prescription of **opioids** without adequate doses of laxatives.
- Other **drugs** (anticholinergics, antihistamines, NSAIDs, phenothiazines, tricyclics, diuretics, iron, vincristine).
- Low-fiber **diet.**
- **Dehydration.**
- **Inactivity.**
- Weakness.
- Inconvenient, unfamiliar, or unphysiologic toilet arrangements.
- Hypercalcemia, hypokalemia.
- Compression of bowel or invasion of neural plexus by tumor.

Clinical Findings

History

- *Symptoms* that may be associated with constipation:
  - Anorexia.
  - Nausea and vomiting.
  - Abdominal pain (usually colicky), which can radiate to chest, back, and upper legs; pain in right iliac fossa.
  - Bloating.
  - Tenesmus.
  - Diarrhea (caused by liquid feces leaking past the hard fecal obstruction).
- *Ask the patient:*
  - When did you last move your bowels? When was the time before that?
  - What is the *consistency* of your bowel movements (hard, soft, liquid)?
  - What is the *volume* of your bowel movements (normal, increased, decreased)?
  - Do you have *pain* or difficulty in moving your bowels?
  - Do you sometimes pass your bowels before you can get to the toilet (*incontinence*)?
  - Do you feel a need to defecate but find that you cannot do so (*tenesmus*)?
  - Have you passed any *blood* or *mucus* in your stools?
  - Do you use *laxatives*? If so, what laxatives? What dosage? How often?
  - Do you use *suppositories*? Which ones and how often?

- Do you use *enemas*? How often?
- What other things help you to move your bowels?

Physical Examination

- On *abdominal* examination, look for
  - Distention.
  - Mild to moderate tenderness, especially over the cecum (right lower quadrant).
  - Fecal masses—distinguish from tumor:
    - Fecal masses are most often palpable in the descending colon (left lower quadrant), are usually movable, and will indent on pressure.
    - Fecal masses disappear after constipation is relieved.
- On *rectal* examination, look for
  - Hard, impacted feces.
  - An empty, dilated rectum (may be a sign of more proximal fecal impaction).
  - Hemorrhoids, painful fissures, fistulas.
  - Intraluminal tumor.
  - Extrinsic compression on the rectum by an abdominal mass.
  - Scarring or stenosis.

General Measures in the Management of Constipation

Contributing Cause	Remedial Measures
Opioids given without adequate laxative dosage	Change laxative regimen (see below).
Drugs	Review the patient's *entire* medication regimen, and switch to less constipating drugs where possible (e.g., change antiemetic from ondansetron to metoclopramide).
Low-fiber diet	To the extent feasible, add fruits and vegetables to the patient's diet (often not practical). Addition of bran, psyllium, and other fibers to the diet are theoretically possible but not usually well-tolerated. (Addition of fiber contraindicated in patients with structural blockage of the bowel.)

continued

Contributing Cause	Remedial Measures
Dehydration	Encourage oral fluids.
Inactivity	Encourage patient to increase activity level.
Inconvenient, unfamiliar, or unphysiologic toilet arrangements	Use bedside commode rather than a bedpan wherever possible, to enable optimal benefit from the patient's abdominal muscles and from gravity. Exploit the gastrocolic reflex by encouraging use of the commode 30–60 minutes after eating. Establish a regular bowel regimen based on what is normal and convenient for the *patient*.
Hypercalcemia	Increase patient's fluid intake; consider intravenous fluids and biphosphonates.
Hypokalemia	Give fresh fruits and vegetables if tolerated; otherwise oral potassium supplements.

Specific Measures for the Constipated Patient

Clinical Findings	Recommended Intervention
Soft fecal masses in abdomen that indent on pressure; no evidence of distal impaction	Stimulant laxative, such as bisacodyl (Dulcolax). Osmotic cathartic, such as lactulose (Chronulac). If no response, may need to give oil retention enema (to soften feces) followed by phosphate enema to stimulate peristalsis.
Rectum filled with soft feces	Give a peristalsis-stimulating laxative (e.g., senna, bisacodyl) with or without a microenema.
Large fecal mass in rectum (too large to pass through anal sphincter)	Digital piecemeal disimpaction after premedication with morphine and diazepam. For hard stool, administer olive oil retention enema (120 ml) overnight before disimpaction. Follow by high enema.
Empty, distended rectum with a history of constipation	High enemas.
Hemorrhoids or anal fissures	Bulk-forming agents (e.g., psyllium). Stool softener (docusate). Analgesic anal suppositories (Anusol, Xyloproct).

Clinical Findings	Recommended Intervention
Intraluminal or extrinsic mass compressing the rectum	Surgical consultation before giving bowel stimulants.
Signs and symptoms of bowel obstruction	Avoid laxative drugs. See Chapter 21.

Drugs Used in the Treatment of Constipation

Drug	Dosage	Mechanism and Comments
Contact cathartics		
Anthraquinones		
Senna (Senokot)	**Senokot** tabs qd hs or bid	Act directly on colon wall to stimulate peristalsis. Must undergo conversion to active metabolite in colon → effective only in distal colon.
Cascara	**Cascara**, 0.3– 0.6 gm PO hs	May cause colicky abdominal pain (dose-related).
Diphenylmethanes		
Bisacodyl (Dulcolax)	**Dulcolax**, 5 mg tab PO hs	Safe and well tolerated; effective within 12– 24 hours.
Phenolphthalein (Dialose Plus)		
Castor oil		Seldom used, except in management of acute, self-limited constipation.
Osmotic cathartics		Draw fluid into bowel lumen → decrease transit time of stool. May cause abdominal cramps (dose-related).
Lactulose (Chronulac)	10–30 ml bid–qid	More effective for chronic use. (May take several days to have an effect.) Useful in hepatic encephalopathy. Causes nausea in some patients, and may produce gaseous distention. May be more palatable if mixed with fruit juice.

continued

Drug	Dosage	Mechanism and Comments
Magnesium salts	1-2 tsp in at least ½ cup of water in the morning	Harsh laxative, producing rapid (3-6 hours) evacuation; use for severe constipation resistant to other laxatives; should be followed by large oral fluid intake. Should not be used in renal failure or CHF.
Stool softeners Docusate sodium (Colace)	100 mg bid-qid	Wetting agent that lowers surface tension, thereby allowing water to penetrate hard feces. Also promotes secretion of fluid into small and large bowel. Weak if any effect on peristalsis. Mild laxative. Acts in 1-3 days. Most useful for preventing passage of hard stool (e.g., in patient with anal fissure). Do not use together with mineral oil.
Lubricants Mineral oil	10 ml PO qd	Lubricate the stool, allowing easier passage (do not use in obtunded patients → risk of lipid aspiration); useful in acute Rx of fecal impaction.
Fiber Psyllium (Metamucil)	5 gm qd-tid	Increase stool bulk and soften consistency by increasing mass and water content; effective only after 2-4 days of daily use. Indications: colostomy, ileostomy, hemorrhoids, anal fissure. Do *not* give to debilitated patients whose fluid intake is < 1.5-2 L/day. Do *not* give to patients with suspected intestinal stricture or signs of bowel obstruction.

Drug	Dosage	Mechanism and Comments
Suppositories		Draw fluid into the rectum
Glycerin	2.35 gm PR prn	and act as stimulant to
Bisacodyl	10 mg PR hs	defecation.
Enemas		Useful for treatment of
Sodium biphosphate	1 prn when 3	acute constipation or
(Fleet)	days pass with-	management of fecal
Sodium lauryl sulfo-	out a bowel	impaction.
acetate + sodium	movement	
citrate + glycerol		
(Microlet)		

Strategy for Drug Treatment of Constipation

- Start with a colonic stimulant (e.g., bisacodyl) and stool softener (e.g., docusate sodium).
- If bowel movements are soft but infrequent, give additional contact cathartics (senna, more bisacodyl) to stimulate peristalsis.
- If bowel movements are hard, give an osmotic cathartic (e.g., lactulose for a mild effect; magnesium sulfate for a stronger action).
- If 3 days go by without a bowel movement, do a rectal examination and give a suppository or microenema if not contraindicated.

Summary: Important Points About Constipation

- Constipation can occur even in patients who have no oral or enteral intake.
- Always start a stool softener and a bowel stimulant in adequate dosages *at the same time* that you start opioids. Do not wait for constipation to occur.
- The management goal is a soft bowel movement every 3 days or less. If 3 days pass without a bowel movement, perform a rectal examination and prescribe a suppository or enema, as required.
- Suspect fecal impaction when there is new-onset diarrhea and incontinence.

Points of Emphasis in Patients Taking Opioid Drugs

- A large majority of cancer patients receive opioid medication during the advanced stages of their disease.
- **Opioids create special problems** in the evacuation of stool:
  - Increase sphincter tone (ileocecal valve; anal sphincter).
  - Increase segmentation (pyloric, small intestine, colon).
  - Increase the absorption of water and electrolytes from the small and large bowel → drier, harder stool.
  - Decrease the defecation reflex (rectum less sensitive to distention).
- Prevention and treatment of constipation in patients taking opioids:
  - Always **start a bowel stimulant and osmotic cathartic** in adequate dosages *at the same time* **that you start opioids**.
    - Do not wait for constipation to occur.
    - If lactulose produces gastric distention, give a simethicone/charcoal preparation to relieve gas rather than stopping the lactulose.
  - If despite the above measures the stool is still hard and difficult to pass, **add a stool softener** (docusate).
  - If constipation persists despite triple therapy (i.e., bowel stimulant, osmotic cathartic, stool softener), continue triple therapy but in addition open the bowels ("uncork") with a **suppository**, Fleet **enema**, or standard enema.

References and Further Reading

Bruera E, Suarez-Almazor M, Velasco A, et al. The assessment of constipation in terminal cancer patients admitted to a palliative care unit: A retrospective review. *J Pain Symptom Manage* 9:515, 1994.

Curtis E, Krech R, Walsh T. Common symptoms in patients with advanced cancer. *J Palliative Care* 7:25, 1991.

Glare P, Lickiss N. Unrecognized constipation in patients with advanced cancer: A recipe for therapeutic disaster. *J Pain Symptom Manage* 7:369, 1992.

Portenoy RK. Constipation in the cancer patient. *Med Clin North Am* 71:301, 1987.

Sykes NP. A clinical comparison of laxatives in a hospice. *Palliative Med* 5:307, 1991.

20 Fecal Impaction

*This disease occurs when a thick mass of feces is burnt
together in the intestine ... and the intestine, inasmuch as
these masses become hardened, swells around them. The
patient accepts neither the medications drunk from above,
vomiting them up instead, nor enema administered from
below. The disease is acute and dangerous.*

HIPPOCRATES, *AFFECTIONS,* 21

Definition

The accumulation of compacted fecal material in the rectum (most
often) or colon (generally the distal colon, but impaction may occur
anywhere along the length of the large bowel).

Etiology and Pathophysiology

- The same **factors that** lead to constipation **predispose to fecal
  impaction,** especially
- Debility and immobility (bedridden patient).
- Prescription of opioids without adequate doses of laxatives.
- Other drugs (anticholinergics, antihistamines, iron, sucralfate,
  NSAIDs, phenothiazines, tricyclics, diuretics).
- Dehydration.
- Diet low in fiber.
- Mental impairment.

- Tumor interfering with passage of feces.
- Cord compression from spinal metastases.
- Painful lesions in the anal area (fissures, hemorrhoids, perirectal abscess).
- Metabolic abnormalities (hypercalcemia, hypokalemia).
- Once **stool begins to accumulate** in the rectum or colon, for whatever reason →
  - **Salt and water** continue to be **absorbed** across the colonic mucosa → hardening of the stool.
  - **Peristaltic activity** continues → **compacting** of the stool → enlarging of the fecal mass → **fecal mass** becomes **too large to pass** the anal sphincter.

Clinical Findings

History

The history may be nonspecific:
- History of **previous** fecal **impaction**.
- **Frequency of bowel movements decreases** to less than one every other day or bowel movements cease altogether, *but*
- **Paradoxical diarrhea** with **incontinence** may occur if fecal mass acts as a ball-valve to allow seepage of liquid stool.

> THE PASSAGE OF SOME STOOL DOES NOT RULE OUT THE PRESENCE OF FECAL IMPACTION.

- **Anorexia**
- Nausea and vomiting
- Crampy abdominal pain
- **Urinary frequency**, retention, overflow incontinence

Physical Examination

Findings on physical examination depend somewhat on the location of the impaction:
- Most commonly, there is a **fecal mass in the rectal vault**, usually hard (but may be of any consistency).

> AN EMPTY RECTUM DOES NOT RULE
> OUT FECAL IMPACTION.

- More proximal impaction may be detected as an **abdominal mass**.
  - Differentiate from tumor mass: A fecal mass is usually **nontender**, **moveable**, and can be **indented with pressure**.
  - Obtain x-ray confirmation with plain film of the abdomen (look for masses of stool, colonic dilatation, or air-fluid levels in the small bowel).
- **Signs of obstruction** (distention, tenderness) occur late.
- Nonspecific signs that may be present: **fever**, dysrhythmias.

Potential Complications of Fecal Impaction

- Fecal incontinence →
  - Decubitus ulcers.
  - Urinary tract infections.
- Large bowel obstruction.
- Ischemic necrosis and ulceration of the colonic wall (stercoral ulceration) → perforation.

Management of Established Fecal Impaction

Impaction Within the Reach of the Examiner's Fingers

- Soft stool → bisacodyl suppository daily until rectal vault is empty.
- Hard stool → manual **disimpaction**:
  - **Oil retention enema** (120 cc) overnight, then:
  - **Premedicate** with IV midazolam (start with 1 mg, titrate up by 0.5-mg increments until adequate sedation has been achieved) + morphine (start with 4 mg). In rare cases, saddle block anesthesia may be required.
  - **Position patient** on left side with upper knee flexed.
  - Place incontinent **pad** beneath patient's buttocks.
  - Don gloves, and lubricate index finger with **lidocaine jelly**. Spread lidocaine jelly on surface of anus, and insert lubricated finger into anus.
  - Instill 10 ml of 1% lidocaine jelly into the rectum, and wait 10 minutes.

- Perform gentle, progressive **dilatation** of the anal sphincter, first with one finger, then two fingers.
- Use two fingers to **fragment** the impacted feces **and remove** piecemeal.
- Follow by high sodium phosphate or tap water **enema**.

Impaction Beyond the Reach of the Examiner's Finger

- Lavage under endoscopic visualization.
- Fluoroscopically directed enema with water-soluble contrast material (e.g., Gastrografin).

Prevention of Recurrent Impaction

Once impaction is resolved, take measures to prevent recurrent impaction:

- Establish regular bowel regimen based on what is convenient for the patient.
- Improve laxative regimen.
- Review *all* the patient's medications, and switch to less constipating drugs where possible.
- Encourage oral fluids.
- Encourage consumption of fruits and vegetables.
- Use bedside commode rather than bedpan whenever possible.
- Correct hypercalcemia, hypokalemia.

References and Further Reading

Cefalu CA, McKnight GT, Pike JI. Treating impaction: A practical approach to an unpleasant problem. *Geriatrics* 36:143, 1981.

Dresen KA, Dratzer GL. Fecal impaction in modern practice. *JAMA* 170:644, 1959.

Gupta KL. Intestinal obstruction due to constipation in the elderly. *Br J Clin Pract* 37:155, 1983.

Portenoy RK. Constipation in the cancer patient: Causes and management. *Med Clin North Am* 71:303, 1987.

Young RW. The problem of fecal impaction in the aged. *J Am Geriatr Soc* 21:383, 1973.

21 Bowel Obstruction

Definition

Situation in which normal transit through the intestinal tract is abnormally delayed or prevented altogether.

Incidence

- Intestinal obstruction occurs in approximately **3% of all patients** admitted to hospice.
- Obstruction is particularly common in
  - **Ovarian** cancer (25–40%).
  - **Colorectal** cancer (10–15%).
  - Less frequently: cancers of the pancreas, stomach, endometrium, bladder, prostate.

Causes of Bowel Obstruction in Patients with Advanced Cancer

Bowel obstruction in patients with cancer is due to
- The original tumor (65% of patients).
- Nonmalignant causes, such as adhesions (25%).
- A new primary tumor, which may be surgically resectable (10%).

Category	Specific Causes of Obstruction
Cancer-related problems	Tumor mass exerting *external pressure* on intestine. Obstructing mass *within the bowel lumen* ("apple core" lesions of the colon). Invasion by tumor of the neural plexus of the intestine → *ileus* and pseudo-obstruction (common in ovarian cancer). Intussusception (melanoma, polypoid lesions of the right colon).
Consequences of treatment for cancer or its symptoms	Adhesions after abdominal surgery. Radiation injury to small bowel. Chemotherapy: Neurotoxicity from vinca alkaloids → high fecal impaction. Narcotic bowel syndrome. Effects of other drugs on GI motility (e.g., tricyclics, anticholinergics, neuroleptics). Fecal impaction due to drugs, debility.
Nonmalignant lesions	Adynamic ileus (e.g., electrolyte disturbances, pneumonia). Diverticulitis. Bowel infarction. Hernia. Adhesions. Pancreatitis.

Pathophysiology

- **Obstruction** occurs at some point along the length of the intestine →
- **Fluid accumulates** in the intestinal lumen proximal to the point of obstruction from
  - Ingested fluids.
  - Swallowed saliva.
  - Gastric, biliary, and pancreatic secretions.
  - Failure of efflux of sodium and water from the distended area of bowel.
  - Subsequently, movement of water and sodium *into* the bowel lumen.
- **Intraluminal pressure rises** → colicky pain, nausea, vomiting.

Clinical Findings

Symptoms

Symptoms tend to be intermittent early in the course of obstruction and to increase with time.

- **Pain** may be of two types:
  - **Colicky** (in 75% of obstructed patients):
    - Crampy pain occurring in paroxysms, with relatively pain-free intervals in between.
    - The higher the obstruction, the more severe the pain.
    - Episodes of colicky pain associated with audible borborygmi.
    - Colic is absent in adynamic ileus.
    - Colic poorly relieved by opioids (but can be relieved with antispasmodics).
  - **Continuous** (in 90%):
    - Steady pain produced by pressure from tumor, stretching of the liver capsule, or abdominal distention.
    - Very severe steady pain may signal strangulation of bowel.
    - Usually responsive to morphine.
- **Nausea**.
- **Vomiting** (occurs in a majority of patients with obstruction).
  - Find out *how often* the patient vomits, what is the *volume* of the vomitus, and what is the *character of the vomitus*. The higher the obstruction, the earlier and more profuse the vomiting:
    - Vomiting large volumes of undigested food → suspect duodenal obstruction.
    - Fecal vomitus → suspect obstruction of distal ileum.
  - Establish whether vomiting occurs *with or without nausea* (the patient may be able to tolerate occasional vomiting if nausea is not present).
- Most patients progress slowly from partial or intermittent to complete bowel obstruction, and it is often difficult to distinguish clinically between partial and complete obstruction. Depending on the stage of obstruction, the patient may have
  - **Constipation** (in more advanced obstruction), or
  - **Diarrhea**.

Signs

Signs of intestinal obstruction depend on the location of the obstruction.
- Abdominal **distention** becomes more prominent as the obstruction is lower (more distal).
- Hyperactive bowel sounds and **borborygmi** characterize low obstruction; bowel sounds are quiet or absent in adynamic ileus.
- Be sure to examine the rectum for **signs of fecal impaction**!

Summary of Clinical Findings in Intestinal Obstruction

High Obstruction (Duodenum)	Low Obstruction (Colon)	Adynamic Ileus
Severe colicky pain, usually epigastric. Vomiting occurs early: profuse, contains bile and mucus. Abdomen not distended. Bowel sounds may be normal. Succussion splash.	Lower-intensity colicky pain, usually suprapubic. Vomiting occurs late, if at all; rarely feculent. Abdomen very distended and tympanitic. Bowel sounds hyperactive (borborygmi).	Colicky pain absent (there may be discomfort from distention). Vomiting frequent but rarely profuse (gastric contents + bile). Hiccups common.

Radiologic Findings

In patients in the terminal stages of cancer, abdominal films are indicated only when

- The patient may be a candidate for palliative surgery to relieve the obstruction (see next section), or
- It is important to distinguish between mechanical obstruction and severe constipation.

Findings in Obstruction	Findings in Paralytic Ileus	Findings In Constipation
Proximal to obstruction: bowel distended with gas and fluid. Distal to obstruction: bowel is empty. Upright film: air-fluid levels with "hairpin" loops or "stepladder" distribution.	Diffuse fluid and gaseous distention of small and large bowel. Upright film: balanced air-fluid levels in long loops.	Ground-glass appearance of retained feces throughout the colon.

Management of Intestinal Obstruction in the Terminally Ill Patient

Surgery

Surgery should be considered in the management of every patient with intestinal obstruction.

- In 35% of cases, *obstruction* is *due to a benign cause or a new primary* tumor that may be resectable.
- Surgical management is almost always warranted in patients with unproven intra-abdominal malignancy.
- Patients who are good candidates for surgery:
  - Life expectancy > 2 months.
  - Performance status (ECOG) = 2 or better.
  - The patient does *not* have malignant ascites, palpable abdominal masses, distant metastases (especially to lung), pleural effusion, or laboratory studies suggesting hepatic failure.
  - The patient has not undergone radiation to the abdomen.
  - The patient has undergone no more than one surgical procedure for obstruction in the past year (and that procedure provided good palliation for > 4 months).
- Even with careful patient selection, *surgical morbidity and mortality are high*:
  - Mortality: 18% to 35%.
  - Potential complications:
    - Fecal fistula (7–10%).
    - Reobstruction (30–40%).
    - Dehiscence.
    - Sepsis.

Nasogastric Suction and Intravenous Fluids

Nasogastric suction and IV fluids are useful in preparing patients for surgery but are **not generally recommended** for management of terminally ill patients.

- Disadvantages of nasogastric intubation:
  - Interferes with cough.
  - Can lead to aspiration, esophagitis.
  - Uncomfortable for the patient.
  - The nasogastric tube creates a barrier between the patient and the family.
- Sometimes, however, when pharmacologic measures (see below) fail and vomiting is intractable (> 2 episodes/8 hr), nasogastric decompression and parenteral hydration are preferable to the suffering produced by unremitting emesis.
- If nasogastric intubation will be required over a long time (> 2 weeks), consider percutaneous venting gastrostomy.

Nonsurgical Management

- The majority of terminally ill cancer patients with intestinal obstruction can be managed medically without nasogastric suction or IV fluids.
- Conservative management does not shorten survival.
- The preferred route of administration for giving drugs to patients with intestinal obstruction is continuous subcutaneous infusion via syringe driver.

Symptom/Problem	Management Measures
Nausea and vomiting	Goal is to eliminate nausea altogether and to reduce vomiting to once or twice a day at most: - *High obstruction*: **haloperidol**, 1.5 mg ± **hydroxyzine**, 25 mg ± **octreotide**, 0.3 mg by continuous SQ infusion (syringe driver) over 24 hours. - *Low obstruction*: **haloperidol**, 1.5 mg, *or* **metoclopramide**, 60 mg ± **hydroxyzine**, 25 mg ± **octreotide**, 0.3 mg, by continuous SQ infusion (syringe driver) over 24 hours. - **Dexamethasone**, 8 mg qam PO/IM. Allow patients to eat and drink ad libitum. Give small meals, low residue, liquid diet.
Colicky pain	**Discontinue** colonic **irritant laxatives** (e.g., bisacodyl, senna). **Discontinue gastrokinetic agents** (metoclopramide, cisapride). Give antispasmodic: - If the patient is able to take oral medications, try **loperamide**, 2 mg PO qid. - If the patient is unable to keep down oral medications, use a **scopolamine transdermal patch**, 1.5 mg, applied behind the ear every 3 days.
Steady, abdominal pain	**Morphine sulfate** PO or by continuous SQ infusion (mixed with other medications in the syringe driver).
Constipation	**Docusate tabs**, 200 mg bid PO. High-phosphate **enema**. For fecal impaction, treat as described in Chapter 20.
Diarrhea	**Loperamide**, 2 mg PO qid prn, *or* **tincture of opium**, 15–20 gtt PO tid prn.
Obstruction due to gastric cancer or cancer of the head of the pancreas	Add **dexamethasone**, 4–8 mg to the 24-hour infusion. If vomiting remains intractable, consider venting gastrostomy.

- Typical regimen for 24-hour SQ infusion for a patient with intestinal obstruction:

24-Hour Infusion by Syringe Driver
Morphine sulfate, 60 mg
Haloperidol, 1.5 mg
Octreotide, 0.3 mg
Hydroxyzine, 25 mg

Narcotic Bowel Syndrome

Pathophysiology

- Opioids affect GI function in several ways:
  - Increase muscle tone in the gastric antrum, small intestine, and colon.
  - Increase segmental (nonpropulsive) contractions of the bowel.
  - Produce contraction of GI sphincters (ileocecal valve, sphincter of Oddi).
  - Increase water and electrolyte absorption from the gut lumen.
- The net effect is to reduce stool volume and frequency.

Clinical Findings

- Anorexia.
- **Nausea and vomiting**.
- **Constipation**.
- Vague abdominal **pain**.
- Episodes of **pseudo-obstruction** (tympanitic abdominal distention, tenderness).

Management of Narcotic Bowel Syndrome in Terminally Ill Patients

- In patients who are not suffering from cancer, the treatment of choice is to stop the narcotic, under cover of clonidine to prevent withdrawal symptoms.

- In patients with cancer, the option of stopping narcotics is usually not practical, since the patient needs opioids to maintain pain control.
- Symptomatic relief can be obtained without stopping narcotics by giving **metoclopramide, 60 mg/24 hr by continuous SQ infusion.**

References and Further Reading

Ashby MA, Game PA, Devitt P, et al. Percutaneous gastrostomy as a venting procedure in palliative care. *Palliative Med* 5:147, 1991.

Baines M, Oliver DJ, Carter RL. Medical management of intestinal obstruction in patients with advanced malignant disease. *Lancet* ii:990, 1985.

Beattie GJ, Leonard RCF, Smyth JF. Bowel obstruction in ovarian carcinoma: a retrospective study and review of the literature. *Palliative Med* 3:275, 1989.

Bruera E, Brenneis C, Michaud M, MacDonald N. Continuous SC infusion of metoclopramide for treatment of narcotic bowel syndrome. *Cancer Treat Rep* 71:1121, 1987.

Chan A, Woodruff RK. Intestinal obstruction in patients with widespread intraabdominal malignancy. *J Pain Symptom Manage* 7:339, 1992.

Fainsinger RL, Spachynski K, Hanson J, Bruera E. Symptom control in terminally ill patients with malignant bowel obstruction. *J Pain Symptom Manage* 9:12, 1994.

Gallick HL, Weaver DW, Sachs RJ, Bouwman DK. Intestinal obstruction in cancer patients. *Am J Surg* 52:434, 1986.

Ibister WH, Elder P, Symons L. Non-operative management of malignant intestinal obstruction. *J R Coll Surg Edinb* 35:369, 1990.

Khoo D, Hall E, Matson R, et al. Palliation of malignant intestinal obstruction using octreotide. *Eur J Cancer* 30:28, 1994.

Khoo D, Riley J, Waxman J. Control of emesis in bowel obstruction in terminally ill patients (letter). *Lancet* 339:375, 1992.

Mercadante S, Spoldi E, Caraceni A, et al. Octreotide in relieving gastrointestinal symptoms due to bowel obstruction. *Palliative Med* 7:295, 1993.

Osteen RT, Guyton S, Steele G, Wilson RE. Malignant intestinal obstruction. *Surgery* 67:611, 1980.

Riley J, Fallon MT. Octreotide in terminal malignant obstruction of the gastrointestinal tract. *Eur J Palliative Care* 1(1):23, 1994.

Ripamonte C. Malignant bowel obstruction in advanced and terminal cancer patients. *Eur J Palliative Care* 1(1):16, 1994.

Sandgren JE, McPhee MS, Greenberger NJ. Narcotic bowel syndrome treated with clonidine. *Ann Intern Med* 101:331, 1984.

22 Diarrhea and Rectal Discharge

Definition

Diarrhea: Passage of more than three to four loose or fluid stools in 24 hours.

Incidence

- Diarrhea occurs in 5% to 10% of patients with advanced cancer.
- Diarrhea is far less common than constipation in cancer patients.

Pathophysiology of Diarrhea

- The fluid load presented to the small intestine is normally 7 to 9 L/day.
  - Fluid consists of oral intake plus salivary, gastric, pancreatic, and biliary secretions.
  - The normal small intestine absorbs large quantities of fluid with moderate efficiency (75%).
  - The normal colon is more efficient and absorbs 90% of the fluid presented to it.

- Absorption of sodium (and therefore fluid) from the gut involves active transport (sodium pump), neutral sodium-chloride absorption, glucose-stimulated absorption, and solvent drag.
- **Mechanisms** of diarrhea:
  - Impaired reabsorption of fluids from damaged bowel (malnutrition).
  - Hypersecretion of fluids into bowel lumen (endotoxins, hormones).
  - Hypermotility of the bowel (stimulant laxatives).
  - Increased osmotic load within the bowel lumen (sorbitol, osmotic laxatives).

Causes of Diarrhea in Advanced Cancer

Cause of Diarrhea	Comments
Fecal impaction	Particularly common among the **elderly, debilitated,** and patients taking **opioids** without adequate laxative coverage. Diarrhea may come on without warning and is usually preceded by several days without a bowel movement. Rectal examination typically reveals impacted feces (but rectum may be empty). See Chapter 20 for details.
Intermittent bowel obstruction	Diarrhea occurs in 34% of patients with malignant bowel obstruction (most commonly in cancers of the ovary or colon); may or may not alternate with constipation. Other symptoms of obstruction (nausea, vomiting, distention) likely to be present.
Effects of cancer treatments	**Radiation** enteritis: usually starts after second week of radiation therapy and continues for 2–3 weeks after completion of radiation. **Chemotherapy**, especially 5-FU, produces diarrhea at the time of the white blood cell nadir. **Surgery:** ▪ Gastrectomy → dumping syndrome. ▪ Ileal resection → ↓bile acid resorption → watery diarrhea. ▪ Total colectomy → ↓distal water reabsorption → excess water and salt loss through the ileostomy.
Medications	Laxatives. Antibiotics. Iron preparations. Sorbitol (in cough syrups or other elixirs). NSAIDs (especially diclofenac, mefenamic acid).

Cause of Diarrhea	Comments
Pancreatic insufficiency	May occur in the context of cancer of the head of the pancreas or after gastric or ileal resection. Signaled by **steatorrhea** (loose, pale, foul-smelling feces that tend to float in the toilet bowl).
Malnutrition	Starvation (cancer cachexia) produces changes in the bowel mucosa that promote malabsorption and diarrhea.
Rectal incontinence	Rectal tumor → mucus discharge. Neurogenic rectum from spinal cord compression; there is usually perianal numbness. General debility.
Infection	Overgrowth of bacteria or *Candida* in immuno-compromised patients or after antibiotic treatment.
Carcinoid tumors	Slow-growing tumors usually of the small bowel that secrete **serotonin** → profuse, watery diarrhea.
Concurrent medical conditions	Ulcerative colitis or Crohn's disease. Diabetes.

Clinical Findings

History

In taking the history, ask:
- How long has diarrhea been present? Was there a preceding period of constipation?
- How frequent are the patient's bowel movements?
- Is the patient continent?
- Are the stools formed, unformed, or liquid altogether?
- What color are the stools?
- Do the stools have a bad smell?
- Do the stools float in the toilet bowl?
- Is the passage of stool preceded by crampy pain?
- What medications is the patient taking?

Physical Examination

On physical examination, pay particular attention to:
- Examination of the abdomen:
  - **Bowel sounds**: Present or absent? If present, hypo- or hyperactive?
  - Palpable **masses** or feces.

- Rectal examination:
  - Anal **sphincter tone** and intactness of perianal **sensation**.
  - Is the rectal **ampulla** filled with feces?
  - Are there signs of rectal **discharge** (maceration of the perianal skin, bad odor)?

Laboratory Studies

- Stool anion gap will sometimes distinguish secretory from nonsecretory diarrheas:

  Stool anion gap = stool osmolality − 2(stool sodium + stool potassium).

  - Anion gap > 50 mmol/L → osmotic diarrhea.
  - Anion gap < 50 mmol/L → secretory diarrhea.
- Stool examination for ova and parasites.

Management of Diarrhea in Advanced Cancer

General Measures

- **Stop laxatives!**
- **Rest the bowel**:
  - Clear liquid diet with mostly carbohydrates (toast, rice).
  - Avoid proteins, fats, and milk products until diarrhea abates, then reintroduce slowly.
- **Avoid severe** degrees of **dehydration**:
  - Rehydrate orally if possible: WHO rehydration fluid or add **2 gm of salt + 50 gm of sugar** to **1 L of water** (flavor with lemon juice if preferred by patient).
  - If patient is severely dehydrated and symptomatic and unable to take fluids by mouth, give intravenous Ringer's lactate to match losses.
- **Review** the patient's **medications**, and wherever possible, stop medications that may be contributing to diarrhea (e.g., iron, sorbitol-containing syrups).
- For diarrhea resistant to conservative measures, give
  - **Loperamide**, 4 mg initially, then 1 capsule (2 mg) after each loose stool (maximum = 16 mg/24 hr).
  - **Tincture of opium**, 15 to 20 gtt PO q4h prn.

Specific Measures

Cause of Diarrhea	Specific Management
Fecal impaction	Manual disimpaction under sedation, as described in Chapter 20.
Intermittent bowel obstruction	Symptomatic treatment, as described in Chapter 21.
Radiation enteritis Post-5-FU enteritis	Usually self-limiting. Eliminate fiber and milk products from the diet while patient is symptomatic. NSAIDs (aspirin, ibuprofen) effective in radiation enteritis. Give tincture of opium as needed. For severe chemotherapy-induced enteritis, consider octreotide, 100 μg SQ bid.
Postgastrectomy dumping syndrome	Frequent, small meals. If severe, consider octreotide, 300 μ/day by continuous SQ infusion.
Pancreatic insufficiency	Pancreatic enzymes (Creon, Donnazyme, Entozyme): 2 tabs with meals and with snacks + Famotidine, 20 mg PO bid, to increase fat absorption + Loperamide, 2 mg PO, with each loose stool to slow peristalsis and increase water reabsorption (maximum dosage = 16 mg/day).
Carcinoid syndrome	Octreotide, 150-300 μg SQ bid or over 24 hours by continuous SQ infusion.

Rectal Discharge in Patients with Advanced Cancer

Most Common Causes in Patients with Advanced Cancer

- Rectal tumor.
- Fistulas.
- Fecal impaction.
- Radiation proctitis.

Symptoms and Signs

- Pruritus ani.
- Foul odor.

- Mucous or bloody discharge from the rectum.
- Damage to the perianal skin.

Management of Rectal Discharge

General Measures

- **Protect the skin**:
  - Wash the anal area thoroughly with warm water (no soap) as necessary, and dry gently with a soft cloth (no toilet paper, no rough towels).
  - Protect unbroken skin with zinc oxide paste.
  - For skin that is already inflamed or macerated, use a corticosteroid cream for 1 to 2 days.
- Give sedating **antihistamines for pruritus** (e.g., promethazine, 6.25–12.5 mg PO hs). Add a locally acting agent, such as Proctofoam or Nupercainal as needed.
- For foul-smelling discharge, give **metronidazole**, 500 mg PO tid.

Specific Measures

- For rectal tumors:
  - Consider palliative radiation therapy or endoscopic laser therapy.
  - Hydrocortisone foam, 1 applicator PR bid.
- For acute radiation proctitis: prednisolone suppositories bid.

References and Further Reading

Binder HJ. The pathophysiology of diarrhea. *Hosp Pract* 19(10):107, 1984.

Cascini S, Fedeli A, Fedeli S, Catalano G. Control of chemotherapy-induced diarrhea with octreotide in patients receiving 5-fluorouracil. *Eur J Cancer* 28:482, 1992.

Grady GF, Keusch GT. Pathogenesis of bacterial diarrheas. *N Engl J Med* 285:831 & 285:891, 1971.

Mennie AT, Dalley VM, Dinneen LC, Collier HO. Treatment of radiation-induced gastrointestinal distress with acetylsalicylate. *Lancet* ii:942, 1975.

23 Ascites

Definitions

- *Ascites*: Effusion of fluid into the peritoneal cavity.
- *Chylous ascites*: Effusion of chyle (lymph plus emulsified fat taken up from the intestine by the lacteals) into the peritoneal cavity.

Incidence

- Estimates vary:
  - Fifteen percent to 50% of patients with malignancy may suffer from ascites at some time in their course.
  - Six percent of patients entering hospices have ascites.
- Ascites occurs most commonly in patients with primary malignancy in
  - **Ovary** (35% have ascites at presentation; 60% have ascites at the time of death).
  - **Breast**.
  - Endometrium.
  - Colon.
  - Stomach.
  - Pancreas.
  - Bronchus.

Pathophysiology

- **Peritoneal carcinomatosis** probably accounts for more than 50% of cases.
  - Tumor cell deposits on visceral or parietal peritoneum → mechanical obstruction to lymphatic drainage.
  - Most common in ascites due to GI and ovarian cancers.
- Tumor **invasion** (primary or metastatic) **of liver parenchyma** accounts for 15% of cases →
  - Hepatic venous obstruction → ↑hydrostatic pressure→ ascites develops rapidly.
  - Patient has tender hepatomegaly.
- **Chylous ascites**:
  - Caused by obstruction of or leakage from abdominal lymphatics.
  - Most cases of malignant chylous ascites due to abdominal lymphoma.

Clinical Findings

History

- **Increasing abdominal girth** (ask about change in clothing or belt size).
- Ask about recent **weight gain** and **ankle swelling**.
- Elevation of the diaphragm produces:
  - Symptoms of esophageal reflux: **heartburn, regurgitation—** worse in recumbent position.
  - Symptoms of squashed stomach syndrome: **bloating, early satiety, nausea**.
  - Dyspnea and **orthopnea**.

Physical Examination

- Abdominal signs:
  - Very small amounts (140 ml) of ascitic fluid can be detected by aficionados of physical diagnosis using the **puddle sign** (Guarino, 1986), but such small volumes are unlikely to cause the patient discomfort and are not, therefore, relevant to palliative care of the terminally ill.
  - **Bulging flanks** may become apparent when there is more than 500 ml of fluid in the abdomen.

- To distinguish bulging flanks caused by ascites from those caused by obesity, percuss for **flank dullness**, then **shifting dullness** and/or **fluid wave.**
- Tense ascites may produce abdominal **hernias.**
- Ascites due to extensive liver invasion may be accompanied by abdominal **bruits** and/or **engorgement of the abdominal veins.**
- Extra-abdominal signs that may accompany ascites:
  - Signs of **pleural effusion** (e.g., dullness to percussion), usually on the *right.*
  - Upward and lateral displacement of the cardiac point of maximal impulse.
  - **Edema** of the legs, genitalia, lower abdomen.

Management of Malignant Ascites in the Terminally Ill Patient

Mild Ascites or Ascites that Is Not Causing Distressing Symptoms

- Start diuretics:
  - **Spironolactone, 100 mg PO qam** (may increase stepwise to 200 mg bid as needed), together with:
  - **Furosemide, 40 mg PO qam** (may increase stepwise to 240 mg qam as needed). *Note:* Furosemide given by bolus IV reduces GFR in patients with ascites, but continuous infusion of IV furosemide (100 mg over 24 hours) has been reported to produce significant diuresis and marked relief of ascites.
- Dietary salt and water restriction, used in the treatment of cirrhotic ascites, causes unnecessary discomfort to the dying patient.

Tense Ascites or Ascites Causing Distressing Symptoms (e.g., Pain, Tachypnea)

- Perform abdominal **paracentesis**:
  - With patient semirecumbent, and after he has voided, choose a **puncture site** in the midline caudal to the umbilicus and caudal to the level of percussible dullness (alternatively, in the flank at the anterior axillary line). Avoid areas of surgical scars.
  - **Prep** the skin with povidone-iodine. Local anesthesia for thick abdominal wall.

- With a gloved hand, **retract the skin caudad,** and insert a 14- to 16-gauge needle or **Intracath** that has been attached to an IV extension tube. (Place the distal end of the extension tube in a collection bottle or urine collection bag.)
- **Drain to dryness** over 6 hours.
- Rapidly **withdraw needle,** allowing skin to return to position (creating Z-track). If puncture was on one of the flanks, the patient should lie with that side *up* for several hours. If there is leakage around the puncture site, an ostomy bag may be placed over the site for 24 to 48 hours.
- Send ascitic fluid for
  - Total protein, LDH.
  - White blood cell count to rule out bacterial peritonitis (WBC > 500-750/mm^2 suggests infection).
  - Gram's stain and culture (> 30% of patients have culture-positive ascitic fluid).
- *Note:* Single or even repeated paracentesis in patients with advanced cancer does *not* significantly lower serum protein.

Ascites that Recurs Rapidly

- Consider **intracavitary therapy** (40-60% have partial or complete response for > 2 months).
  - Paracentesis to drain the abdomen dry.
  - Dilute 60 to 120 mg of **bleomycin** in 100 ml of saline, and inject into the paracentesis catheter. Flush with an additional 100 ml of saline.
  - Have patient change position every few minutes for 1 hour, to disperse the drug.
  - Potential side effects: fever and abdominal tenderness.
- For patients with life expectancy > 1 month (especially with primary tumor in breast or ovary), consider **peritoneovenous shunt** (LeVeen or Denver).
  - Shunt exploits 5 to 15 cm H_2O pressure gradient between the full peritoneal cavity and the central venous circulation (gradient increases further on inspiration): When pressure gradient > 3-5 cm H_2O, one-way flow valve opens and ascitic fluid flows from abdominal cavity into central vein.
  - Operation can be performed under local anesthesia.
  - In 15 reported series comprising 372 patients, nearly 70% had excellent symptomatic relief (in contrast to patients with cirrhotic ascites, in whom shunting has not been very useful).

References and Further Reading

Amiel SA, Blackburn AM, Rubens RD. Intravenous infusion of frusemide as treatment for ascites in malignant disease. *Br Med J* 288:1041, 1984.

Frakes JT. Physiologic considerations in the medical management of ascites. *Arch Intern Med* 140:620, 1980.

Greenway B, Johnson PJ, Williams R. Control of malignant ascites with spironolactone. *Br J Surg* 69:441, 1982.

Guarino JR. Auscultatory percussion to detect ascites. *N Engl J Med* 315:1555, 1986.

Lacy JH, Wieman TJ, Shively EH. Management of malignant ascites. *Surg Gynecol Obstet* 159:397, 1984.

Lifschitz S. Ascites, pathophysiology and control measures. *Int J Radiat Oncol Biol Phys* 8:1423, 1982.

Paladine W, Cunningham TJ, Sponzo R, et al. Intracavitary bleomycin in the management of malignant effusions. *Cancer* 38:1903, 1976.

Ostrowski MJ. An assessment of the long term results of controlling the reaccumulation of malignant effusions using intracavitary bleomycin. *Cancer* 57:721, 1986.

Reinhold RB, Lokich JJ, Tomashefski J, Costello P. Management of malignant ascites with peritoneovenous shunting. *Am J Surg* 145:455, 1983.

Rubinstein D, McInnes I, Dudley F. Morbidity and mortality after peritoneovenous shunt surgery for refractory ascites. *Gut* 26:1070, 1985.

Runyon BA. Care of patients with ascites. *N Engl J Med* 330:337, 1994.

Sharma S, Walsh D. Management of symptomatic malignant ascites with diuretics: Two case reports and a review of the literature. *J Pain Symptom Manage* 10:237, 1995.

Souter RG, Tarin D, Kettlewell MGW. Peritoneovenous shunts in the management of malignant ascites. *Br J Surgery* 70:478, 1983.

Respiratory

24 Dyspnea

Definition

- An unpleasant sensation of shortness of breath.
- By definition, dyspnea is *subjective*, and its severity can be gauged only by the patient.
  - The degree of dyspnea may not be related to the severity of the underlying problem.
  - Dyspnea in patients with advanced cancer is almost invariably attended by anxiety and fears of choking or suffocation.
  - Dyspnea is frightening to the patient according to the *meaning* the patient has assigned to it (e.g., that it is a sign of serious illness or a harbinger of death); hence part of the treatment of dyspnea may be to alter its meaning for the patient.

Incidence

- Dyspnea occurs in **70%** of terminal cancer patients at some time during the last 6 weeks of life and tends to correlate inversely with the length of survival.
- **Risk factors** for dyspnea in cancer patients:
  - Lung or pleural involvement by the tumor.
  - Presence of underlying pulmonary or cardiac disease.
  - Poor performance status.
- However, 24% of dyspneic cancer patients have none of the above risk factors. Their dyspnea is ascribed to the "debility of terminal cancer" (general muscle weakness, medical complications).

Causes of Dyspnea in Patients with Cancer

Cancer-Related Causes

- Obstruction of bronchus by tumor.
- Replacement of lung parenchyma by tumor.
- Pleural effusion.
- Lymphangitic carcinomatosis.
- Superior vena cava syndrome.
- Ascites, causing pressure on the diaphragm and restriction of pulmonary excursion.

Treatment-Related Causes

- Pneumonectomy.
- Radiation fibrosis in the lung.
- Chemotherapy-induced damage (bleomycin).

General Medical Conditions with a High Incidence Among Cancer Patients

- COPD/asthma.
- Pulmonary embolism.
- Left heart failure.
- Pneumonia.
- Anemia.

General Measures for the Treatment of Dyspnea

- Allow the patient to assume a **position of comfort** (which will usually be sitting or semisitting).
- Provide **reassurance**. Determine what meaning the patient attaches to the dyspnea, and try to help the patient find a less frightening significance for the symptom.
- For patients who are receptive to such methods, teach **relaxation techniques** to forestall respiratory panic attacks.
- Make sure the patient's room is **well-ventilated**. Use a **fan** if necessary to create a breeze over the patient's face.

- Give **nebulizer treatments**:
  - Start with **morphine, 2.5 mg + dexamethasone, 2.0 mg in 2.5 ml of saline** q4h and prn.
    - Increase morphine dosage as needed to achieve relief of dyspnea.
    - Nebulized morphine may benefit even patients taking very large doses of oral or parenteral morphine for pain (probably acts directly on receptors in the lung).
    - Probably less then 5% to 15% of inhaled morphine is absorbed systemically.

> THE MOST EFFECTIVE TREATMENT
> FOR DYSPNEA IN ADVANCED CANCER IS
> INHALATION OF NEBULIZED MORPHINE.

  - Add **albuterol, 0.5 ml**, if wheezing is heard on auscultation of the chest and is not relieved by corticosteroids.
  - Many patients prefer to take nebulizer treatments by mouthpiece rather than by mask.
  - Always use **0.9% saline** as the diluent for nebulizer treatments and *not* sterile water, because nebulized water provokes bronchoconstriction. (Use normal saline intended for injection and not bacteriostatic saline, which has preservatives that may also cause pulmonary complications.)
- If the patient is dyspneic at rest, try **oxygen** by nasal cannula at 4 L/min for short periods (10–20 minutes) every few hours.
- For **respiratory panic**:
  - Make sure someone is with the patient at all times.
  - Respiratory sedatives
  - **Midazolam**, 5 to 10 mg IM/slowly IV, *or*
  - **Morphine**, 5 to 10 mg by nebulizer or IV, *or*
  - **Chlorpromazine**, 25 mg PO or IM.

Additional Specific Measures for Management of Dyspnea

Contributing Cause	Treatment
Obstruction of bronchus by tumor	**Radiation** therapy (will relieve dyspnea in up to to 90% of cases). **Dexamethasone:** Start at 8–12 mg PO qam → taper rapidly to 4 mg PO qam.
Replacement of lung parenchyma in SCLC	**Chemotherapy** (etoposide).
Pleural effusion	**Drain** up to 1.5 L (see Chapter 27). **Furosemide,** 40 mg PO qam + **spironolactone,** 100 mg PO qam.
Lymphangitis	**Dexamethasone,** 4 mg PO qam. Consider radiation.
Superior vena cava syndrome	**Dexamethasone,** 24 mg IV stat. **Radiation** therapy. Possible further oncologic treatment. (See Chapter 28.)
Ascites	**Furosemide,** 40 mg PO qam + **spironolactone,** 100 mg PO qam (see Chapter 23).
Congestive heart failure	**Oxygen.** **Furosemide,** 40-240 mg PO/IV. If patient is not taking opioids, **morphine,** 5–10 mg IV. Consider ACE inhibitor.
COPD/Asthma	**Beclomethasone** by metered-dose inhaler.
Pneumonia	If producing distressing symptoms (fever, cough, pleuritic pain), give **antibiotic,** as per culture results.
Pulmonary embolism	**Oxygen.** Treat for respiratory panic, if present.
Anemia	For alert patient with hemoglobin < 9, consider **transfusion** of packed red blood cells.

References and Further Reading

Beauford W, Saylor TT, Sansbury DW, et al. Effects of nebulized morphine sulfate on the exercise tolerance of the ventilatory limited COPD patient. *Chest* 104:175, 1993.

Booth S, Kelly M, Adams L, Cox N. The treatment of dyspnoea in hospice patients—does oxygen help? (abstract). *Palliative Med* 8:71, 1994.

Bruera E, deStoutz N, Velasco-Leiva A, et al. Effects of oxygen on dyspnoea in hypoxaemic terminal-cancer patients. *Lancet* 342:13, 1993.

Bruera E, MacMillan K, Pither J, MacDonald N. Effects of morphine on the dyspnoea of terminal cancer patients. *J Pain Symptom Manage* 5:341, 1990.

Collins TM, Ash DV, Close HJ, Thorogood J. An evaluation of the palliative role of radiotherapy in inoperable carcinoma of the bronchus. *Clin Radiol* 39:284, 1988.

Cowcher K, Hanks G. Long-term management of respiratory symptoms in advanced cancer. *J Pain Symptom Manage* 5:320, 1990.

Davis CL. Use of nebulized opioids for breathlessness (letter). *Palliative Med* 9:169, 1995.

DeConno F, Spoldi E, Caraceni A, Ventafridda V. Does pharmacological treatment affect the sensation of breathlessness in terminal cancer patients? *Palliative Med* 5:237, 1991.

Farncombe M, Chater S, Gillin A. The use of nebulized opioids for breathlessness: A chart review. *Palliative Med* 8:306, 1994.

Heyse-Moore LH, Ross V, Mullee MA. How much of a problem is dyspnoea in advanced cancer? *Palliative Med* 5:20, 1991.

Krech RL, Davis J, Walsh D, Curtis EB. Symptoms of lung cancer. *Palliative Med* 6:309, 1992.

Light RW, Muro JR, Sato RI, et al. Effects of oral morphine on breathlessness and exercise tolerance in patients with chronic obstructive pulmonary disease. *Ann Rev Respir Dis* 139:126, 1989.

O'Neill PA, Morton PB, Stark RD. Chlorpromazine—a specific effect on breathlessness? *Br J Clin Pharmacol* 19:793, 1985.

Regnard C, Ahmedzai S. Dyspnoea in advanced cancer—a flow diagram. *Palliative Med* 4:311, 1990.

Reuben DB, Mor V. Dyspnea in terminally ill cancer patients. *Chest* 89:234, 1986.

Rogers DF, Barnes P. Opioid inhibition of neurally mediated mucus secretion in human bronchi. *Lancet* 335:930, 1989.

Schwartzstein RM, Lahive K, Pope A, et al. Cold facial stimulation reduces breathlessness induced in normal subjects. *Am Rev Respir Dis* 136:58, 1987.

Stone P, Kurowska A, Tookman A. Nebulized frusemide for dyspnoea (letter). *Palliative Med* 8:258, 1994.

Twycross RG. Symptom control: the problem areas. *Palliative Med* 7(Suppl 1):1, 1993.

Young IH, Daviskas E, Keena VA. Effect of low dose nebulised morphine on exercise endurance in patients with chronic lung disease. *Thorax* 44:387, 1989.

25   Cough

Incidence

Cough occurs in 30% to 50% of all patients with terminal cancer and approximately 80% of patients with cancer of the lung.

Physiology

- Cough is a physiologic mechanism to clear the airways of foreign materials or excessive secretions. Most people cough 1 to 2 times an hour while awake to maintain a clear airway; coughing more often is abnormal.
- Cough usually results from stimulation of sensory nerves in the upper airway.
- A cough consists of a deep inhalation → closure of the glottis → ↑intrathoracic pressure → violent exhalation producing high flow rates.
  - Cough reflex is suppressed by most agents that depress consciousness.
  - Requires intact abdominal and thoracic musculature and sufficient strength to deploy those muscles.

Most Common Causes of Cough in Terminally Ill Patients

- Primary or metastatic involvement of the lung or pleura by the **malignancy**:
  - Endobronchial invasion by tumor.
  - Pleural effusion.
- Underlying chronic **airways disease** (asthma, COPD).
- Respiratory **infection**.
- Esophageal **reflux**.
- Left **heart failure**.
- Nasal **sinusitis** with postnasal drip.
- Medications (e.g., ACE inhibitors).

Workup of Cough in Terminally Ill Patients

- A careful history will enable clinical diagnosis of the source of cough in 80% of patients.

Symptom	Possible Cause(s)
Cough precipitated by re-cumbency or cough that is worse at night	Esophageal reflux Left heart failure
Nasal stuffiness	Postnasal drip with or without sinusitis
Purulent sputum; afebrile	Decompensation of COPD Bronchiectasis
Purulent sputum; febrile	Pneumonia, lung abscess
Copious frothy, pink sputum	Left heart failure (Rarely) alveolar cell carcinoma
Hemoptysis	Malignant involvement of lung
Dry, hacking cough	Endobronchial spread of cancer Pleural effusion Asthma ACE inhibitors
Bovine cough with hoarseness	Vocal cord paralysis

- **Diagnostic tests** to determine source of cough are not warranted in the terminally ill but may be useful for patients still undergoing active anticancer treatment:

If you suspect	Test(s) indicated
Malignant involvement of lung or pleura	Chest x-ray; CT of the chest
Sinusitis/postnasal drip	Examination of nares, pharynx Sinus x-rays
Esophageal reflux	Barium swallow and/or endoscopy
Asthma	Spirometry before and after bronchodilator
Left heart failure	Echocardiogram
Pneumonia	Chest x-ray, sputum cultures

Medications Used to Treat Cough

Class	Examples	Comments
Demulcents	**Simple linctus** Most proprietary cough medications that contain mainly sugar	Sugar solutions have a soothing effect, possibly by (a) increasing saliva production→ ↑swallowing; (b) coating sensory nerve endings; or (c) acting as a protective barrier to cough receptors.
Opioids	**Codeine, morphine, etc.** **Dextromethorphan**	Opioids probably work both centrally and on sensory nerve endings that initiate cough. μ-Receptor stimulation may also reduce mucus production. *Note:* Meperidine is not an antitussive.
Antihistamines	**Diphenydramine**	Antihistamines may help at night because of sedative effects and/or reduction of postnasal drip.
Expectorants	**Ipecacuanha, ammonium chloride, guaifenesin, potassium iodide, terpin hydrate, normal saline**	Some drugs in this class work by stimulating chemoreceptor trigger zone and therefore also produce nausea and vomiting; have not been shown to be effective.
Mucolytics	**Bromhexine, *N*-acetylcysteine**	Act by changing the viscosity of mucus. Clinically important effects on cough have not been demonstrated.

continued

Class	Examples	Comments
Bronchodilators	**Ipratropium bromide** β_2**-agonists** (e.g., albuterol)	Act on bronchial smooth muscle; may reduce input from stretch receptors → ↓cough reflex; have been most effective for postinfective cough or cough due to chronic bronchitis.
Local anesthetics	**Lidocaine**	Prevent sensory nerve traffic in fibers in the pharynx that mediate cough. Most effective when given by nebulizer. Abolish protective reflexes in the lung and may induce bronchospasm, so must be used with caution. Effects are short-lived. Patients must be NPO for 1 hour after administration to prevent aspiration. Indicated for cough due to endobronchial malignancy.

Approach to the Treatment of Cough in the Terminally Ill Patient

- General measures:

Situation	General Measures
Dry, hacking cough	- Simple demulcent antitussive such as **simple linctus**, 5-10 mg qid to soothe pharynx. - For patients not already taking opioids, **codeine**, 30-60 mg PO q4h, *or* **morphine**, 5-20 mg PO q4h. - For patients already taking opioids: **morphine**, 2.5-5 mg + **dexamethasone**, 2 mg by nebulizer. Administer via mouthpiece (rather than face mask) when possible. - In severe cases, 2 ml of **2% lidocaine** in 1 ml of normal saline by nebulizer for 10 minutes tid (NPO for 1 hour afterward).
Wet cough; patient able to raise sputum	- Humidification via steam inhalations or nebulizer. - **Albuterol**, 0.5 ml in 2.5 ml of normal saline via nebulizer tid. - Chest physiotherapy.

Situation	General Measures
Wet cough; patient too weak to raise sputum	▪ Centrally-acting cough suppressant (see dosages of **opioids** for dry, hacking cough, above). ▪ **Atropine**, 1-2 mg + **morphine**, 2.5-5 mg ± **dexamethasone**, 2 mg by nebulizer qid. ▪ Anxiolytic such as **midazolam**, 2.5-5 mg IM. ▪ Avoid suctioning; use suction only for bleeding into throat, for fulminant pulmonary edema, or in tracheostomy with copious secretions. ▪ For terminal bubbling, **atropine**, 1-2 mg IM/IV, *or* **scopolamine**, 0.3-0.6 mg IM/SQ q4h.

▪ *When the precipitating cause* of cough *is known*, treat according to the underlying mechanism:

Cause of Cough	Recommended Treatment
Extension of bronchial cancer	Palliative **radiotherapy**. **Dexamethasone**, 4 mg PO qam. **Lidocaine 2%** by nebulizer for 10 minutes qid; keep patient NPO for 1 hour after each treatment.
Pleural effusion	Patient should lie on the side of the pleural effusion (i.e., healthy lung up). As soon as possible: **Drain dry**. Consider installing a sclerosing agent (tetracycline, talc).
Esophageal reflux	**Raise head of bed**. **Metoclopramide**, 10 mg PO tid. **Famotidine**, 20 mg PO hs.
Left heart failure	Raise head of bed. **Oxygen**. **Furosemide**, 40 mg qam; titrate upward as needed. **Morphine**, 5-10 mg IV for acute CHF.
Sinusitis and post-nasal drip	**Diphenhydramine**, 25-50 mg tid and hs. **Beclomethasone** aerosol, 1 dose to each nostril qid. For documented sinusitis, **amoxicillin**, 500 mg tid × 10-21 days.
Pulmonary infection	**Antibiotics** as per culture results. Chest physiotherapy. Nebulized normal saline.*
COPD or asthma	By nebulizer: **albuterol**, 0.5 ml + **dexamethasone**, 2 mg in 2.5 ml of normal saline* by nebulizer tid-qid.

*Always use 0.9% saline in the nebulizer and *not* water because water provokes bronchoconstriction. Use normal saline that does not contain bacteriostatic agents, since such agents may lead to inflammatory changes within the lungs.

continued

Cause of Cough	Recommended Treatment
ACE inhibitors	Change to a different antihypertensive drug. If that is not feasible, give: **Sulindac**, 100 mg PO tid.
Vocal cord paralysis	Injection of Teflon into affected vocal cord (ENT consultation).

References and Further Reading

Collins TM, Ash DV, Close JH, Thorogood J. An evaluation of the palliative role of radiotherapy in inoperable carcinoma of the bronchus. *Clin Radiol* 39:284, 1988.

Cowcher K, Hanks G. Long-term management of respiratory symptoms in advanced cancer. *J Pain Symptom Manage* 5:320, 1990.

DiSilva I, Garrett J. Cough in adults. *Patient Manage* 22(8):55, 1993.

Eddy NB, Friebel H, Hahn K-J, Hallbach H. Codeine and its alternatives for pain and cough relief: 3. The antitussive action of codeine—mechanism, methodology, and evaluation. *Bull WHO* 40:425, 1969.

Eddy NB, Friebel H, Hahn K-J, Hallbach H. Codeine and its alternatives for pain and cough relief: 4. Potential alternatives for cough relief. *Bull WHO* 40:639, 1969.

Fuller RW, Jackson DM. Physiology and treatment of cough. *Thorax* 45:425, 1990.

Hagen N. An approach to cough in cancer patients. *J Pain Symptom Manage* 6:257, 1991.

Louie K, Bertolini M, Fainsinger R. Management of intractable cough. *J Palliative Care* 8(4):46, 1992.

Lowry RH, Higenbottam TW. Antitussive properties of inhaled bronchodilators on induced cough. *Chest* 93:1186, 1988.

Reynolds RD, Smith RM. Nebulized bacteriostatic saline as a cause of bronchitis. *J Fam Pract* 40:35, 1995.

Rogers DF, Barnes PJ. Opioid inhibition of neurally mediated mucus secretion in human bronchi. *Lancet* 335:930, 1989.

Trochtenberg S. Nebulized lidocaine in the treatment of refractory cough. *Chest* 105:1592, 1994.

Walsh TD. Symptom control in patients with advanced cancer. *Am J Hospice Palliative Care* 9(6):32, 1992.

Zervanos NJ, Shute KM. Acute disruptive cough. *Postgrad Med* 95(4):153, 1994.

26 Hemoptysis

Definitions

- *Hemoptysis*: Coughing up of blood.
- *Massive hemoptysis*: Expectoration of between 200 and 1000 ml of blood in 24 hours.

Incidence

- Occurs in up to 10% of patients admitted to hospice facilities.
- In patients with primary lung neoplasms, hemoptysis is present in 30% to 50% at diagnosis.

Causes of Hemoptysis in Patients with Cancer

- Bleeding from a vessel in the bronchus, secondary to malignant invasion.
- Pulmonary embolism.
- Pneumonia.
- Bronchitis.
- Bleeding from an extrapulmonary source (epistaxis, mouth or throat).

Management of Hemoptysis in Patients with Cancer

Degree of Hemoptysis	Steps to Take
Specks of blood in sputum	In patient receiving active treatment, seek source of bleeding (chest x-ray, lung CT scan, endoscopy), and treat accordingly (e.g., antibiotics for pneumonia). In the terminally ill patient, no treatment is necessary except reassurance. Can give **cough suppressant**, such as codeine, 30–60 mg PO q4h.
Streaks or small globs of blood in sputum	Oral hemostatic agent: **tranexamic acid**, 500 mg PO bid. Watchful waiting; minor hemoptysis may be the prelude to massive bleeding. Have strong opioid and anxiolytic on hand at bedside.
Hemoptysis persisting or increasing despite oral hemostatic agents	External beam **radiation therapy** (will control hemoptysis in 88% of cases), *or* **Laser therapy**.
Massive projectile hemoptysis (very rare)	Trendelenburg position to decrease symptoms of suffocation. If side of the lesion is known, patient should lie with the bleeding side down to minimize bleeding into the good lung. **Morphine**, 10–15 mg IV push. **Midazolam**, 5 mg IM. Colored towels and blankets to cover blood, so that it will not alarm patient and family.

References and Further Reading

Collins TM, Ash DV, Close JG, Thorogood J. An evaluation of the palliative role of radiotherapy in inoperable cancer of the bronchus. *Clin Radiol* 39:284, 1988.

Hetzel MR, Smith SGT. Endoscopic palliation of tracheobronchial malignancies. *Thorax* 46:325, 1991.

Jones DK, Davies RJ. Massive haemoptysis. *Br Med J* 300:889, 1990.

Lung Cancer Working Party. Inoperable non-small cell lung cancer (NSCLC): a Medical Research Council randomised trial of palliative radiotherapy with two fractions or ten fractions. *Br J Cancer* 63:265, 1991.

27 Pleural Effusions

Definitions

Pleural effusion: Abnormal volume of fluid in the pleural space.
Exudate: Fluid with total protein > 3.0 gm/dl (or pleural-serum protein > 0.5); LDH > 225 (or pleural-serum LDH > 0.6); or WBC > 2500/ml.
Transudate: Fluid whose total protein, LDH, and WBC count is lower than the figures cited above for an exudate.

Incidence and Significance of Pleural Effusions in Cancer Patients

- Malignant pleural effusions most likely to occur in (listed in decreasing order of frequency)
  - **Bronchogenic** carcinoma (especially adenocarcinoma).
  - **Breast** carcinoma (up to 50% of breast cancer patients will develop a pleural effusion).
  - **Ovarian** carcinoma.
  - Gastric carcinoma.
  - Lymphoma.
  - Melanoma.
  - Sarcoma.
- Malignant pleural effusion is a sign of **advanced, widespread disease**.

Cancer Type	Mean Survival*
All types	3 months
Lung cancer	2 months
Ovarian cancer	3 months
Breast cancer	7–15 months

*From detection of pleural effusion.

Pathophysiology of Malignant Pleural Effusions

- Normally 500 to 700 ml of fluid moves through the pleural space each day → 80% to 90% is reabsorbed, leaving a normal volume of 10 to 20 ml to act as a lubricant between the visceral and parietal pleura.
- Mechanisms leading to abnormal pleural fluid collections in malignancy:
  - Inflammation of pleural surface by tumor ("peripheral" effusions) → ↑capillary permeability → transudation of fluid into the pleural space.
  - Infiltration of mediastinal lymph nodes ("central" effusions) → impaired lymphatic drainage → impaired efflux from the pleural space →
  - Malignant exudate starts to collect → ↑pleural osmotic pressure → ↓outflow of pleural fluid.
  - Pleural effusion may also occur from spillover from ascites via right-sided peritoneopleural channels (→ right pleural effusion).

Symptoms and Signs of Pleural Effusion

Symptoms

- Dry, nonproductive **cough** caused by compression of the bronchi by fluid.
- Progressive **dyspnea** due to compression of the lungs and consequent restriction of pulmonary excursion.
- Pain:
  - Metastases to the parietal pleura → **dull**, continuous, deep **chest pain**.
  - Inflammation of the parietal pleura → **pleuritic chest pain** (remits as fluid separates the pleural surfaces from one another).

- Irritation of the diaphragmatic parietal pleura → **sharp ipsilateral shoulder pain.**
- The *severity* of symptoms depends on how quickly the fluid accumulated rather than on the total amount of fluid present in the intrapleural space.

Signs

- Tachypnea.
- Labored breathing.
- Possible tracheal shift (to the side opposite the effusion).
- Decreased respiratory excursion.
- Dullness to percussion.
- Undetectable diaphragmatic excursion.
- Muffled breath and voice sounds with whispered pectoriloquy.
- Decreased vocal fremitus.
- Egophony.

Radiographic Findings

- Upright PA film can detect as little as 200 ml of fluid, as **blunting of the costophrenic angle.**
- Lateral decubitus film will detect as little as 100 ml of fluid.
- Most important determination to make on x-ray is *whether the fluid is loculated,* for that will determine feasibility of pleurodesis (vide infra).

Management of Malignant Pleural Effusions

Asymptomatic Pleural Effusions

- In *patients still undergoing active treatment,* diagnostic thoracentesis is warranted. Send samples for
  - Lactate dehydrogenase, protein, specific gravity, pH, glucose.
  - Cell count.
  - Cytology.
  - Culture and stain for bacteria (including tuberculosis), fungi.
- In *patients no longer receiving oncologic treatment,* there is no reason to perform thoracentesis for asymptomatic pleural effusion.

Pleural Effusion Producing Distressing Symptoms

First presentation → **simple aspiration** under local anesthesia:
- Assemble equipment:

Equipment for Thoracentesis

Skin prep (sponges, povidone-iodine solution)

Fenestrated drape and sterile cloth on which to place equipment

Sterile gloves

10-ml syringe for local anesthetic, with 25-gauge and 2-inch 22-gauge needle

Lidocaine 1% or bupivacaine 0.25%, 5–10 ml, for local anesthesia

10-ml syringe

14-gauge Intracath

2 curved clamps

Sterile intravenous tubing

Plasma vacuum bottle

Sterile sponges and adhesive tape

- **Review** patient's current **chest x-ray** to confirm location of pleural effusion.
- **Position the patient:** sitting up, arms supported on bedside table.
- **Choose site** for puncture:
  - Confirm fluid level by percussion.
  - Use the first or second intercostal space *below* the fluid level in the posterior axillary line (but no lower than the eighth intercostal space).
- **Prep** area with povidone-iodine.
- Don sterile **gloves**.
- Place sterile **drape** over chest with window over selected puncture site.
- **Infiltrate** local **anesthetic**, and confirm presence of intrapleural fluid.
  - Inject 5 to 10 ml of local anesthetic at the *superior* rib margin.
  - Infiltrate through the pleura (you should feel a "pop"), and **aspirate** to confirm presence of fluid.
  - Clamp needle at the skin to mark the depth of penetration, and withdraw needle.
- **Wait** 5 to 10 minutes for local anesthetic to take full effect!

- Meanwhile, **prepare equipment** for drainage:
  - Clamp proximal end of tubing.
  - Insert distal end of tubing into vacuum bottle.
  - Place 10-ml syringe onto Intracath needle.
  - Apply clamp to Intracath needle at same depth as clamp on needle used for anesthesia, to prevent excess depth of penetration.
- **Insert Intracath needle** at anesthetized puncture site, at the superior rib margin, to depth marked by clamp.
- **Remove syringe**, and immediately **occlude** the **needle** with your finger (to prevent air entry).
- **Insert cannula** into needle, and **advance** the cannula **into** the **pleural space.**
- **Slide the** *needle* **back** over the cannula, and attach the protective clip to prevent cannula shear.
- **Release the clamp** on the intravenous tubing to start drainage.
- **Do not remove more than 1 to 1.5 L** (rapid reexpansion of the lung may cause severe pain and ipsilateral pulmonary edema).
- When drainage is complete, **remove the cannula**, and apply a **sterile dressing** to the puncture site.
- If patient shows respiratory distress *after* the procedure, obtain a **chest x-ray** to rule out pneumothorax.

Note: When thoracentesis is for any reason not feasible, one may try to reduce the volume of the pleural effusion with diuretics: **furosemide**, 40 mg PO qam + **spironolactone**, 100 mg PO qam.

Pleural Effusion that Reaccumulates After Thoracentesis

- In 90% of patients, pleural effusion will recur 1 to 30 days after thoracentesis.
- Treatment options:
  - For metastatic tumors sensitive to chemotherapy (breast, lymphoma, ovary), **chemotherapy** may give dramatic results, especially relatively early in disease.
  - For central pleural effusions, **radiation therapy**
  - For other recurring pleural effusions, consider **pleurodesis** (symphysis of the visceral and parietal pleura to obliterate the pleural space).*

---

*Little-known fact: Elephants do not have a pleural space at all but seem not to suffer any disadvantage in respiratory dynamics as a consequence.

- **Selection criteria** for pleurodesis:
  - Pleural effusion that *reaccumulates* rapidly (1–3 days) or repeatedly (after two or three needle aspirations).
  - The patient is *symptomatic,* and *aspiration* of the effusion previously *relieved* the patient's *symptoms.*
  - The patient's *life expectancy* is estimated at *more than 1 month.*
  - The effusion is *peripheral* rather than central.
  - The effusion is freely moving, not loculated.
- **Pleurodesis procedure:**
  - A **chest tube** (28 or 32 French) is inserted in the anterior axillary line in the sixth or seventh intercostal space and attached to a water-seal gravity drainage system with negative suction of 15 to 20 cm H_2O.
  - The pleura is allowed to **drain dry** (this may take 2–3 days), so that the visceral and pleural parietal surfaces will be in apposition.
  - When drainage is < 50 ml/24 hr, obtain a chest film to be certain all the fluid is evacuated.
  - Instillation of the sclerosing solution:
    - **Premedicate** the patient with morphine, 5 to 10 mg IM/IV ½ hour before instillation.
    - Inject the sclerosing agent into the chest tube.
      - In *palliative care,* the sclerosing agent of choice is **tetracycline,** 1 gm in 30 ml of normal saline (tetracycline has a high success rate with fewer side effects than with any other agent). Add 150 mg of **lidocaine** to the mixture to minimize pleuritic pain.
      - Flush chest tube with another 50 ml of saline after the sclerosing agent is injected.
    - Keep chest tube clamped for 6 hours.
  - Unclamp tube, and allow pleural fluid to drain (with negative suction of 15–20 cm H_2O for the first 24 hours, then by gravity).
  - When drainage is less than 50 ml/24 hr, the chest tube is removed and the site closed with a 3-0 silk suture.

References and Further Reading

Fentiman IS. Effective treatment of malignant pleural effusions. *Br J Hosp Med* 37:42, 1987.

Hausheer FJ, Yarbro JW. Diagnosis and treatment of malignant pleural effusion. *Semin Oncol* 12:54, 1985.

Leff A, Hopewell PC, Costello J. Pleural effusion from malignancy. *Ann Intern Med* 88:532, 1978.

Tattersall MHN, Boyer MJ. Management of malignant pleural effusions. *Thorax* 45:81, 1990.

28 Superior Vena Cava Syndrome

Definition

Clinical syndrome arising from obstruction to the superior vena cava (SVC).

Etiology and Incidence

- Today, malignant disease accounts for the vast majority (> 80%) of cases of SVC syndrome.
- Among malignant etiologies:
  - **Bronchogenic** carcinoma, almost always involving the *right* lung (usually small cell lung cancer) accounts for 80% of cases.
  - Non-Hodgkin's **lymphoma** accounts for 15%.
  - Metastatic disease (usually from **breast** or testicular cancers) accounts for 5%.
  - In the majority of patients (nearly 60%), SVC syndrome develops before a primary diagnosis has been established; therefore, SVC syndrome tends to be seen more often in oncology settings than in terminal care settings.

Pathophysiology

The SVC is the principal vessel draining venous blood from the head, neck, upper thorax, and upper extremities.

- Thin walled, easily compressed.
- Encircled by chains of lymph nodes.
- Adjacent structures include trachea, right bronchus, and perihilar and paratracheal nodes.
- Other mediastinal structures that may become involved by a mass compressing the SVC include the esophagus and spinal cord.
- Mechanisms of obstruction of the SVC:
  - Usually extrinsic pressure from bronchogenic tumor or enlarged lymph nodes.
  - Sometimes direct invasion of the vein by tumor.
  - Intraluminal thrombosis secondary to low-flow states often responsible for acute onset of symptoms.

Clinical Findings in Superior Vena Cava Syndrome

- Symptoms:

Symptom	% of Cases
Dyspnea	63%
Facial and neck **swelling** ("tight collar")	50%
Sensations of **fullness** in head	50%
Cough	24%
Arm swelling	18%
Chest pain	15%
Dysphagia	9%

Adapted from Yahalom J. In deVita VT, et al. *Cancer: Principles & Practice of Oncology* (3rd ed). Philadelphia: Lippincott, 1989, p. 1972.

- Sensations of choking and headache (worse on bending) are also frequent presenting complaints.
- Symptoms that suggest involvement of other mediastinal structures:
  - **Hoarseness** suggests involvement of recurrent laryngeal nerve.
  - **Dysphagia** suggests involvement of esophagus.
  - **Dyspnea** suggests involvement of trachea.
  - Coexistence of **backache** suggests spinal cord compression (usually lower cervical and upper thoracic).

- Signs:

Sign	% of Cases
Venous distention of the neck	66%
Venous distention of chest wall	54%
Facial edema	46%
Cyanosis	20%
Plethora of the face	10%
Edema of the arms	14%
Vocal cord paralysis	3%
Horner's syndrome	3%

Adapted from Yahalom J. In de Vita VT et al. *Cancer: Principles & Practice of Oncology* (3rd ed). Philadelphia: Lippincott, 1989, p. 1972.

- Antecubital veins distended and do not collapse when the arm is raised above the level of the heart.
- On funduscopic examination, retinal veins may be dilated.
- Findings on chest x-ray:
  - **Widening of superior mediastinum** (60–75%).
  - Hilar **lymphadenopathy** (50%).
  - **Pleural effusion** (25%), nearly always on the *right* side.
  - Chest film is normal in 16% of patients with SVC syndrome.

Management of Superior Vena Cava Syndrome

Contrary to previous conceptions, SVC syndrome does *not* in itself constitute *an immediate threat to life* (except when other mediastinal structures, such as the trachea or pericardium, are also compromised).
- If the patient presents with SVC syndrome before there is a histologic diagnosis, priority goes to establishing a tissue diagnosis in order to identify malignancies that may be amenable to cure (e.g., histiocytic lymphoma, seminoma) or improved survival with chemotherapy (e.g., small cell lung cancer).
- **Emergency treatment** indicated only **when** there is evidence of
  - **Airway compromise.**

- **Decreased cardiac output.**
- **Cerebral dysfunction.**

General Supportive Measures

- Bed rest, with head of bed elevated.
- Oxygen administration.
- Diuretic therapy: **furosemide**, 40 mg + **spironolactone**, 100 mg PO qam.
- Corticosteroids are commonly given, especially when there is cerebral edema, although they are of unproven value. **Dexamethasone**, 24 mg IV stat, then PO qam, tapering by one-third every 3 to 4 days.

Specific Treatment Measures

Cause of SVC Syndrome	Specific Treatment
Small cell lung cancer Non-Hodgkin's lymphoma	Chemotherapy with or without adjuvant radiation therapy (do not use arm veins for chemotherapy infusion). Resolution of symptoms occurs within 7–10 days.
Non-small cell lung cancer	Radiation therapy: 2–4 large initial fractions (300–400 cGy), followed by usual fractionation to total dose of 3000–4000 cGy.

References and Further Reading

Ahman FRA. A reassessment of the clinical implications of the superior vena caval syndrome. *J Clin Oncol* 12:961, 1984.

Nieto AF, Doty DB. Superior vena cava obstruction: Clinical syndrome, etiology and treatment. *Curr Probl Cancer* 10:44, 1986.

Schraufnagel DE, Hill R, Leech JA, Pare JAP. Superior vena caval obstruction: Is it an emergency? *Am J Med* 70:1169, 1981.

Sculier JP, Feld R. Superior vena cava obstruction syndrome: Recommendation for management. *Cancer Treat Rev* 12:209, 1985.

Urinary

29 Urinary Incontinence, Frequency, and Retention

Physiology of Voiding

- Normal voiding of urine requires
  - An intact nerve supply to the bladder and urethra.
  - Open urinary passages.
  - An intact bladder wall (detrusor muscle).
- Innervation of the urinary tract:
  - The **bladder** receives both sympathetic and parasympathetic innervation:

	Sympathetic (Adrenergic)	*Parasympathetic (Cholinergic)*
Source	Hypogastric nerves	Pelvic nerves
Action on detrusor muscle	Relaxes	Contracts
Action on bladder sphincter	Contracts	Relaxes
Net effect	Stops urination	Enables urination

continued

	Sympathetic (Adrenergic)	Parasympathetic (Cholinergic)
Inhibited by	Damage to sympathetic nerves (cord compression)	Anticholinergic drugs (phenothiazines, haloperidol, tricyclics, antihistamines)

- The **urethral sphincter** is innervated by the pudendal nerve.

Incontinence in Patients with Advanced Cancer

- **Incidence:** Incontinence occurs in about 20% of patients with advanced cancer.
- **Classification:**

Type	Causes	Clinical Features
Overflow incontinence	Bladder outlet obstruction (by tumor, fecal impaction, or Rx) or detrusor failure (anticholinergic drugs) → bladder unable to empty normally → overdistention → leakage.	Suprapubic discomfort. Urgency. Feeling of inability to void. Urinary frequency (small volumes). Palpable bladder. Large postvoid residual.
Urge incontinence	Bladder irritation (infection, tumor, radiation, chemotherapy). Spinal cord lesion → neurogenic bladder.	Patient senses urge to void but cannot control leakage long enough to reach toilet. Frequency, nocturia.
Stress incontinence	Damage or dysfunction of bladder sphincter → leakage of urine when intra-abdominal pressure is raised.	Incontinence on coughing, lifting, bending, laughing, sneezing. Normal urine volumes.
Functional incontinence	Immobility or severe cognitive impairment (GU tract intact).	Patient unaware that he or she has voided.

- Principal **causes of urinary incontinence** in patients with advanced cancer:

- Due to the cancer itself:
  - **Tumor invasion** of the bladder or urethra or surrounding structures.
  - Vesicovaginal **fistula**.
  - Spinal **cord compression** → hypotonic bladder → overflow obstruction.
- Due to treatment of cancer or its symptoms:
  - **Chemotherapy:** cyclosphosphamide → bladder wall fibrosis → contraction and stiffening of bladder wall.
  - **Surgery** → fibrosis and scarring.
  - **Radiation** → bladder wall fibrosis.
  - Anticholinergic **drugs** → bladder outlet obstruction.
  - **Opioids** → bladder outlet obstruction.
  - **Fecal impaction** from any cause (e.g., opioids).
- Infection: **cystitis**.

- **Evaluation** of the patient with urinary incontinence:

History	Have you had problems in controlling your urine? If yes, How often are you incontinent?
	Do you feel an urge to void before urine leaks out?
	Does coughing, sneezing, laughing, or lifting heavy objects cause you to lose control of your urine?
	When was your last bowel movement?
	What medications are you taking?
	What treatments have you received for your tumor?
Physical examination	Is the bladder palpable?
	Is there inflammation of the periurethral or perineal skin?
	Is there stool impacted in the rectum?
	Neurologic: Is there loss of sensation over T10–L2 dermatomes, or are there other sensory/motor deficits?
Tests	Urinalysis.
	Insertion of catheter to measure postvoid residual.

- **Management** of urinary incontinence in patients with advanced cancer:
  - **General measures:**
    - Make it **easy** for the patient **to reach toilet facilities** quickly (urinal, bedpan, bedside commode as necessary).
    - For patients able to cooperate, consider establishing a **regular voiding schedule** (e.g., q2h).

- **Avoid fluid loading** in uncatheterized patients who are prone to incontinence, particularly in the evening.
- **Avoid diuretics** and foods with diuretic action (coffee, tea, alcohol, parsley).
- For nocturnal incontinence in patients with normal urine output, consider **desmopressin** (DDAVP), 20 µg by intranasal spray at bedtime.
- **Treat fecal impaction**, and institute measures to prevent recurrence.
- For patients with minimal incontinence (e.g., women with stress incontinence), use **absorbent pads** and undergarments.
- In male patients, consider **condom drainage**, preferably intermittently (e.g., during the nights).
- To minimize odor and skin irritation, use absorbent underpads, with underlying waterproof sheets and mattress protectors; change bedding whenever it is wet.
- Give particular attention to **perineal skin care**: cleansing with mild soaps, barrier creams.
- Consider an indwelling urinary catheter (see below).
- Specific measures:

Cause of Incontinence	Management
Overflow incontinence	Review medications and **stop** as many **anticholinergic drugs** as possible. Check for fecal impaction, and treat if present. Trial of **bethanechol** (Urecholine), 10 mg PO tid (titrating upward to a maximum of 50 mg PO tid). For overflow incontinence due to detrusor instability, **flurbiprofen**, 50-100 mg bid, may reduce urgency and frequency. When overflow incontinence is due to mechanical obstruction of bladder neck or urethra, an indwelling **catheter** may be the only solution.
Urge incontinence	When due to bladder irritation: ▪ Treat infection. ▪ Partially deflate balloon of indwelling catheter. ▪ Give **phenazopyridine**, 100-200 mg PO tid. Try anticholinergic therapy: **oxybutynin**, 2.5-5 mg PO tid-qid. For neurogenic bladder: ▪ **Imipramine**, 10-20 mg PO hs, *or* ▪ **Propantheline** bromide, 7.5 mg PO tid, titrating up to a maximum of 30 mg PO tid.

Cause of Incontinence	Management
Stress incontinence	Scheduled voiding. Trial of imipramine, 10–20 mg PO hs. Ring pessary for women with pelvic relaxation; penile clamp for men. Use of incontinence pads.
Vesicovaginal fistula	Catheter drainage of the bladder to promote spontaneous closure. For patients with life-expectancy > 2–3 months, consider surgery (e.g., ileal conduit or bilateral nephrostomies). Otherwise, use incontinence pads (vaginal tampons are usually *not* effective).

Use of Indwelling Catheters

Indications

- Urinary **retention**.
- Maceration of skin from constant urinary leakage.
- **Patient comfort**, when discomfort is caused by urinary frequency, incontinence, or pain from bladder distention.
- Technical or other problems in carrying out intermittent clean catheterizations.

Important Considerations

- Discuss the matter with the patient and his or her family:
  - Find out what they know about catheters and what anxieties or questions they have.
  - Provide factual information about the pros and cons of catheterization.
  - Respect the patient's wishes.
- Catheter type:
  - When long-term catheterization is anticipated, a **silicone catheter** is preferred (less likely to form concretions → requires less frequent changes, only every 6–8 weeks).
  - For patients with hematuria, use a **triple-lumen catheter**, to permit continuous irrigation (see Chapter 30).
- Catheterization procedure:
  - Observe **aseptic technique**.
  - Use a small-diameter (**12–16F**) catheter with a small-volume (**5 ml**) **balloon**.
  - Lubricate the catheter with lidocaine jelly.

- Catheter maintenance:
  - The catheter drainage **tubing** should be **looped** and taped to the patient's thigh to prevent traction on the catheter.
  - The urine collection **bag** should always be **below** the level of the **bladder**. (Use a covered leg-bag for ambulatory patients.)
  - The catheter should be **changed only if it becomes blocked** or encrusted. A well cared-for catheter can usually stay in place for 4 to 6 weeks. Routine catheter changes are unnecessary and potentially harmful.
  - The catheter should *not* be routinely irrigated. Catheter **irrigation**, with sterile saline, is indicated **only when there is blockage** or near blockage.
  - Virtually all catheterized patients develop bacteriuria. There is **no necessity to treat asymptomatic bacteriuria**. Give antibiotics only to catheterized patients who develop urinary symptoms (dysuria, fever, bladder spasms).
- If debris is a problem, acidify the urine (ascorbic acid, 500 mg PO bid).

Urinary Frequency

Definition: Passage of urine more than 7 times during the day and twice at night.

Cause of Urinary Frequency	Clinical Features	Management
Cystitis	Dysuria Cloudy urine (WBCs on microscopic examination) Bacteriuria	Obtain culture. Pending results, give a 3-day course of trimethoprim-sulfamethoxazole, 2 tabs PO bid.
Fecal impaction	Anorexia Crampy abdominal pain ↓Bowel movements ± diarrhea	Disimpaction (see Chapter 20).
Increased urine volume Diuretics Hypercalcemia	Large volumes of urine passed with each void.	Stop unnecessary diuretics. Measure serum calcium, and treat for hypercalcemia.

Cause of Urinary Frequency	Clinical Features	Management
Diabetes mellitus Diabetes insipidus		Measure blood-urine sugar; treat to keep blood sugar < 300 mg/dl. Treat diabetes insipidus with desmopressin, 40 μg intranasally hs.
Atrophic vaginitis	Elderly women Dysuria Sometimes incontinence	Ethinyl estradiol, 0.02 mg PO qam (do not give to patients with cancer of the breast, cervix, or endometrium).

Urinary Retention

- Urinary retention often occurs at the initiation of opioid therapy. Tolerance to this side effect usually develops within days to weeks.
- Determine whether the patient is truly in retention or has decreased urine output from other causes (e.g., dehydration):
  - Palpate the abdomen for a distended bladder.
  - In-and-out bladder catheterization may be necessary to assess residual urine volume.
- Principal causes of urinary retention in patients with advanced cancer:

Cause	Management
Fecal impaction	Disimpact.
Benign prostatic hypertrophy	Have patient void sitting down, with manual pressure on bladder. Trial of terazosin HCl, 1 mg PO hs. For patients with prognosis > 3 months, consider transurethral resection of the prostate or finasteride (Proscar), 5 mg PO qam.
Anticholinergic drugs (including opioids)	Try to find substitute medication that does not disturb urinary function.
Tumor compressing bladder neck	Trial of corticosteroids to reduce peritumor inflammation. Urethral catheterization if possible. Suprapubic catheterization may be necessary if bladder neck obstruction is complete.

References and Further Reading

Breitenbucher RB. Bacterial changes in the urine samples of patients with long-term indwelling catheters. *Arch Intern Med* 144:1585, 1984.

Consensus Conference. Urinary incontinence in adults. *JAMA* 261:2685, 1989.

Fainsinger RL, MacEachern T, Hanson J, Bruera E. The use of urinary catheters in terminally ill patients. *J Pain Symptom Manage* 7:333, 1992.

Moul JW. Benign prostatic hyperplasia: New concepts in the 1990s. *Postgrad Med* 94(6):141, 1993.

Regnard CFB, Mannix KA. Urinary problems in advanced cancer—a flow diagram. *Palliative Med* 5:344, 1991.

Stamm WE, Hooton TM. Management of urinary tract infections in adults. *N Engl J Med* 329:1328, 1993.

Williams ME, Pannill FC. Urinary incontinence in the elderly: Physiology, pathophysiology, diagnosis, and treatment. *Ann Intern Med* 97:895, 1982.

30 Hematuria

Definition

Blood in the urine.

Causes of Hematuria in Patients with Advanced Cancer

- Cystitis.
- Invasion of bladder or prostate by tumor.
- Coagulopathies.
- Chemotherapy (cyclophosphamide, ifosfamide).
- Renal tumor.
- Too rapid drainage of obstructed bladder.

Management of Hematuria in Patients with Advanced Cancer

Degree of Hematuria	Management
Mild (hemoglobin stable; no clots in urine)	Reassurance. Exclude infection as a source. (If cystitis is present, treat with antibiotics as indicated by culture.) Maintain good urine output.

continued

Degree of Hematuria	Management
Moderate to heavy (hemoglobin falling; clots in urine)	Insert Foley catheter, and start **bladder washouts** bid–tid with 1% alum solution.* If bleeding does not stop, replace standard Foley catheter with **triple-lumen catheter,** and institute continuous bladder irrigation with cold water or saline. If bleeding still does not stop, consider palliative **radiation therapy.** Consider **transfusion** when patient is severely symptomatic from blood loss, level of function is otherwise good, and patient desires transfusion. Do *not* give tranexamic acid (leads to hard clots that are difficult to evacuate from the bladder).

*To prepare alum solution, add 100 mg of alum to 1000 ml of sterile water. For each irrigation, take 50 ml of the prepared solution and dilute it in 500 ml of sterile saline.

References and Further Reading

DeVries CR, Freih FS. Hemorrhagic cystitis: A review. *J Urol* 143:1, 1990.

Bullock N, Whitaker RH. Massive bladder haemorrhage. *Br Med J* 291:1522, 1985.

Mariani AJ, Mariani MC, Macchioni C, et al. The significance of adult hematuria: 1,000 hematuria evaluations including a risk-benefit and cost-effectiveness analysis. *J Urol* 141:350, 1989.

31 Dysuria and Bladder Spasms

Dysuria

Definition

Pain on voiding.

Causes

- Bacterial cystitis or urethritis.
- Tumor infiltration into the bladder wall.
- Radiation therapy.
- Chemotherapy (cyclophosphamide).

Investigations

- Urinalysis.
- Urine culture.

Management

- Treat urinary tract infection when present.
- Provide pain relief.
  - Opioids are generally *not* very effective for dysuria.
  - Try **phenazopyridine** (Pyridium), **100–200 mg PO qid**. Warn the patient that his urine will turn orange or red!
  - If pain is not relieved, try **lidocaine rinse** in catheterized patients: Draw up 10 ml of 2% lidocaine, add to 50 ml of saline, irrigate the catheter, clamp for 20 minutes, and then unclamp and allow to drain.

Bladder Spasm

Definition

Intermittent, painful, paroxysmal contractions of the detrusor muscle, leading to tenesmoid suprapubic pain and urgency.

Causes

- Urinary tract infection.
- Fecal impaction.
- Tumors of the bladder and prostate.
- Indwelling urinary catheter, especially with a large-volume balloon.
- Radiation cystitis.
- Morphine may exacerbate existing bladder spasm (by increasing detrusor tone).

Investigations

- Urinalysis; urine culture.
- Rectal examination.

Management

- Treat reversible causes:

Cause	Management
Cystitis	Antibiotics, as per urine culture. Oral fluids. If catheterized, change catheter.
Irritation by indwelling catheter	Change catheter. Partially deflate balloon. Saline irrigations.
Fecal impaction	Disimpact.

- Symptomatic management of bladder spasm:
  - Start with **imipramine, 10–20 mg PO hs**, or **amitriptyline, 25–50 mg PO hs**; if that does not control spasm,
  - Add **oxybutynin, 2.5–5 mg PO tid** (anticipate anticholinergic side effects, such as dry mouth). For the elderly, 2.5 mg PO bid may be sufficient.

- Also potentially helpful:
  - **Belladonna and opium (B & O) suppositories**, 1 suppository PR q2-4h.
  - **Naproxen**, 250-500 mg PO bid.

Neurologic and
Neuropsychiatric

32 The Mental Status Examination

Reasons for Performing a Mental Status Examination

- A significant percentage of patients with advanced cancer develop changes in mental status during the course of their illness, especially during hospitalizations.
- Early, subtle changes in mental status are apt to go unnoticed, especially if the patient is not causing a disturbance.
- Changes in mental status may be the first sign of a treatable medical complication (e.g., hypoglycemia, hypercalcemia).

A well-documented mental status examination at admission permits serial assessment of the patient and early detection of delirium.

Components of the Mental Status Examination

- There are several systems for evaluating mental status, for example:
  - Mini-Mental State Exam (MMSE) of Folstein et al. (1984).
  - Cognitive Capacity Screening Examination (CCSE) of Jacobs (1977).
- Whatever system is used, certain parameters must be assessed. Those parameters can be summarized by the mnemonic **COASTMAP**:

C	Consciousness	Note the patient's level of *alertness*, ability to pay *attention* and to *concentrate*.
O	Orientation	To *person*: Ask the patient his name. To *place*: Ask the patient where he is (country, region, state, city, hospital, ward, floor) To *time*: Ask the patient what is the year, season, month, date, day of the week, time of day.
A	Activity	Is the patient unusually *quiet? agitated?* Is he making any unusual or repetitive movements?
S	Speech	Note rate, volume, articulation, and intonation. Is there pressure of speech? Is the speech slurred (dysarthria)? Is there difficulty in finding words (aphasia)?
T	Thought	Is the patient making sense? Is his reasoning logical? Is his thinking circumstantial or tangential? Is he expressing apparently false ideas (*delusions*)? Test *cognitive function* with serial sevens or other simple arithmetical exercises. *Insight, judgment,* and *reasoning* may be assessed in the course of taking the history: How much does the patient know about his illness, the treatment he received, etc.?
M	Memory	Form a general impression of the patient's memory as he reconstructs the story of his illness. To test memory formally, ask the patient's permission to administer a little quiz. Then name three objects (e.g., apple, pencil, dog). Ask the patient to repeat them back (to test *registration*). A few minutes later, ask the patient if he can remember the three words you named earlier (to test *retention* and *recall*).
A	Affect and Mood	The patient's mood may be most apparent in his body language. Does he appear happy, sad, irritable, angry, fearful? Is his affect appropriate to the situation? Does he express feelings of guilt, worthlessness, anger toward family or staff, fear of specific events, free-floating anxiety?
P	Perceptions	Is the patient misinterpreting perceptions (*illusions*)? Does he see or hear things that are not present (*hallucinations*)? Since patients may be hesitant to volunteer such information, ask directly, "Do you ever hear or see things that other people can't hear or see?"

Note that the majority of the mental status examination can be accomplished within the context of standard history taking and, except for assessment of memory, does not require special tests that would tire the patient.
- **Record your findings** in detail! Note the date and time of the examination.

References and Further Reading

Folstein MF, Fetting JG, Lobo A, et al. Cognitive assessment of cancer patients. *Cancer* 53(Suppl May 15): 2250, 1984.

Folstein MF, Folstein SE, McHugh PR. "Mini-mental state," a practical method for grading the cognitive state of patients for the clinician. *J Psychiatr Res* 12:189, 1975.

Jacobs JW. Screening for organic mental syndromes in the medically ill. *Ann Intern Med* 86:40, 1977.

33 Brain Metastases

Epidemiology

- Metastases to brain are *common*.
  - One reason: The most common primary cancers (lung, breast, melanoma) have a high incidence of brain metastases.
  - Occur in **25% to 35% of all cancer patients**.
  - More common than brain primaries.
  - Usually occur by *hematogenous spread*.
    - Often not directly from primary but from metastatic site ("metastasis of a metastasis"), hence **signals advanced disease**.
    - **Metastases to skull** (from breast, prostate) or neuroblastoma may penetrate intracerebrally.
- Most common **sites of origin** (in order of frequency):
  - **Lung**:
    - Accounts for 40% to 60% of all brain metastases.
    - Ten percent of patients with SCLC have brain metastases at presentation.
    - Eighty percent of SCLC patients who survive 2 years develop brain metastases unless given prophylactic cranial radiation.
  - **Breast**.
  - **Gastrointestinal**.
  - **Urinary**.
  - Unknown primary.
  - **Melanoma** (65% of melanomas metastasize to brain).
- Average age of onset of brain metastases: male: 56 years; female: 48 years.

▪ Brain metastases are **multiple** in 60% of cases.
  • *Solitary metastases* more common in renal, ovarian, and breast carcinomas and osteosarcoma.
  • *Multiple metastases* more common in cancer of lung, in melanoma, and in seminoma.

Clinical Findings

▪ In 80% of cases, signs of brain involvement occur *after* diagnosis of primary tumor.
▪ Median interval from diagnosis of primary to discovery of cerebral metastases is 17 months.
  • Briefer intervals: lung, melanoma, renal.
  • Longer intervals: breast, colon, sarcoma.
▪ **Signs and symptoms** usually develop insidiously → progress to disability over a few weeks (but onset may be sudden).
  • **Mechanisms**:
    - Mechanical distortion, herniation by enlarging mass.
    - Increases in intracranial pressure, especially if rapid.
    - Decreases in cerebral blood flow.
    - Worsening of vasogenic *cerebral edema*.
    - Derangement of metabolic processes in the brain.

Symptoms	*Frequency*	*Signs*	*Frequency*
Headache	53%	**Impaired cognition**	70%
Weakness, focal	40%	**Hemiparesis**	66%
Mental disturbance	31%	Sensory loss, unilateral	27%
Gait disorder	20%	Papilledema	26%
Seizures	15%	Ataxia	24%
Visual disturbance	12%		
Language disturbance	10%		

  • **Headache**: most common presenting symptom.
    - Usually present before arising from bed in morning, disappears during the day, recurs the next morning.

- Gradually increases in frequency/duration/severity.
- When unilateral, of localizing value.
- **Ataxia** particularly common with cerebellar metastases.
- **Seizures** are the most common acute onset → **Todd's paralysis** (transient hemiparesis after seizure)—especially in melanoma.
- Papilledema may be reflected in blurred vision.
- **Differential diagnosis**:

Category	Diagnosis
Neoplastic	Primary brain tumors (glial) Meningioma
Infectious	Abscess (pyogenic, TB*) Meningitis Fungal Toxoplasmosis, etc.
Cardiovascular	Cerebral infarct Cerebral hemorrhage Acute or chronic subdural/epidural hematoma
Toxic	Radiation necrosis Drug overdose (review patient's medications)
Metabolic	↓Sodium, magnesium, phosphate Hypoglycemia Hypercalcemia Hypoxemia, hypercapnia, acid-base disturbance Hypo/hyperthyroid (after radiation therapy to neck) Azotemia or liver failure

*Occurs more frequently in immunosuppressed patients.

Diagnostic Workup in the Terminally Ill

- Meticulous history and physical examination, including
  - Funduscopic examination for papilledema.
  - Careful neurologic examination.
- Complete blood count.
- Serum electrolytes, glucose, calcium, BUN, liver function tests.

Management

Aggressiveness of management will depend on the patient's overall condition.

Condition of Patient	Treatment Indicated
Ambulatory patient (performance status = 2 or better) with rapidly evolving, symptomatic cerebral metastases	**Steroids:** Start with **dexamathasone**, 16–36 mg IV push (if impending herniation), then 4 mg q6h → increase as needed up to 100 mg/day if not responsive at that dose. • Effects noticeable within 6–24 hours, maximal in 3–7 days. • Will temporarily resolve symptoms in 60–80% of patients. • Relieve generalized symptoms (headache, confusion) better than focal signs (hemiparesis). **Osmotherapy** if steroids alone not effective. • Mannitol, 100 gm IV, then 25 gm IV if needed. • Requires an intact blood-brain barrier. Keep **head elevated** > 20 degrees to facilitate venous return from brain. Anticonvulsants for patients with seizures (*not* for prophylaxis). General supportive measures (e.g., airway protection, ventilatory support). **Radiation therapy** is the basis of treatment of all patients. • Port encompasses **whole brain**, since metastases assumed to be multiple. • 20 Gy over 5 days to whole brain. • Taper **dexamethasone** after radiation is completed. • 80% of patients show good initial response: • Headache completely relieved in 69% of patients after radiation. • Confusion, motor/sensory deficits respond in > 50%. • Main toxic side effect is alopecia. • No appreciable gain in survival from radiation treatment; palliation only.
Bedridden patient (performance status = 3–4)	**Steroids:** Start with **dexamethasone, 16–36 mg PO qam**, then decrease dosage by 2 mg every 3 days until minimal effective dosage is reached. If symptoms worsen while tapering steroids, increase the dosage again by 4 mg/day.

Prognosis

▪ Survival rates

Treatment Modality	Median Survival
Untreated	1-2 months
Steroids	2-5 months
Radiation therapy (± steroids)	3-6 months
Surgery/steroids/radiation	> 6 months

▪ Prognostic indicators:
  • **Neurologic status** and **extent of systemic disease.**
  • Intrinsic malignant behavior of primary.
  • **Interval from detection of primary** to development of symptomatic cerebral metastasis.
  • Some surgical patients have long survivals (with or without radiation therapy), especially those with brain metastases from melanoma.

References and Further Reading

Bell G, Glynne-Jones R, Vernon CC. Cerebral metastases and dexamethasone: psychiatric aspects. *Palliative Med* 1:132, 1987.

Grossman SA, Moynihan TJ. Neoplastic meningitis. *Neurol Clin North Am* 9:843, 1991.

Posner JB. Neurologic complications of systemic cancer. *Med Clin North Am* 63:783, 1979.

Wilson CB, Fulton DS, Seager ML. Supportive management of the patient with malignant brain tumor. *JAMA* 244:1249, 1980.

34 Seizures

Incidence

Seizures occur in approximately 1% of patients with advanced cancer.

Causes of Seizures in Patients with Advanced Cancer

Most Common Causes

- Primary or metastatic **tumor** in the brain.
- **Stroke.**
- Preexisting seizure disorder.

Less Common Causes

- Hypoxemia.
- Metabolic: uremia, hypoglycemia, hyponatremia.
- Sepsis.
- Withdrawal from drugs or alcohol.

General Considerations

- In the patient with advanced cancer known to have brain metastases, it is *not* **necessary to give routine prophylaxis** against seizures.
- Only 15% of patients with primary or metastatic brain tumors will experience seizures at any time during their course.

- All antiseizure medications have side effects that should not be incurred without good cause.
- Seizure prophylaxis can and should be instituted after the first seizure, if such an event occurs.
- **Seizures are frightening**—to the patient and the family.
- When a seizure has occurred, particularly if it is the patient's first seizure, take time afterward to explore the concerns of the patient and family and to offer honest reassurance.
- Typical concerns, often unstated, include
  - Will the patient swallow his tongue or choke to death during a seizure?
  - Will there be permanent brain damage from a seizure?
  - Will seizures hasten death?
- In the patient being cared for at home, provide practical advice to the family on what to do (and what not to do) if a seizure occurs when medical personnel are not present:

What to Do if the Patient Has a Seizure: Advice to the Family

- Try to make sure that the patient does not fall or bump into any sharp objects.
- Do not attempt to restrain the patient.
- Do not try to force anything into the patient's mouth.
- When the seizure stops, it is a good idea to turn the patient onto his or her side.
- The patient will be sleepy for a while after a seizure.
- If the seizure does not stop by itself in about 5 to 10 minutes, or if another seizure occurs soon after the first, call for medical assistance.

Management of Seizures in Patients with Advanced Cancer

Management of the Isolated Grand Mal Seizure

- Prevent the patient from injuring himself by clearing the area around him of hard or sharp objects.
- Maintain the **airway** manually, by lifting up the patient's chin.
- When the seizure is over, place the patient in the stable side position until he or she is alert.
- Send blood tests for laboratory investigations (see p. 258).

- Start oral anticonvulsive medication as prophylaxis against further seizures:
  - *Loading dose* of **phenytoin**, 400 mg PO → 300 mg PO 3 hours later → 300 mg PO 3 hours later.
  - Thereafter, continue *maintenance dose* of **phenytoin, 300 mg PO hs.**
  - In patients with renal or hepatic insufficiency, dispense with loading dose and start with maintenance dose.
  - Check serum phenytoin level after 10 to 14 days of therapy and again if seizures recur.
- For **focal seizures**, the prophylactic drug of choice is **carbamazepine**, starting with a dosage of 100 to 200 mg bid and titrating upward, as needed, to a maximum of 400 mg qid.

Management of Status Epilepticus

- **Definition:** Status epilepticus occurs when there is continuous seizure activity for more than 30 minutes or when two or more seizures occur, one after the other, without full recovery of consciousness in between.
- Status epilepticus should be controlled, even in the unconscious patient near death, because of the distress that continuous seizures cause to the patient's family.
- **Steps in management:**
  1. Protect the patient's **airway** by backward tilt of the patient's head.
  2. Administer **oxygen** by two-pronged nasal cannula.
  3. If possible, establish an **IV line**.
  4. Draw blood for laboratory investigations (see p. 258).
  5. **Drug therapy:**

Patient Who Has IV Line	*Patient Without IV Line*
▪ Give **lorazepam**, 4 mg IV over 2–4 minutes. ▪ Start an **infusion of phenytoin**, 20 mg/kg at 25 mg/min. (This will take up to 40 minutes.) Do not use a glucose-containing solution. ▪ If seizures persist, give additional doses of phenytoin, 5 mg/kg to a maximal total dose of 30 mg/kg. ▪ If seizures still persist, give **phenobarbital**, 20 mg/kg IV at a rate of 100 mg/min.	▪ **Diazepam**, 10-mg solution may be given PR and repeated q5–10 min × 3 prn. ▪ For maintenance, start a SQ infusion of **midazolam**, 30 mg/24 hr. May increase dosage up to 60 mg/24 hr if necessary.

6. If a metabolic source of seizures is ruled out by laboratory tests, the presumption is that the seizures are due at least in part to intracranial edema, and a trial of corticosteroids is worthwhile. Start with **dexamethasone, 16 to 36 mg PO/IV qam.**
7. When the acute situation is under control, start maintenance anticonvulsant therapy with **phenytoin, 300 mg PO qhs.**

▪ **When the patient is no longer able to take oral medications:**
  • If the patient is deeply comatose and seizures have not been a major problem up to that point, stop the anticonvulsants.
  • If the patient has been taking anticonvulsants for an established seizure disorder and survival for more than a few days is likely, **switch to parenteral phenobarbital:**
    – Intravenous phenytoin is very hard to maintain because of its sclerosing effect on peripheral veins.
    – Give **phenobarbital, 100 to 200 mg IM qd** or **200 to 300 mg/ 24 hr** by continuous **SQ infusion.** (Do not mix phenobarbital with any other drug. If the patient is receiving other medications by continuous SQ infusion, use a separate syringe driver for the phenobarbital infusion.)
    – Alternatively, **valproic acid syrup** may be given rectally in doses of **250 to 500 mg PR tid.**

Laboratory Investigations

When seizures occur in the context of advanced cancer, easily diagnosed and treatable causes should be ruled out with the following tests:
▪ Blood **glucose.**
▪ Serum **sodium, potassium, calcium,** and **magnesium.**
▪ Serum **urea.**
▪ Arterial **oxygen** saturation (pulse oximetry).
▪ Plasma **phenytoin levels** in patients already taking anticonvulsant medication (**therapeutic range for plasma phenytoin = 10–20 mg/L** = 40-79 µmol/L).

References and Further Reading

Mitchell WG, Crawford TO. Lorazepam is the treatment of choice for status epilepticus. *J Epilepsy* 3(1):7, 1990.

Shaner DM, McCurdy SA, Herring MO, Gabor AJ. Treatment of status epilepticus: A prospective comparison of diazepam and phenytoin versus phenobarbital and optional phenytoin. *Neurology* 38:202, 1988.

Working Group on Status Epilepticus. Treatment of convulsive status epilepticus. *JAMA* 270:854, 1993.

35 Spinal Cord Compression

Incidence

- The vertebral column is the *most common site* of skeletal metastasis; 70% of patients dying from cancer have spinal metastases at autopsy.
- Cord compression occurs in 5% of all patients with malignancy.
- Cord compression may be the presenting complaint of a cancer.
- Average age of occurrence: 58 years.
- Sources:

Primary Tumor	% of Patients
Lung	16
Breast	12
Unknown primary	11
Lymphoma	11
Myeloma	9
Sarcoma	8
Prostate	7
Kidney	6

- **Distribution**:
  - Cervical spine: 10%.
  - Thoracic spine: 70%.
  - Lumbosacral spine: 20%.
  - Multiple contiguous levels: 10% to 38%.

Pathogenesis

- Spinal involvement is almost always **extradural**; usually tumor in the vertebral body (85% of cases) presses on the *anterior* aspect of the dural sac.
- Paraspinal tumors (e.g., lymphoma) may invade through intervertebral foramen and compress cord without bony involvement.
- Signs and symptoms probably not due solely to compression of cord; ischemia secondary to vascular involvement may also be a factor (especially when cord compression develops suddenly over a few hours).

Natural History

- Rates of progression vary:
  - *Slow*, with pain for several months before neurologic signs: breast cancer, lymphoma.
  - Very *rapid* (hours) progression to complete, irreversible cord damage: lung cancer, renal cancer, myeloma.
- Usual sequence of events:
  - **Pain** →
  - Limb **weakness** and gait difficulties; DTRs brisk, extensor plantar →
  - **Sensory changes** →
  - Loss of **sphincter control**.
- Prognostic factors: The most important single factor determining **prognosis** is the **level of neurologic function at the beginning of therapy**:

Favorable Prognosis (> 50%*)	Intermediate Prognosis (30%*)	Worst Prognosis (< 15%*)
Diagnosis before onset of motor weakness or incontinence. Slowly progressive neurologic symptoms and signs. Patients who are ambulatory. Myeloma or lymphoma.	Early neurologic abnormalities in breast or prostate cancer. Paresis before treatment. Lesions affecting vertebrae above T5.	Lung or renal cancer. Sphincter incontinence (< 5%*). Neurologic function deteriorates in < 72 hours (< 5%*). Paraplegia (0%*).

*Chance of recovering neurologic function.

Clinical Findings

Symptoms

- **Pain** is the **presenting symptom in 95% of patients.**
- May be the only symptom in 10% of patients.
- Two types of pain:
  - **Local back pain** (midline/paravertebral) nearly always present.
    - Usually *constant*, close to site of lesion.
    - *Relieved by sitting or standing* up (contrast disc disease).
    - Exacerbated by any *increase in intrathoracic pressure* (sneeze, cough, Valsalva, straining at stool).
    - Above historic points may be only clue to impending spinal cord compression.
  - **Radicular pain** from spinal root compression occurs in 66% of patients.
    - More common with cervical (79%) and lumbosacral (90%) metastases than with thoracic metastases (55% of cases).
    - Patients complain of a band or girdle of pain/tightness radiating from back to front; in extremities, radicular pain usually *unilateral*.
    - Exacerbated by recumbency, movement, cough, sneeze, Valsalva.
    - Worse at night.
    - Improved by sitting or standing.
    - Radiates in a dermatomal pattern.
    - May produce *numbness and tingling* (cervical or lumbar root).

- ○ May resemble pain from intervertebral disc disease, pleurisy, cholecystitis, pancreatitis.
- ○ Distinguish from brachial or lumbosacral plexus involvement.
- ○ Localizes the lesion within one or two vertebral segments.
- EARLY DIAGNOSIS ESSENTIAL TO PREVENT NEUROLOGIC DAMAGE:
  - – Must have high index of suspicion when patient reports back pain or radicular pain.
  - – Patient with many pains may neglect to mention new pain in back. (**Instruct patients to report new pains promptly.**)
  - – In most patients, pain is present for weeks to months before onset of neurologic symptoms; without treatment, the next symptom is
- **Weakness** in legs (76% of patients).
- Experienced as stiffness, dragging of a limb, unsteadiness.
- May be accompanied (or preceded) by
- **Sensory disturbances** (51% of patients).
- Numbness usually *begins in the toes*, gradually ascends to level of cord compression (usually *without* paresthesias).
- Sensation of coldness.
- Upper limit of sensory level often one to two vertebral bodies below site of compression.
- Sensory loss → **ataxia** (3% of patients).
- **Autonomic dysfunction** (57% of patients).
- Early signs: Loss of bladder control, hesitancy, urgency.
- Late signs: Urinary retention, overflow incontinence.
- Constipation.
- *Loss of sweating* below level of the lesion.

Signs Due to Progressive Encroachment of Epidural Space by Tumor

- **Tenderness to percussion** over involved vertebrae.
- Pain over involved vertebrae on neck flexion or straight-leg raising.
- Weakness, spasticity, **hyperactive DTRs, extensor plantar**.
- **Sensory loss** below involved cord segment, most marked distally.
  - All modalities equally affected (pinprick, vibration, position).
  - Perianal anesthesia to pinprick in cauda equina lesions.
- Palpable bladder, large postvoid residual.
- Decreased anal sphincter tone.

Diagnostic Evaluation

- Administer **dexamethasone** *immediately* when history and physical examination suggest spinal cord compression, *before* continuing workup: 100 mg IV → 4 to 24 mg q6h (see below).

  Extent of diagnostic workup indicated in any given case **depends on overall condition of patient.** In patients expected to live more than 1 to 2 months and who are not already paraplegic, the following tests are indicated (listed in increasing order of complexity and discomfort to patient):

- **Spine radiographs** predict presence or absence of epidural metastases in 85% of patients. Findings diagnostic of spinal tumor:
  - Erosion and **loss of pedicles.**
  - Partial/complete **collapse of vertebral bodies** associated with osteoblastic or osteolytic lesions.
  - Presence of > 50% collapse on plain radiograph in patient with severe back pain = 87% chance of spinal epidural cord compression.
  - **Paraspinous** soft tissues **masses.**
  - *But* normal spine films do not exclude epidural metastases (60% of patients with epidural metastases from lymphoma may have normal spine films).

- **Magnetic resonance imaging (MRI)** to define level of lesion(s) (sensitivity = 93%; specificity = 97%).
  - Advantages of MRI:
    - Noninvasive; no contrast material injected.
    - Images the whole spine—sagittal, parasagittal, transverse.
    - Distinguishes extradural, intradural, extramedullary, etc.
    - Avoids risk of neurologic deterioration after lumbar puncture.
  - Disadvantages:
    - Not universally available.
    - Necessity for patient to lie still in one position.

- **Myelography** is essential to determine proximal and distal extent of block if MRI is not available.
  - DO NOT perform lumbar puncture before myelography when cord compression suspected.
    - Take CSF sample at the time of myelography for protein, etc.
    - Cerebrospinal fluid findings usually nonspecific.
    - If complete block, do not remove more than 1 ml of CSF.

- Bone scans are not useful—too nonspecific.

Differential Diagnosis

Diagnosis	Distinguishing/Suggestive Features
Epidural hematoma	Usually more than one vertebral segment involved on myelography; patient on anticoagulants or low platelets.
Epidural abscess	Fever; more than one segment on myelography.
DJD spine	Pain usually low cervical or lumbar; recumbency alleviates pain; no masses on MRI.
Disc disease	No masses on MRI; usually lower lumbar.

Treatment

Principles

- **Rapid diagnosis and therapeutic intervention is essential.**
- Paraplegia from malignant spinal cord compression is always irreversible and is not an emergency.

Corticosteroids

Corticosteroids should be started immediately.

- In patients with short prognosis or poor performance status, corticosteroids may be the *only* treatment feasible.
- Shown to improve neurologic function and relieve pain; not known whether steroids have any effect on ultimate neurologic recovery.
- Reduce edema and have a direct oncolytic effect.
- **Dexamethasone, 100 mg IV stat** → 4 to 24 mg q6h →
- Taper over 10 to 14 days after improvement or irreversibility: Reduce dosage one-third every 3 to 4 days.

Radiation Therapy

Radiation therapy (RT) provides definitive treatment in most patients.
- Indications:
  - Known radiosensitive tumor.
  - No spinal instability.
- Response is best in patients with radiosensitive tumors.
  - Best results: seminoma, lymphoma, myeloma, Ewing's sarcoma, neuroblastoma.

- Fair to good results: breast, prostate, renal cancers.
- Poor results: lung cancers.
- Radiation therapy alone gives equivalent results to laminectomy plus adjuvant RT.
- Radiation therapy should be started immediately after diagnosis.
- Radiation portal includes site of myelographic block and extends *two vertebral bodies above and below block*: 3000 to 4000 cGy over 2 to 4 weeks.

Surgery

Surgery may be warranted in selected cases with good performance status.

- Excision and fusion for vertebral body tumor, laminectomy for posterior tumor.
- Indications:
  - Relapse at site of previous radiation.
  - Failure to respond to radiation; deterioration during RT.
  - Pathologic fracture with spinal instability or compression of spinal cord by bone (surgery plus adjuvant RT).
  - Radiation-resistant tumor with neurologic deficit (surgery plus adjuvant RT).
  - Unknown tissue diagnosis (surgery plus adjuvant RT).

Chemotherapy

Indications:

- Adjuvant therapy in adult patients with responsive tumors (e.g., lymphoma, germ cell tumor, neuroblastoma).
- Relapse of responsive tumor at site of previous surgery/RT.
- Paraplegia due to prostate cancer may respond to hormonal therapy without RT.

References and Further Reading

Byrne TN. Spinal cord compression from epidural metastases. *N Engl J Med* 327:614, 1992.
Gilbert RW, Kim J-H, Posner JB. Epidural spinal cord compression from metastatic tumor: Diagnosis and treatment. *Ann Neurol* 3:40, 1978.
Harries B. Spinal cord compression. *Br Med J* 1:611–614 and 1:673–676, 1970.

Ingham J, Beveridge A, Cooney NJ. The management of spinal cord compression in patients with advanced malignancy. *J Pain Symptom Manage* 8:1, 1993.

Kramer JA. Spinal cord compression in malignancy. *Palliative Med* 6:202, 1992.

Latini P, Maranzano E, Ricci S, et al. Role of radiotherapy in metastatic spinal cord compression: Preliminary results from a prospective trial. *Radiother Oncol* 15:227, 1989.

Sorenson PS, Borgesen SE, Rohde K, et al. Metastatic epidural spinal cord compression: Results of treatment and survival. *Cancer* 65:1502, 1990.

36 Confusional States

If [the patient] is slightly raving, does not recognize his friends, and cannot hear or understand, it is a mortal symptom.

HIPPOCRATES, *APHORISMS*, VII:87

Definitions

Delirium: An *acute* confusional state resulting from *global* impairment of mental function.

Dementia: Chronic, progressive loss of intellectual abilities, memory, and other higher functions.

Distinguishing Delirium from Dementia

Feature	Delirium	Dementia
Onset	Sudden, over hours to days.	Gradual, over months or years.
Diurnal course	Usually gets worse at night ("sundowning").	Usually stable throughout 24 hours.
Sleep-wake cycle	Severely disordered.	May be normal.

continued

Feature	Delirium	Dementia
Level of consciousness	Impaired; fluctuates over 24 hours.	Normal.
Hallucinations	Frequent; often vivid and frightening.	Rare.
Orientation	Disoriented to time and sometimes to place.	May be impaired.
Level of activity	Abnormally reduced or increased; agitation is common.	Usually normal.

This chapter will be concerned primarily with the evaluation and management of *delirium*, that is, *acute* confusional states.

Incidence

- Acute confusional states (delirium) occur commonly in patients with advanced cancer, especially during hospitalization for active or palliative treatment.
  - Estimates of prevalence range from 20% to 70%.
  - The incidence of delirium approaches 90% to 95% as the patient nears death.
- Dementia is considerably less common than delirium.
- In ill elderly patients, delirium and dementia may be present together.

Risk Factors for Delirium

- Advanced disease.
- Hospitalization.
- Advanced age.

Causes of Delirium in Patients with Advanced Cancer

- In patients with advanced cancer, the cause of delirium is often **multifactorial**.
- Nonetheless, a **search** should be made **for treatable causes** that are easily diagnosed (e.g., hypoglycemia, full bladder).

Category	Examples
Direct tumor effects	**Brain** primary or **metastases**. Meningeal carcinomatosis.
Side effects of anticancer therapy	Chemotherapy, especially with high-dose methotrexate, cisplatin, vinca alkaloids, bleomycin, procarbazine. Cranial irradiation → dementia.
Drugs used in palliative care	Corticosteroids (see below). Opioids. Cimetidine. Anticholinergics. Antiemetics. Acyclovir.
Withdrawal	Cessation of medications or alcohol intake.
Pain or discomfort	Uncontrolled pain. Full bladder. Fecal impaction.
Metabolic derangements	Blood glucose fluctuations (especially with steroids). Fluctuations of sodium and potassium.
Failure of vital organs	Uremia. Hepatic encephalopathy. Hypoxemia from respiratory or cardiac failure. Stroke. Thyroid or adrenal dysfunction.
Infection	CNS, urinary, respiratory tract, or generalized sepsis. Signs of infection may be masked by steroids and debility.
Nutritional deficiencies	Thiamine deficiency → Wernicke-Korsakoff syndrome. Folate/B_{12} deficiency → progressive dementia.

- Behavioral effects of **corticosteroids**:
  - Usually produce sense of well-being, but may cause insomnia, restlessness, agitation, depression, or frank steroid psychosis.
  - Adverse behavioral effects may be seen *at any dosage* and *at any time* during treatment, but
    - More common with higher dosage.
    - Usually occur during first 2 weeks of treatment.

- Severe mental and behavioral disturbances are most likely to occur when the *dosage* of corticosteroid is *abruptly changed* (upward or downward).
- Corticosteroids mask the signs of sepsis, which may also be a factor in a patient's delirium.

Diagnostic Workup of the Patient with Delirium

Review the Patient's Chart

- Nursing notes regarding patient's behavior, sleep.
- Medication chart:
  - What drugs is the patient receiving?
  - Is there a temporal relationship between the introduction of a new medication or change in a dosage and the onset of the patient's delirium?

Mental Status Examination

- Early changes in mental status may go unnoticed if not specifically sought → the mental status examination should be performed at admission, carefully documented, and repeated periodically.
- Signs of delirium (adapted from Fleishman and Lesko, 1990):
  - *Early* signs:
    - Disordered sleep, "sundowning."
    - Withdrawal, with refusal to talk to staff or family.
    - Irritability, bad temper.
    - New forgetfulness.
    - New onset of incontinence.
  - *Later* signs approach those of a psychotic state, with severe behavior disturbance:
    - Outbursts of anger, hostility, abusiveness.
    - Refusal to cooperate.
    - Psychomotor agitation.
    - Illusions, delusions, and hallucinations, often with paranoid content.

Physical Examination

Pay particular attention to the following:

Region Examined	*Look for*	*Suggests*
Vital signs	Tachycardia + hypotension	Internal bleeding, hypoglycemia, hypocalcemia, cardiac failure, sepsis.
	Bradycardia + hypertension	Increased intracranial pressure.
	Tachypnea + hyperpnea	Hypoxemia, acidosis.
Skin	Cold, clammy skin	Internal bleeding, hypoglycemia, hypocalcemia, cardiac failure, sepsis.
	Hot, red skin	Anticholinergic toxicity.
Face	Chvostek's sign	Hypocalcemia.
Extraocular motions	Ophthalmoplegia (sixth cranial nerve)	Wernicke's encephalopathy (thiamine deficiency).
Sclerae	Icterus	Hepatic encephalopathy.
Pupils	Constricted	Opioid toxicity.
	Dilated	Anticholinergic toxicity.
Ocular fundus	Papilledema	Increased intracranial pressure.
Mouth	Smooth, shiny, sore tongue	Folate deficiency.
	Odors on breath: fetor hepaticus	Hepatic failure, etc.
Neck	Stiffness	Meningitis or meningeal carcinomatosis.
Chest	Rales	Heart failure.
	Egophony	Pneumonia.
Heart	S_3 gallop	Heart failure.
Abdomen	Palpable bladder	Urinary retention.
Rectum	Palpable feces	Fecal impaction.
Extremities	Trousseau's sign	Hypocalcemia.
	Tender, swollen calf muscles	Thiamine deficiency.
	Asterixis	Hepatic failure.
Neurologic	Mental status examination	See above.
	Hemiparesis/hemiplegia	Stroke.
	Proximal myopathy	Corticosteroid toxicity.
	Symmetric foot drop	Thiamine deficiency.
	Loss of position/vibration sense and ataxia	Thiamine or B_{12} deficiency (with B_{12} deficiency, difficulty in walking is worse in the dark).

Useful Laboratory Examinations

- Blood glucose.
- Serum electrolytes, urea, calcium.
- Bilirubin.
- Enzymes: LDH, SGOT, SGPT.
- Arterial blood gases for oxygenation and acid-base status (pulse oximetry is a noninvasive method of obtaining information about arterial oxygen saturation).
- Urine culture.

Management of Delirium in Patients with Advanced Cancer

- **Correct metabolic abnormalities**, where possible (hypoglycemia, hypercalcemia, abnormalities of serum sodium and potassium).
- **Discontinue as many drugs as possible**; decrease dosage of drugs that cannot be discontinued.
  - Opioids: Consider switching to another opioid.
  - Corticosteroids: Taper dosage. (If dosage was recently changed, return to previous dosage.)
  - For withdrawal syndrome, resume responsible drug (e.g., alcohol), and taper slowly.
- **Treat urinary retention and fecal impaction**, as needed.
- Take simple **measures to calm and orient the patient**:
  - Verbal reassurance, to patient and family.
    - Confusion can be very frightening to both the patient and the family.
    - Explain the cause(s) of confusion.
    - Reassure the patient that he is not "losing his mind."
  - Frequent orientation.
  - Correct misperceptions. ("Yes, that does look like a snake, but actually it's just the cord from the television.")
  - Quiet, well-lit room (night-light in the evenings and night); avoid frequent comings and goings or excessive sensory input.
  - Familiar objects in patient's visual field (family photos, personal articles).
  - Visible calendar and clock.
  - Frequent contact with familiar people (family, staff).
  - Encourage activity, if the patient is physically able.

- **Pharmacologic treatment**:
  - If the patient is known or suspected to have brain metastases and serum chemistries are normal (thereby ruling out a metabolic source of delirium), a **trial of corticosteroids** is worthwhile: **dexamethasone, 16 to 36 mg PO qam.**
  - For agitated delirium of unknown cause, the drug of choice is **haloperidol**:
    - For mild delirium, 1 mg PO tid may be sufficient.
    - For severe delirium with psychosis, start with parenteral dosing, 1 to 2 mg IV or IM; repeat q30-60 min × 2 prn until acute agitation is under control → switch to oral dosing (start at one half the parenteral dose; titrate up to 1.5 times the parenteral dose).
  - At the same time, start **diphenhydramine**, 25 mg PO tid, to prevent extrapyramidal reactions from haloperidol and to provide mild sedation.
  - If more sedation is required, one may add:
    - **Midazolam**, 30 mg/24 hr by continuous infusion, especially when agitation and restlessness are pronounced; *or*
    - **Methotrimeprazine**, 12.5 to 25 mg q4-6h.

> NOTE: DEPRESSED PATIENTS ARE AT INCREASED RISK OF SUICIDE DURING PERIODS OF DELIRIUM.

References and Further Reading

Bruera ES, Chadwick A, Weinlick A, MacDonald RN. Delirium and severe sedation in patients with terminal cancer. *Cancer Treat Rep* 71:787, 1987.

Bruera E, Miller L, McCallion J, et al. Cognitive failure in patients with terminal cancer: A prospective study. *J Pain Symptom Manage* 7:192, 1992.

Caraceni A, Martini C, DeConno F, Ventafridda V. Organic brain syndromes and opioid administration for cancer pain. *J Pain Symptom Manage* 9:527, 1994.

De Stoutz ND, Tapper N, Fainsinger R. Reversible delirium in terminally ill patients. *J Pain Symptom Manage* 10:249, 1995.

Engel G, Romano J. Delirium: A syndrome of cerebral insufficiency. *J Chronic Dis* 9:260, 1959.

Fainsinger R, Tapper M, Bruera E. A perspective on the management of delirium in terminally ill patients. *J Palliative Care* 9(3):4, 1993.

Fleishman SB, Lesko LM. Delirium and Dementia. In Holland J, Rowland J (eds). *Handbook of Psychooncology*. New York: Oxford University Press, 1990, Chap. 30.

Francis J, Martin D, Kapoor WN. A prospective study of delirium in the hospitalized elderly. *JAMA* 263:1094, 1990.

Lipowski ZJ. Delirium (acute confusional states). *JAMA* 258:1789, 1987.

Massie MG, Holland J, Glass E. Delirium in terminally ill cancer patients. *Am J Psychiatry* 140:1048, 1983.

Posner JB. Neurologic complications of systemic cancer. *Med Clin North Am* 63:783, 1979.

Stedeford A, Regnard C. Confusional states in advanced cancer: A flow diagram. *Palliative Med* 5:256, 1991.

Steifel F, Fainsinger R, Bruera E. Acute confusional state in patients with advanced cancer. *J Pain Symptom Manage* 7:94, 1992.

37 Depression and Suicide

Definition

Depression is a psychiatric syndrome of dysphoric mood and related symptoms (see below) present for a significant period of time.

Incidence

- Depression occurs in **15% to 25% of patients with cancer** overall (compared with a prevalence of 6% in the general population).
- The prevalence of depression among cancer patients varies inversely with the Karnofsky performance status:
  - In patients with advanced cancer and Karnofsky performance status < 40, the prevalence of depression is 75%.
  - In patients who are in better physical condition (Karnofsky score > 60), the prevalence of depression is 23%.
- Depression is particularly common in pancreatic cancer and may precede other symptoms of the disease by several months.

- Depression is *not* more common in severely ill cancer patients than in equally ill patients with other medical diagnoses.

Risk Factors for Depression in Patients with Advanced Cancer

- Advanced stage of cancer.
- Poorly controlled pain or other symptoms.
- History of depression in the past.
- History of alcoholism.
- Medications:
  - Corticosteroids.
  - Chemotherapeutic agents (vinca alkaloids, procarbazine, interferon).
  - Cimetidine, ranitidine.
  - β-Blockers.
  - Benzodiazepines.
  - Neuroleptics.
  - Levodopa.
- Endocrine disorders (thyroid, adrenal).
- Neurologic conditions, such as
  - Stroke.
  - Parkinson's disease.
- Nutritional deficiencies (Folate, B_{12}).

Diagnosing Depression in Patients with Advanced Cancer: General Considerations

Somatic Symptoms of Depression

Somatic symptoms of depression are **less useful** for diagnosing depression in cancer patients than in patients who are not medically ill because the same symptoms may be the result of the terminal illness itself:

- Anorexia.
- Weight loss.
- Fatigue and loss of energy.
- Insomnia.
- Decreased libido.
- Constipation.

Psychological Symptoms of Depression

- Some psychological symptoms ordinarily associated with depression may be an appropriate response of the patient with advanced cancer to the illness:
  - Sadness.
  - Withdrawal from friends and family.
- The **most accurate markers of depression in patients with advanced cancer** are
  - Feelings of **worthlessness**.
  - Exaggerated feelings of **guilt**.
  - Thoughts of **suicide**.

Evaluating the Depressed Patient

Depressed affect is not always obvious. Sometimes the only indication is that the clinician feels sad while talking to the patient.

History

Ask specifically about
- Past psychiatric illnesses.
- Family history of depression or suicide.
- Current and recently withdrawn medications.
- Do you feel sad a lot of the time? Do you cry a lot?
- Has your ability to concentrate changed since you became ill?
- Do you find yourself thinking a lot about things you've done that you wish you had done differently?
- Do you ever feel that you are a burden to other people?
- Have you ever thought that it might be better just to end it all?

Physical Examination

Pay particular attention to
- Appearance, dress, and grooming.
- Level of activity (is there agitation or psychomotor retardation?).
- Attention span.
- Affect.
- Speech (retardation, dysarthria, aphasia).
- Orientation and memory.

- Neurologic deficits (e.g., hemiparesis).
- Peripheral neuropathy suggestive of B vitamin deficiency.
- Stigmata of endocrine syndromes (e.g., lid lag, striae).

Worthwhile Laboratory Investigations

- Serum electrolytes, calcium.
- Complete blood count, including RBC indices.
- Thyroid function tests, when indicated by clinical findings.

Management of Depression in Patients with Advanced Cancer

Pharmacologic Management of Depression

Pharmacologic management is the mainstay of treatment.

Class of Drug	Drug and Dosage	Most Useful When	Drawbacks/ Precautions
Tricyclic anti-depressants	**Amitriptyline**: Start with 10–25 mg hs; increase by 10–25 mg q3 days until the desired effect is achieved or a maximum dose of 125 mg is reached.	Sedation is desir-able (e.g., agi-tated depres-sion). Adjuvant analge-sic effect is required. When parenteral (IM) medica-tion is required.	Strong anticho-linergic side effects → caution in elderly pa-tients. Cardiac effects: orthostatic hypotension; aggravation of heart block. Like all tri-cyclics, has a delayed on-set of anti-depressant action.
	Doxepin: Start with 25–50 mg hs; in-crease dosage by 25 mg q3 days to a total dose of 75–150 mg as needed.	Patient has a sei-zure disorder (other tricyc-lics lower the seizure thresh-old). Sedation is desir-able.	Strong anti-cholinergic side effects (although somewhat less than ami-triptyline).

Class of Drug	Drug and Dosage	Most Useful When	Drawbacks/ Precautions
Tricyclic anti-depressants *cont.*	**Desipramine**: Start with 25 mg hs, increase by 25 mg q3 days to a total dose of 75–150 mg as needed.	Anticholinergic effects must be avoided (prostatism, stomatitis). Sedation is undesirable (patient with psychomotor retardation).	
Sympatho-mimetic stimulants	**Methylphenidate**: 10 mg PO at 0800 and 5 mg at noon, *or* **Dextroamphetamine**: 2.5–5 mg qam; titrate upward to a maximum of 30 mg, *or* **Pemoline**: 18.75 mg PO at breakfast and lunch.	Expected life span < 2 weeks. Opioids produce excess sedation. Tricyclics are contraindicated. Rapid onset of action is needed. Adjuvant analgesia is needed. Withdrawn, apathetic, elderly patients.	May suppress appetite. Sometimes produce tremor, tachycardia, and other symptoms of sympathetic overstimulation. Tolerance and dependence
Benzodiazepines	**Alprazolam**: Start with 0.25 mg tid; increase to 1–2 mg tid. (The only benzodiazepine with antidepressant activity.)	Anxiety accompanies depression. Nausea and vomiting are present.	
Lithium carbonate	**Lithium**: 300–600 mg bid	Patient is already taking lithium for preexisting bipolar depression.	Therapeutic levels must be monitored frequently. Toxicity to nerves, thyroid, heart.

- Important points in using **tricyclic antidepressants**:
  - The total **dose required** to manage depression in patients with advanced cancer is usually considerably **lower** than in patients who do not have cancer. Maximum effective doses in cancer patients are usually in the range of **75 to 150 mg/day**.
  - An adequate **therapeutic trial requires** that the patient be maintained at therapeutic dosage for **2 to 3 weeks**. If the patient's life expectancy is less than 3 to 4 weeks, there is no point in starting tricyclic antidepressants.
  - Patients showing a therapeutic response to tricyclic antidepressants should be maintained on the drug for at least 4 months from the time that depression remits (or until death).
  - Tricyclic antidepressants **should not be stopped abruptly**.
    - In patients who were on chronic tricyclic therapy, decrease the dose by 50% for at least 1 month, then taper to zero.
    - In patients who have been taking tricyclics for only a few weeks, taper by 50% every 3 days.
- **Other antidepressive medications are less suitable** for use with terminally ill patients:
  - *Monoamine oxidase (MAO) inhibitors* require dietary restrictions and caution with the concomitant use of opioids.
  - *Fluoxetine* (Prozac), despite its wide popularity among the general public, has side effects that limit its usefulness in patients with advanced cancer:
    - Anorexia and sometimes weight loss.
    - Mild nausea.
    - Sometimes increased nervousness and insomnia.

Nonpharmacologic Management of Depression

- Short-term *supportive psychotherapy*—goals:
  - To discover and mobilize the patient's strengths and coping strategies.
  - To help the patient regain self-esteem.
  - To help the patient make peace with the past.
- General strategies:
  - Encourage the patient to talk about the past and important life experiences.
  - Be receptive to questions about matters that may be worrying the patient, including questions about death.

- Messages that should be conveyed, explicitly and implicitly, to the patient in interaction with the doctor and other staff:
  - You will remain in control. Nothing will be done to you against your wishes.
  - There is almost no symptom you can develop that we cannot control or ameliorate.
  - You will not be abandoned.

Suicide in Patients with Advanced Cancer

Incidence

Suicide is relatively uncommon among cancer patients, but the incidence is higher than among the general population. (Different studies have given widely varying results.)
- As in the general population, completed suicide is more common among men than women.
- Most cancer suicides take place at home.
- Suicide is more frequent among patients with oral, pharyngeal, and lung cancers (perhaps because of heavy use of alcohol and tobacco generally associated with those cancers) and Kaposi's sarcoma with AIDS.

Risk Factors for Suicide Among Patients with Cancer *

- **Advanced disease** and perceived poor prognosis.
  - In one study, 86% of suicides in cancer patients took place during the terminal stages of illness despite physical debility.
  - Patients with advanced disease are more likely to have other risk factors (pain, fatigue, depression).
- **Depression** and **hopelessness** figure in at least half of all suicides.
- Inadequately controlled **pain** is a factor in the majority of suicides among cancer patients.
- Feelings of **helplessness** and **loss of control**.
  - Patients who need to feel in control are the most vulnerable.
  - Cancer and its treatment present many assaults on a person's sense of control:
    - Loss of bowel and/or bladder control from tumor, radiation, surgery, spinal cord compression.

*Adapted from Breitbart, 1990.

- Loss of mobility from weakness, neurologic deficits.
- Loss of mental control from sedating medications, brain metastases, delirium.
- **Exhaustion** from a long sickness and protracted dying process.
- **Delirium** → loss of impulse control.
- **Preexisting psychopathology,** especially alcohol/drug abuse, personality disorders, psychosis.
- **Previous suicide attempts.**
- **Family history** of suicide.

Evaluation and Management of the Cancer Patient at Risk of Suicide

- Establish **rapport** with the patient. Sit down, and be prepared to spend time listening.
- Determine **what the patient knows or believes** about his or her illness and prognosis.
- Assess for **risk factors,** as listed above.
- **Ask** specifically **about suicidal thoughts,** for example:
  • Have you ever thought that it wasn't worth living any more?
  • Have you ever considered ending your own life? (If the answer is affirmative:)
  • Have you thought about how you would go about it?
- Assess the *meaning* of the patient's suicidal thoughts.
  • Some patients talk about suicide as a means of trying to assert some control over their own life and death when they feel that control has been taken from them.
  • The physician should acknowledge the legitimacy of the patient's concerns and need for control.
- **Address the patient's specific fears** with specific information.
- **Treat uncontrolled symptoms** to the degree possible.
  • Pay particular attention to pain and insomnia.
  • Allow the patient to make choices regarding symptom control (e.g.,"Do you prefer to be nearly pain-free but very drowsy, or would you rather be more awake at the price of somewhat more pain?").
- Treat depression, agitation, delirium, and psychosis as needed with the appropriate pharmacologic agents.

Physician-Assisted Suicide and Euthanasia

The goal of intervention should not be to prevent suicide at all costs, but to prevent suicide that is driven by desperation. Prolonged suffering due to poorly controlled symptoms lead[s] to such desperation, and it is our role to provide effective management of such problems as an alternative to suicide in the cancer patient.

BREITBART, 1990

- Requests for help in hastening death are not uncommon, and the physician working with cancer patients can expect to receive such requests, from patients or family members, with increasing frequency because of increased public discussion of the issue.
- Each physician must come to his own resolution of this issue, consistent with his own moral convictions and religious beliefs.
- It is the conviction of these authors and the policy of the Tel Hashomer Hospice *not* to participate in assisted suicide or any other form of euthanasia by any other name.
  - In the vast majority of cases, it is possible to deal with the patient's hopelessness and despair through other means:
    - Building trust.
    - Providing good symptom control.
    - Enabling the patient to talk about painful things.
    - Helping to repair damaged family relationships.
    - Restoring the patient's sense that he or she is a valued person.
  - Jewish religious strictures forbid hastening the death of another person.
  - The family that requests or consents to assisted suicide may be left afterward with a burden of unresolved (and unresolvable) guilt.
  - The medical staff that participates in measures to hasten death often suffers as well from guilt and internal recriminations, with a net negative impact on staff morale.
  - Willingness of the medical staff to assist in hastening death creates ambiguity of professional roles and thereby undermines trust in the professional staff ("Is the doctor/nurse holding that syringe coming to give me something that will help me or that will kill me?"). **Patients must be able to have absolute faith that the doctor will never do anything to harm them.**

- Approach of the Tel Hashomer Hospice to requests to hasten death:
  - We explain to the patient or family that we respect their point of view, but that they must also respect ours and that our moral and professional codes do not permit us to undertake such an action.
  - We explain that we shall give any medication necessary to alleviate pain and discomfort, but that we will not give a medication with the intention of shortening life.
  - All such discussions are documented in the medical record.
  - Decisions in these matters are not taken in a matter of minutes or hours, but over days to weeks.
  - In the rare instances where symptoms cannot be adequately controlled with analgesics and other medications, or where existential suffering is intense, **we offer the patient the option of sedation**.
    - As opposed to assisted suicide or euthanasia, **sedation is potentially reversible**; the patient can be allowed to awaken from time to time to reconsider his decision or for important contacts with family members.
    - Although it is recognized that sedation may hasten death, it is not given with the *intent* to hasten death (cf. the ethical "**principle of double effect**," which distinguishes between the intended effect of an action and the unintended, even if foreseen, effects).
    - Sedation is achieved with
      ○ When there is pain, the highest dose of **opioids** that does not produce unacceptable side effects (myoclonus, respiratory depression), given by continuous SQ infusion ±
      ○ **Midazolam, 30 mg/24 hr** by continuous SQ infusion, *or*
      ○ **Methotrimeprazine, 25 mg/24 hr** by continuous SQ infusion.
      ○ Other centers prefer barbiturates to benzodiazepines or phenothiazines and give **thiopental sodium, 20 to 80 mg/hr IV**.

References and Further Reading

Beck AT, Kovacs M, Weissman A. Hopelessness and suicidal behavior: An overview. *JAMA* 234:1146, 1975.

Billings A, Block S. Depression. *J Palliative Care* 11(1):48, 1995.

Breitbart W. Suicide. In Holland JC, Rowland JH. *Handbook of Psychooncology*. New York: Oxford University Press, 1990, pp. 291–299.

Breitbart W, Bruera E, Chochinov H, Lynch M. Neuropsychiatric syndromes and psychological symptoms in patients with advanced cancer. *J Pain Symptom Manage* 10:131, 1995.

Brown JH, Henteleff S, Barakat S, Rowe CJ. Is it normal for terminally ill patients to desire death? *Am J Psychiatry* 143:208, 1986.

Bukberg J, Penman D, Holland J. Depression in hospitalized cancer patients. *Psychosomatic Med* 46:199, 1984.

Cherny NI, Portenoy RK. Sedation in the management of refractory symptoms: Guidelines for evaluation and treatment. *J Palliative Care* 10(2):31, 1994.

Cody M. Depression and the use of antidepressants in patients with cancer. *Palliative Med* 4:271, 1990.

Cohen SR, Steiner W, Mount BM. Phototherapy in the treatment of depression in the terminally ill. *J Pain Symptom Manage* 9:534, 1994.

Greene WR, Davis WH. Titrated intravenous barbiturates in the control of symptoms in patients with terminal cancer. *Southern Med J* 84:332, 1991.

Kaplitz SE. Withdrawn, apathetic geriatric patients responsive to methylphenidate. *J Am Geriatr Soc* 23:271, 1975.

Massie MJ, Holland JC. Diagnosis and treatment of depression in the cancer patient. *J Clin Psychiatry* 45(3, Sec.2):25, 1984.

Peteet JR. Depression in cancer patients: An approach to differential diagnosis and treatment. *JAMA* 24:147, 1979.

Spiegel D, Sands S, Koopman C. Pain and depression in patients with cancer. *Cancer* 74:2570, 1994.

Truog RD, Berde CB, Mitchell C, Grier HE. Barbiturates in the care of the terminally ill. *N Engl J Med* 327:1678, 1992.

38 Extrapyramidal Drug Reactions

Incidence

In the general population, extrapyramidal drug reactions occur in 39% of patients taking phenothiazines and up to 2% of patients taking antiemetics related to metoclopramide. Among patients with advanced cancer, the incidence is higher (e.g., up to 25% of patients taking metoclopramide), but precise figures are not available.

Drugs Most Likely to Produce Extrapyramidal Reactions

- Neuroleptics:
  - Phenothiazines, especially high-potency forms (e.g., fluphenazine, trifluoperazine).
  - Thioxanthenes (e.g., chlorprothixene).
  - Butyrophenones (haloperidol).
- Metoclopramide (Reglan).
- Some antihistamines, in high doses:
  - Hydroxyzine (Atarax, Vistaril).
  - Promethazine (Phenergan), especially when given parenterally in high doses.
- Methyldopa.

Forms of Extrapyramidal Reaction Seen in a Palliative Care Population

- Akathisia.
- Parkinsonism.
- Acute dystonic reactions.

Akathisia

Incidence

- Most common of the extrapyramidal drug reactions (occurs in 21% of patients taking phenothiazines).
- Twice as common in **women** as in men.
- Most likely among **middle-aged** patients.
- Onset is usually **5 to 60 days after starting** the offending medication.

Symptoms and Signs

- Motor **restlessness**: Patient **cannot sit still** but constantly fidgets or paces the floor.
- When standing, the patient rocks back and forth or shifts his weight from foot to foot.
- Subjective feelings of **anxiety** ("jitters") and of needing to move.

Management

- The key to appropriate treatment is making the correct diagnosis.
  - Akathisia is **apt to be misdiagnosed as severe anxiety or** even psychotic **agitation**.
  - If wrongly diagnosed as psychotic agitation, the dosage of neuroleptic may be *increased* → worsening of the symptoms.
- **Decrease** the offending drug to the minimum effective **dosage**.
- Rapid relief can be provided by **benztropine** (Cogentin), **2 mg IM**, and start on maintenance doses (0.5–4 mg PO bid).
- If severe restlessness persists, give a benzodiazepine, such as **lorazepam, 1 mg tid**.
- If restlessness still persists, add a β-adrenergic blocker, such as **propranolol, 10 to 20 mg bid to tid**.

Parkinsonism

Incidence

- Occurs in approximately 15% of all patients taking phenothiazines; incidence in patients with advanced cancer may be higher.
- Most common in **older** patients (> 60 years old), in whom the incidence approaches 50%.
- Twice as common in **women** as in men.
- Usually occurs **within 5 to 30 days** of starting treatment with the responsible drug.

Symptoms and Signs (Singly or in Combination)

- The earliest, prodromal sign is usually **akinesia**, which is the most common extrapyramidal reaction to phenothiazine and other drugs.
- **Weakness** and muscle fatigue, especially in the legs or the hand used for writing.
- **Joint pains**, most often in the shoulder.
- **Apathy**, lack of initiative, and overall reduction in motor activity.
- **Rigidity** and cogwheeling.
- **Tremor** (3–5 cps), initially often confined to one arm or part of the arm.
- **Mask-like facies.**
- **Drooling.**
- **Festinating gait.**

Management

- If the patient is taking metoclopramide, **switch to cisapride.**
- Decrease the dosage of the neuroleptic drug, *or*
- Add an anticholinergic:
  - **Benztropine** (Cogentin), **0.5 to 4 mg PO bid**, *or*
  - **Diphenhydramine** (Benadryl), **25 mg PO hs**, *or*
  - **Trihexyphenidyl** (Artane), **1 to 5 mg PO tid.**

Acute Dystonic Reactions

Incidence

- Occur in 2% of all patients taking phenothiazines.
- Twice as common in **men** as in women.

- More common in **younger** patients (< 45 years old).
- Onset usually **within 1 to 5 days of starting** the offending medication.

Symptoms and Signs

- **Onset** is usually **abrupt.**
- Symptoms may be frightening and painful.
- Acute spasms affecting the neck, mouth, tongue, axial or appendicular muscles →
  - **Torticollis.**
  - **Grimacing.**
  - **Dysarthria.**
  - **Opisthotonos.**
- **Oculogyric crisis** is one particular form of acute dystonic reaction:
  - Fixed stare → eyes rotate upward and laterally and remain frozen in that position.
  - Head tilted backward.
  - Mouth wide open with tongue protruding.

Management

- Immediate:
  - **Benztropine** (Cogentin), **1 to 2 mg IM or IV**; may be repeated in 30 minutes if symptoms are not completely eradicated, *or*
  - **Diphenhydramine** (Benadryl), **50 mg IM or IV** (not PO).
- Ongoing:
  - If the patient is taking metoclopramide, **switch to cisapride.**
  - Lower the dose of the offending neuroleptic, *or*
  - Give an antiparkinsonian (such as benztropine, 0.5–4 mg PO bid).

> In **patients at high risk** of extrapyramidal reactions (e.g., elderly patients receiving both a neuroleptic and metoclopramide), it is worthwhile starting an anticholinergic (e.g., **benztropine, 2 mg PO bid**) along with the neuroleptic.

References and Further Reading

Arana GW, Goff D, Baldessarini RJ. Efficacy of anticholinergic prophylaxis of neuroleptic-induced acute dystonia. *Am J Psychiatry* 145:993, 1988.

Avorn J, Monane M, Everitt DE, et al. Clinical assessment of extrapyramidal signs in nursing home residents given antipsychotic medication. *Arch Intern Med* 154:1113, 1994.

Ayd FJ. A survey of drug-induced extrapyramidal reactions. *JAMA* 175:102, 1961.

Lipinski JF, Zubenko G, Cohen BM, Barreira P. Propranolol in the treatment of neuroleptic-induced akathisia. *Am J Psychiatry* 141:412, 1984.

Rodgers C. Extrapyramidal side effects of antiemetics presenting as psychiatric illness. *Gen Hosp Psychiatry* 14(3):192, 1992.

Winslow RS, Stillner V, Coons DJ, Robinson MW. Prevention of acute dystonic reactions in patients beginning high-potency neuroleptics. *Am J Psychiatry* 143:706, 1986.

39 Anxiety

Definition

A feeling of deep unease, related to fear, characterized by a particular constellation of symptoms and signs that may include any or all of the following:

Symptoms and Signs of Anxiety

Symptoms	*Signs*
Worrying	Pallor
Insomnia and nightmares	Restlessness
Difficulty in concentrating	Distractibility
Headache	Hypervigilance
Dyspnea	Tremor
Weakness and light-headedness	Sweaty palms
Paresthesias	Diaphoresis
Chest pain or tightness	Tachycardia
Palpitations	Tachypnea/hyperpnea
Anorexia	
"Butterflies" in stomach	
Urinary frequency	

In palliative care, it is useful to **distinguish anxiety from fear**:
- **Fear** has a definable and often realistic referent (e.g., fear of a difficult death, fear of disfigurement, fear of pain).
- **Anxiety** is a state of apprehension and dread whose source the patient cannot identify.

Incidence

Serious anxiety reactions occur in about 35% of patients with advanced cancer.

Causes of Anxiety in Patients with Advanced Cancer

- **Poorly controlled pain.**
- **Reactive anxiety**, reflecting uncertainty about the future.
- **Altered physiologic states**:
  - Hypoxia.
  - Sepsis.
  - Hypoglycemia.
  - Delirium.
  - Hypocalcemia.
  - Bleeding.
  - Pulmonary embolism.
  - Impending heart failure, respiratory arrest, cardiac arrest.
- **Drugs**:
  - Corticosteroids in high dosage.
  - Metoclopramide in high doses.
  - Medications for asthma/COPD (theophylline, albuterol).
  - Neuroleptic medications → akathisia (state of restlessness and agitation that can resemble severe anxiety).
  - Withdrawal from alcohol, narcotics, sedative-hypnotics.
- **Preexisting anxiety disorder.**
- **Hormone-secreting tumors** (e.g., ACTH-secreting lung tumors).

Evaluating the Anxious Patient

History

Ask particularly about
- Specific troubling symptoms.

- Previous personality.
- Previous experience of illness or cancer, and coping strategies used.
- Previous episodes of anxiety (before cancer).
- Knowledge and beliefs about the disease, stage of disease, and prognosis.
- Specific fears.
- Insomnia and nightmares.
- Current and recently discontinued medications.

Physical Examination

Pay particular attention to
- Vital signs: tachycardia, tachypnea, hypertension.
- Skin: flushing, pallor, diaphoresis.
- Head: tense or worried expression.
- Chest: wheezes, rales, egophony.
- Back: muscle tension.
- Abdomen: increased bowel sounds.
- Extremities: fine tremor.
- Neurologic: hypervigilance, distractibility.

Relevant Laboratory Investigations

- Complete blood count.
- Serum electrolytes, glucose, calcium.
- SGOT, SGPT, CK.
- Oxygen saturation (pulse oximetry preferred, as it is noninvasive).
- Thyroid function tests if suggested by physical findings.

Management of Anxiety in the Patient with Advanced Cancer

- **Control the patient's pain**:
  "... One cannot evaluate anxiety until pain has been controlled" (Massie and Holland, 1987).
- Ensure **physical contact** with the patient, by family or staff.
- **Provide rapid relief of anxiety by pharmacologic means**.
  - Rapid relief establishes credibility and enables the patient to talk about fears from an island of relative calm; drug therapy can be discontinued later if other measures added afterward succeed in controlling anxiety.

- There are several pharmacologic approaches to treating anxiety; the choice of a specific drug will depend on what *else* one wants to accomplish:

Drugs for the Treatment of Anxiety and Panic

Class of Drug	Specific Drug and Dosage	When to Use the Drug
Benzodiazepines (usually the first class of drugs to try)	**Lorazepam**, 0.5–2 mg PO/IV/IM q3–6h. **Diazepam**, 2.5–10 mg PO/IM/PR q3–6h. **Midazolam**, starting with 2–10 mg/day IM or continuous SQ. **Clonazepam**: Start with 0.5 mg PO tid, and titrate upward.	Short-acting drug that is safe in patients with hepatic disease. Longer-acting drug. Ideal for continuous SQ infusion. Drug of choice for terminal restlessness. Treatment of anxiety in patients with brain tumors, seizures, mania, or neuropathic pain.
Neuroleptics	**Haloperidol**, 0.5–1.5 mg PO/IM q4–6h. **Thioridazine**: Start with 10 mg PO tid, and titrate up. **Methotrimeprazine**: 6.25–25 mg PO/IM q6–8h or by continuous SQ infusion.	When benzodiazepines are insufficient. When patient has delirium or psychotic symptoms. When insomnia and agitation are prominent. When sedation is desired. When adjuvant analgesic is needed.
Tricyclic antidepressants	**Imipramine**: Start with 10–25 mg tid, and titrate up (may require total dose of 200–300 mg/day).	When anxiety is accompanied by depression or panic disorder.

- **Treat specific problems** detected by history, physical examination, or laboratory studies (e.g., hypoxia, hypoglycemia, hypocalcemia, thyrotoxicosis).
- Wherever possible, **stop drugs that produce symptoms of anxiety** (e.g., anticholinergics, aminophylline, β-adrenergic agents, high-dose metoclopramide).
- **Address the patient's fears**.

- Ask about specific fears (e.g., "What worries you the most?").
- Ask about the content of bad dreams.
- Give the patient an opportunity to ventilate all his or her worries (this takes **time!**).
- Provide factual information and honest reassurance.
- Concrete fears require concrete solutions; do not rush in with major tranquilizers!

At the time a patient is given the bad news, he is also told how much control over the situation he has. I actually use the words, "You have more control over your body than you have any idea." I point out that the enemy of his control is fear. I then try to find out exactly what he is afraid of in the greatest detail. As pointed out earlier, the fears always turn out to be concrete. In equal and explicit detail, I show how each problem can be, or will be, handled. I do my best to be absolutely honest, since I am sure it would be quickly apparent if I dissembled. Honesty here is rarely difficult, inasmuch as misconceptions about the disease, drugs, or dying make up a large number of the fears. On questions I cannot answer, such as "How long will I live?" I am also honest, but I often point out how much of the outcome is within the patient's power. Having promised the control of symptoms or situations, it is absolutely essential that the promise be upheld (Cassell, 1976).

- Teach the patient **relaxation techniques**.
- Breathing exercises, progressive muscle relaxation, self-hypnosis, or similar method.
- Provides the patient with a sense of control.
- For mild to moderate anxiety, relaxation produces results equivalent to those obtained with benzodiazepines.

References and Further Reading

Cassell EJ. *The Healer's Art*. Philadelphia: Lippincott, 1976.
Derogatis LR, Morrow GR, Fetting J, et al. The prevalence of psychiatric disorders among cancer patients. *JAMA* 249:751, 1983.
Holland JC. Anxiety and cancer: The patient and family. *J Clin Psychiatry* 50:20, 1989.
Hollister LE. Pharmacotherapeutic considerations in anxiety disorders. *J Clin Psychiatry* 47:33, 1986.
Massie JG, Holland JC. The cancer patient with pain: Psychiatric complications and their management. *Med Clin North Am* 71:243, 1987.

40 Insomnia

Definition

The subjective perception by the patient that he sleeps poorly. Insomnia may refer to difficulty falling asleep, difficulty maintaining sleep, early morning wakening, wakening without feeling refreshed, or any combination of the foregoing.

Incidence

Insomnia occurs in 29% to 59% of patients with advanced cancer, and nearly half the psychotropic medications prescribed to such patients are sedative-hypnotics.

Importance of Insomnia in Patients with Advanced Cancer

- Sleep deprivation **lowers the pain threshold** → pain interferes with sleep → exhaustion → pain threshold further lowered (vicious cycle).
- Conversely, adequate sleep significantly reduces pain levels in patients with both acute and chronic pain.
- Insomnia also promotes **irritability, hopelessness**, and **loss of energy and will** to cope with problems, physical, emotional, financial, and social.

Causes of Insomnia in Patients with Advanced Cancer

- **Physical symptoms:**
  - **Pain.**
  - **Nausea** and vomiting.
  - **Dyspnea.**
  - Itching.
  - Dyspepsia.
- **Fear and anxiety** are magnified during the quiet, lonely night hours:
  - Fear of dying during sleep.
  - Fear of recurrent nightmares.
  - Practical worries (financial, unfinished business).
  - Anxiety over insomnia itself → vicious cycle.
- **Depression** (insomnia may be a diagnostic marker).
- **Delirium** → disturbances in the normal sleep-wake cycle with reversed circadian rhythms ("sundowning").
- **Medications:**
  - **Corticosteroids.**
  - Stimulant antidepressants (fluoxetine).
  - Methylxanthine bronchodilators (theophylline).
  - **Diuretics** → nocturia.
  - Propranolol, methyldopa → nightmares.
  - Excessive daytime sedation.

Evaluation of Sleep in the Patient with Advanced Cancer

- **How are you sleeping at night?** If the patient indicates there are problems with sleep, take a *detailed sleep history*:
  - When did your sleep problems begin?
  - Do you have trouble falling asleep? If so, what is it that keeps you from falling asleep? Are there particular worries that you can't seem to get out of your head when you try to sleep?
  - Do you wake up several times after you've fallen asleep? If so, are you aware of what has awakened you? (Suggests interference by physical symptoms.)
  - Do you find you waken very early in the morning and then can't get back to sleep? (Suggests depression.)
  - Do you have nightmares? (If so, double-check the patient's current medications.)

- What do *you* think is disturbing your sleep?
- Are you excessively **sleepy during the day**?
- What **medications** (including nonprescription medications) do you take regularly?
- Ask specifically about use of **alcohol, caffeine,** and **tobacco.**

Management of Insomnia in Patients with Advanced Cancer

General Principles of Management

- Try to **restore the normal sleep-wake cycle:**
  - Minimize time in bed during the daylight hours for ambulatory or movable patients.
  - Active daytime schedule even for bedridden patients:
    - Mild exercise where feasible.
    - Social activities.
    - Physiotherapy.
  - Discourage late afternoon or evening naps.
- Encourage patient to **talk of anxieties** ("What kind of thoughts keep you awake at night?"), and address specific fears with specific answers so that the patient does not take his worries to bed with him.
- **Minimize disturbances** to sleep, such as
  - Staff activities in or near the patient's room.
  - Bright lights, noise.

Nonpharmacologic Measures

- Different measures will work with different patients.
- Some patients find it easier to fall asleep if a radio or television is playing in the background.
- Warm milk or carbohydrate snack at bedtime.
- Massage, warm bath.
- Behavioral therapies, such as progressive muscle relaxation.

Specific Pharmacologic Treatment

- **Benzodiazepines** are the hypnotics of choice in advanced cancer:
  - **Temazepam** (Restoril) **capsules, 15 to 30 mg PO 1 to 2 hours before bedtime,** taken on an empty stomach.
  - If anxiety is prominent, use **lorazepam, 0.5 to 1 mg PO hs.**

- **Flunitrazepam**, where available: **0.5 to 1 mg PO/IM hs**.
- Some elderly patients experience paradoxical reactions to benzodiazepines (excitement, agitation). In such cases, use **chloral hydrate** (Notec), **250 to 500 mg PO hs**.
- **Supplement benzodiazepines** with a nighttime opioid, antihistamine, phenothiazine, or sedating antidepressant as required by the patient's other symptoms:

Contributing Cause of Insomnia	Treatment
Pain	Adequate opioid analgesia with controlled-release morphine. Consider amitriptyline, 10–25 mg PO hs.
Itching, nausea	**Hydroxyzine**, 6.25–25 mg PO/IM hs.
Depression	**Amitriptyline**, 25 mg PO 2 hours before bedtime.
Delirium	Try to prevent excessive daytime sleep. Night-light. **Haloperidol**, 0.5–2 mg PO/IM in the late afternoon → increase dosage as needed.
Other drugs	Give corticosteroids and diuretics as a single dose in the morning. Switch from methylxanthines to β_2-selective agents, such as albuterol (Ventolin). Discourage caffeine, alcohol, and cigarettes in the evening hours.

References and Further Reading

Beszierczey A, Lipowski ZJ. Insomnia in cancer patients. *Can Med Assoc J* 116:355, 1977.

Greenblatt DJ, Shader RI. The clinical choice of sedative-hypnotics. *Ann Intern Med* 77:91, 1972.

Lamb MA. The sleeping patterns of patients with malignant and nonmalignant diseases. *Cancer Nurs* 5:389, 1982.

Wittig RM, Zorick FJ, Blumer D, et al. Disturbed sleep in patients complaining of chronic pain. *J Nerv Ment Dis* 170:429, 1982.

Orthopedic

41 Bone Metastases

Incidence

- Thirty percent to 70% of patients with cancer will develop bone metastases at some time during their course.
- Sources of bone metastases:

Primary Tumor in	% of Patients with Bony Metastases
Breast	85
Prostate	85
Thyroid	50
Lung	44
Kidney	37
Rectum	13
Pancreas	13
Stomach	11
Colon	9
Ovary	9

- Bone metastases occur most commonly in the **axial skeleton** and **lower extremities**.

Site of Bone Metastases	% of All Cases	% of Breast Cancer Cases
Vertebrae	69	
Cervical		26
Thoracic		72
Lumbar		68
Pelvis	41	66
Femur	25	44
Skull	14	44
Upper extremities	10-15	14
Ribs		62

Clinical Findings in Patients with Bone Metastases

- **Pain** is considered the hallmark of skeletal metastases.
  - In fact, pain is not universal with bone metastases and is not well correlated with the site of metastases.
  - Twenty percent of patients with cancer of the breast or prostate metastatic to bone do not have bone pain.
  - The most painful site of metastasis in breast/prostate cancer patients is the lumbar spine. (When a patient with cancer complains of increasing back pain, assess immediately for early cord compression!)
  - Metastases to skull, sternum, and arm tend *not* to be symptomatic.
- Symptoms of **hypercalcemia** will develop in up to 50% of patients with skeletal metastases (see Chapter 42).
- Serious **pathologic fractures** occur in about 9% of patients with bone metastases.

Laboratory and Roentgenologic Findings

- **Laboratory tests** are nonspecific but can be useful in following progression:

- **Alkaline phosphatase** is elevated in up to 65% of patients with bone metastases (reflects osteoblastic, or healing, response to tumor) → returns to normal in remission; continued rise indicates disease progression.
- Similarly, continuous rise in serum **LDH** suggests disease progression, especially when there is bone marrow involvement.
- Serum **calcium** and urinary calcium are elevated in at least a third of patients.

- **X-ray findings:**
  - Fifty percent to 70% of invaded bone matrix must be destroyed for a lesion to be visible radiographically.
  - Metastatic bone lesions are **usually multiple**, small (1–3 cm), well demarcated, and rarely extend outside the bone (except in hypernephroma). A single lesion should raise suspicion of primary sarcoma rather than metastatic bone disease.
  - Lesions may be osteolytic, osteoblastic, or mixed:

Type of Bone Lesion	Seen In	Appearance
Primarily osteolytic	Non–small cell lung cancer Hypernephroma Multiple myeloma	May be moth-eaten, infiltrative, or large and expansile (hypernephroma).
Primarily osteoblastic	Small cell lung cancer Prostate cancer Thyroid cancer Hodgkin's disease	Generally smaller than osteolytic lesions.
Mixed osteolytic and osteoblastic	Breast cancer Gastrointestinal cancers Squamous cancers	Combination of the above findings. (Osteoblastic component is a reaction of normal bone to metastasis.)

- **Bone scans** are more sensitive than ordinary x-rays and can detect metastases 2 to 18 months before changes are evident on plain radiographs.

Problems Requiring Palliative Care in Patients with Bone Metastases

- Bone pain.
- Large lytic lesions at risk of fracture.

- Pathologic fracture.
- Hypercalcemia (see Chapter 42).
- Acute spinal cord compression (see Chapter 35).

Bone Pain

Characteristics of Bone Pain Due to Skeletal Metastases

- Classic example of nociceptive somatic pain.
- **Dull, deep, aching, oppressive pain** that is worse at night and not relieved by rest.
- Movement and weight-bearing aggravate pain.

Radiation Therapy

The **treatment of choice** for the pain of bone metastases is external beam **radiation therapy.**

- **A single dose of 8 Gy** gives pain relief equivalent to that from fractionated dosage.
  - Eighty percent of patients will respond within 1 to 2 weeks (50% complete response; 30% partial response).
  - Time to achieve pain relief is longer with slowly proliferating tumors (e.g., prostate).
  - Patients with primary tumors in the breast or prostate are more likely to achieve complete pain relief.
  - Acute *toxicity* depends on the site treated and the volume of tissue in the irradiated area.
    - Toxicity occurs within hours to days of treatment; generally self-limiting.
    - If stomach or liver is in the radiation field → nausea and vomiting.
    - If the small bowel is in the radiation field → crampy abdominal pain and diarrhea.
- For patients with multiple bony metastases, **hemibody radiation** can provide rapid and effective palliation of pain.
  - **Single fraction** of 6 Gy (upper body) or 8 Gy (lower and mid hemibody).
  - Some reduction in pain is seen in 73% to 100% of patients; complete pain relief in up to 57%.
  - The majority of patients experience pain relief within 48 hours, independent of tumor radiosensitivity.
  - In 50% to 86% of those who respond, pain relief lasts for the rest of the patient's life.

- Hemibody radiation—especially upper body radiation—has greater *toxicity* than local irradiation (primarily nausea and diarrhea for 12–24 hours after treatment); patient should be **premedicated** with
  - **Hydrocortisone, 100 mg.**
  - **Metoclopramide, 10 to 20 mg.**
  - Fluids.

Other Treatment Options for Bone Pain

- **Analgesic drugs** should be started early and continued until other modalities (e.g., radiation therapy) provide relief:
  - Start with **acetaminophen**, 1 gm q4h.
  - If that does not control the pain, switch to an NSAID, such as **naproxen**, 500 mg bid. (Gastrointestinal side effects may be a problem.)
  - If the NSAID does not control the pain, add an opioid:
    - Try oxycodone-acetaminophen (**Percocet**), 1 tab q6h; if that isn't strong enough, switch to
    - **Morphine**, 5 to 10 mg q4h titrated upward as needed. (See Chapter 2, on pain management, for technique of dose escalation.)
- Pain from a solitary rib metastasis may be effectively treated with **intralesional injection** of 0.5% bupivacaine (5 ml) plus 80 mg (2 ml) of depot methylprednisolone.
- **Hormonal therapy** may be effective in hormone-responsive tumors, especially of the prostate or breast.

Hormonal Treatment	Breast Cancer		Prostate Cancer
	Premenopausal patient	*Postmenopausal patient*	
First-line	**Tamoxifen**, 20 mg PO qd.	**Tamoxifen**, 20 mg PO qd.	**Orchidectomy**, *or* Goserelin, 3.6 mg q4 weeks, *or* Diethylstilbesterol, 1 mg PO qd.
Second-line	Oophorectomy *or* Goserelin, 3.6 mg q4 weeks.	Megestrol acetate, 160 mg PO qd.	Aminoglutethimide, 250 mg bid–qid + hydrocortisone.

continued

Hormonal Treatment	*Breast Cancer*		*Prostate Cancer*
	Premenopausal patient	*Postmenopausal patient*	
Third-line	Megestrol acetate, 160 mg PO qd.	Aminoglutethimide, 250 mg bid–qid + hydrocortisone.	

- A patient with breast cancer who has had a good response to hormonal therapy in the past is likely to respond well to a second hormone.
- Since hormone therapy may take several weeks to achieve results, analgesic coverage must be provided in the meantime.
- **Biphosphonates** have been used for their analgesic effect in patients with bone metastases from breast cancer. Specifically, **clodronate, 800 mg PO bid**, has shown analgesic effects and also reduces the fracture rate in the axial skeleton.
- **Chemotherapy** may palliate bone pain in patients with breast cancer or multiple myeloma. It is less likely to be effective when the primary is in the prostate, kidney, or lung (non–small cell).
- **Strontium-89** produces pain relief in 37% to 92% of patients with bone metastases from prostate cancer.
  - Can be given as a single intravenous injection.
  - Response takes 2 to 4 weeks.
  - Contraindicated in renal failure and in patients with urinary incontinence.
  - Very expensive.

Large Lytic Lesions at Risk of Fracture

- Large lytic lesions usually **present with pain**.
- Lytic lesions that are 2.5 cm or larger in weight-bearing bones or that cause >50% cortical bone loss → high risk of pathologic fracture.
- Radiation therapy to relieve the pain temporarily weakens the bone → may increase the risk of fracture.
- If the patient's life expectancy is greater than 1 to 2 months, **primary internal fixation** of the lytic area should be considered.
  - It is easier to fix the bone before it has broken than afterward → convalescence and rehabilitation are much shorter.
  - Internal fixation is followed by radiation therapy to inhibit further bone destruction.

Pathologic Fracture

Incidence

Pathologic fracture occurs most commonly in cancers of
- Breast (53% of cases).
- Kidney (11%).
- Lung (8%).
- Thyroid (5%).

Most Common Sites of Pathologic Fracture

- Cervical and trochanteric regions of the femur.
- Shafts of the femur and humerus.

Clinical Findings

- **Pain**.
- **Deformity** and foreshortening of the limb.
- There may be **swelling** and ecchymosis.

Management Objectives

- To relieve pain.
- To preserve as much mobility as possible.
- To facilitate nursing care.

Treatment Measures

- **First aid**: Reduce the fracture manually and splint, under cover of adequate analgesia.
- **Internal fixation** followed by **radiation** therapy (25–40 Gy after wound is healed) is the treatment of choice wherever possible.
- *When the patient is too sick* to undergo surgery:
  - Consider skin **traction** of 5 to 8 pounds to help relieve pain.
  - Palliative radiation, 8 Gy in a single dose to relieve pain.
  - Provide further pain relief with **morphine** as needed.
  - Injection into the fracture site of **methylprednisolone, 80 mg + 0.5% bupivacaine, 10 ml**, may control pain for several days.

References and Further Reading

Aaron AD. The management of cancer metastatic to bone. *JAMA* 272:1206, 1994.

Ashby M. The role of radiotherapy in palliative care. *J Pain Symptom Manage* 6:380, 1991.

Bates TD. The management of bone metastases: radiotherapy. *Palliative Med* 1:117, 1987.

Chalmers J. The management of bone metastases: orthopaedic procedures. *Palliative Med* 1:121, 1987.

Collinson M, Tyrrell C. Treatment of bone pain with biphosphonates. *Eur J Palliative Care* 1(4):175, 1994.

Ernst DS, MacDonald RN, Paterson AHG, et al. A double blind crossover trial of intravenous clodronate in metastatic bone pain. *J Pain Symptom Manage* 7:4, 1992.

Galasko CSB. Skeletal metastases in mammary cancer. *Ann R Coll Surg* 50:3, 1972.

Galasko CSB. Pathologic fractures secondary to metastatic cancer. *J R Coll Surg Edinb* 19:351, 1974.

Galasko CSB. The management of skeletal metastases. *J R Coll Surg Edinb* 25:144, 1980.

Hoskin P. Using radioisotopes for bone metastases. *Eur J Palliative Care* 1(2):78, 1994.

Kirkbride P. The role of radiation therapy in palliative care. *J Palliative Care* 11(1):19, 1995.

Mannix KA, Rawlins MD. The management of bone metastases: nonsteroid anti-inflammatory drugs. *Palliative Med* 1:128, 1987.

Needham PR, Hoskin PJ. Radiotherapy for painful bone metastases. *Palliative Med* 8:95, 1994.

Palmer E, Henrickson B, McKusick K, et al. Pain as an indicator of bone metastasis. *Acta Radiol* 29:445, 1988.

Paterson AHG, Powles TJ, Kanis JA, et al. Double-blind controlled trial of oral clodronate in patients with bone metastases from breast cancer. *J Clin Oncol* 11:59, 1993.

Thurlimann B, Morant R, Jungi WF, Radziwill A. Pamidronate for pain control in patients with malignant osteolytic bone disease: A prospective dose-effect study. *Supportive Care Cancer* 2:61, 1994.

Ventafridda V, Sbanotto A, DeConno F. Pain in prostatic cancer. *Palliative Med* 4:173, 1990.

Metabolic

42 Hypercalcemia

Incidence

- Hypercalcemia is the most frequent metabolic emergency in oncology.
  - Occurs in 10% to 20% of all neoplasms.
  - Almost never a presenting sign of malignancy (except in T-cell lymphoma or multiple myeloma).
  - Most commonly occurs in patients with advanced disease who have failed prior therapy.
- Tumors most often associated with hypercalcemia:
  - Breast (>20%).
  - Lung (25%), usually squamous cell, sometimes adenocarcinoma, rarely small cell.
  - Hypernephroma.
  - Multiple myeloma (40–50%).
  - Squamous cell cancers of the head and neck and esophagus.
  - Thyroid.
- Tumors rarely or never associated with hypercalcemia despite high frequency of bone metastases:
  - Small cell lung cancer.
  - Prostate cancer.
  - Colorectal cancer.

Mechanisms

- In the majority of cases, **bone metastases** → osteoclastic bone resorption.
  - Extent of metastasis does not correlate well with level of Ca^{2+}.

- Hypercalcemia usually suggests disease progression.
- Less frequently, humoral hypercalcemia of malignancy from **PTH-like substances**.
  - Most commonly produced by squamous cell tumors, hypernephromas.
  - Usually have bone-resorbing activity.
- Transient flare of hypercalcemia may occur within 2 weeks of starting **hormone therapy** in breast cancer with widespread bone metastases.
  - Ca^{2+} may rise and bone pain increase within a few days of starting hormone treatment (including tamoxifen).
  - Usually implies patient will respond well to hormonal treatment.
  - Hormone treatment must be temporarily stopped until hypercalcemia is corrected.
- Dietary factors *not* considered important: intestinal absorption of Ca^{2+} is decreased in patients with cancer.

Clinical Findings in Hypercalcemia

Symptoms and Signs

- Severity of symptoms not always related to degree of hypercalcemia.
- Early symptoms and signs:
  - Polyuria, nocturia, polydipsia $\rightarrow$ dehydration.
  - Anorexia.
  - Easy fatigability.
  - Weakness.
  - Hyporeflexia.
  - **Pain** may be precipitated or exacerbated by hypercalcemia.
- Late symptoms:
  - Apathy, irritability, depression, decreased ability to concentrate, obtundation, coma.
  - Profound muscle weakness.
  - Gastrointestinal tract: N/V, abdominal pain, constipation, increased gastric acid secretion, acute pancreatitis.
  - Pruritus.
  - Visual disturbances.
- Sudden death from cardiac dysrhythmias may occur if Ca^{2+} rises fast.

Laboratory Studies

- Elevated **serum calcium**:
  - Ionized calcium = about half of serum calcium.
  - Correct for albumin:

$$\text{Corrected Ca}^{2+} = \text{Ca}^{2+} + 0.8 \,(4 - \text{serum albumin})$$

- **Alkaline phosphatase** usually elevated (except in myeloma).
- Cl⁻ may be elevated in primary hyperparathyroidism.
- Blood urea nitrogen (BUN), creatinine may be elevated from renal damage.
- **Electrocardiogram**: shortened QT, widened T wave, longer PR interval, bradycardia.

Management of Hypercalcemia in the Terminally Ill Patient

Goals of Management

- Promoting urinary calcium excretion (saline diuresis).
- Directly decreasing bone reabsorption (biphosphonates).

Hydration and Saline Diuresis

- The cornerstone of therapy.
- All hypercalcemic patients are dehydrated (polyuria, vomiting).
- Normal saline + KCl (10 mEq/L) at a rate of 2 to 3 L/24 hr, as tolerated.
- No evidence that adding furosemide is of benefit.
  - Increases risk of hypovolemia → decreased GFR → calcium reabsorption.
  - Also induces hypokalemia, alkalosis, hypomagnesemia.
  - May, however, be useful in patients who cannot otherwise tolerate the fluid load required.
- *Monitor*:
  - I&Os, signs of impending CHF.
  - Serum Ca²⁺, K⁺, Mg²⁺.
  - Continue treatment until serum calcium <12 mg/dl.

Biphosphonates

- Inhibit osteoclast activity.
- Especially for breast cancer, myeloma.

- Do not give until the patient is fully rehydrated and has an adequate urine output.
- For the terminally ill, the biphosphonate of choice is **pamidronate** (Aredia), **60 mg in 250 ml of normal saline** infused over at least 4 hours.
  - Maximum effect seen in 4 to 5 days.
  - Advantage over other biphosphonates or gallium: pamidronate can be given in a single infusion; others require daily infusions for 3 to 5 days.
- Best given with **acetaminophen, 500 mg PO/PR** to prevent pamidronate fever.

Other Treatment Measures

Other measures often recommended for hypercalcemia are less relevant for the terminally ill.

- **Corticosteroids** block bone resorption due to osteoclast activating factor.
  - May be useful in myeloma, lymphoma, leukemia, breast cancer (if hypercalcemic flare caused by hormonal treatment).
  - Prednisone, 40 to 100 mg qd for up to 1 week.
- **Gallium nitrate** is at least as effective as pamidronate but must be given by continuous infusion 24 hours a day × 5 days.
  - Directly inhibits bone resorption without toxicity to bone cells.
  - Dosage = **100 to 200 mg/m^2/day**; start only after adequate hydration is achieved.
  - Maintain urine output of 2 L/day.
  - Maximum hypocalcemic effect may occur several days after drug is discontinued.
  - *Nephrotoxicity* is major side effect.
  - Do not give together with aminoglycosides.
- **Mithramycin** directly kills osteoclasts but has potential toxicity (bleeding, hepatic toxicity).
  - Possible indications:
    - Patients in CHF or fluid overload, or
    - Patients not responding to saline diuresis.
  - Contraindicated: thrombocytopenia, hepatic dysfunction.
  - Dosage = **25 µg/kg** by rapid infusion via good IV line (10 µg/kg in renal insufficiency, but calcitonin preferred); may be repeated every 3 to 4 days.
  - Calcium levels fall in 24 to 48 hours.

Summary of Treatment for Acute Hypercalcemia

1. Hydration: **normal saline**, 2-3 L/24 hr as tolerated.
2. Decrease bone resorption: **pamidronate**, 60 mg in 250 ml of saline infused over > 4 hours.

Chronic Hypercalcemia

- Encourage **ambulation** to minimize bone resorption.
- Increased **oral fluid intake** (2-3 L/day) as tolerated.
- **Oral biphosphonates**: etidronate, 200 mg PO bid.
- Avoid thiazide diuretics (which aggravate hypercalcemia).
- Avoid drugs that decrease renal blood flow (ranitidine, cimetidine).
- Avoid vitamins A and D or preparations containing calcium.
- **Glucocorticoids**: prednisone, 20 to 40 mg PO qd (lymphoma, myeloma).
- Avoiding calcium-containing **foods** (e.g., milk products) probably *not* necessary and may exacerbate malnutrition.

References and Further Reading

Heath DA. Hypercalcemia of malignancy. *Palliative Med* 3:1, 1989.

Kovacs OS, MacDonald SM, Chik CL, Bruera E. Hypercalcemia of malignancy in the palliative care setting: A treatment strategy. *J Pain Symptom Manage* 10:224, 1995.

Morton AR, Howell A. Biphosphonates and bone metastases. *Br J Cancer* 58:556, 1988.

Ralston S. Medical management of hypercalcemia. *Br J Clin Pharm* 34:11, 1992.

Ralston S. Management of cancer-associated hypercalcemia. *Eur J Palliative Care* 1:170, 1995.

Warrell RP, Murphy WK, Schulman P, et al. A randomized double-blind study of gallium nitrate compared with etidronate for acute control of cancer-related hypercalcemia. *J Clin Oncol* 9:1467, 1991.

43 Electrolyte Abnormalities

The Approach to Electrolyte Abnormalities in the Terminally Ill: Principles

- **Treat the patient, not the laboratory result**:
  - Treatment of an electrolyte abnormality is warranted when the derangement is producing untoward symptoms.
  - The treatment should not be worse than the symptoms (e.g., draconian fluid restriction, medications that produce nausea).
- In patients whose life expectancy is short, the **aim of treatment is to minimize discomfort**:
  - Frequent venipuncture to obtain blood tests should be avoided → do not give treatments that require hour-by-hour monitoring of blood parameters.
  - Use *initial* laboratory values to calculate the approximate magnitude of the correction required and the rate of correction.
  - Thereafter, to the extent possible, **use** the patient's *clinical* **status to gauge response** to treatment (e.g., disappearance of tetany after infusion of calcium gluconate for hypocalcemia).
  - When death is imminent, electrolyte derangements may serve as a natural anesthetic.

Hyponatremia

Definition

Serum sodium (Na⁺) < **135 meq/L.**

- Mild hyponatremia: Na⁺ = 125 to 134 meq/L.
- Moderate hyponatremia: Na⁺ = 115 to 124 meq/L.
- Severe hyponatremia: Na⁺ < 115 meq/L.

Incidence

Hyponatremia occurs in approximately 20% of cancer patients during the last weeks of life.

Causes of Hyponatremia in Patients with Advanced Cancer

- Syndrome of inappropriate antidiuretic hormone (**SIADH**)—see discussion below.
- **Drugs** used in oncology and palliative care:
  - Diuretics, especially thiazides.
  - Morphine and other narcotics.
  - Chemotherapeutic agents: vincristine, cyclophosphamide.
  - Psychotropics: amitriptyline, phenothiazines.
  - Nonsteroidal anti-inflammatory drugs.
  - Carbamazepine.
- **Renal, hepatic, or cardiac failure.**
- Adrenal failure (usually due to withdrawal of corticosteroid drugs).
- Hyperglycemia (for every 100 mg/dl rise in blood sugar, there is a 1.6 meq/L fall in serum Na⁺).
- Iatrogenic: Volume repletion without adequate salt repletion after fluid losses.

Cause	BUN	Serum Osmolality	Urine Osmolality	Na$^+$	Volume Status
SIADH	↓	↓	↑	N or ↑	N or slightly ↑
Chronic renal failure	↑	↓	Varies	Varies	↑
Edematous state	Varies	↓	↑	↓	↑
Diuretics	N	↓	↑	N or ↑	↓

Syndrome of Inappropriate Antidiuretic Hormone (SIADH)

- Incidence:
  - Occurs in 1% to 2% of all patients with cancer.
  - Most common in patients with **small cell lung cancer** (SCLC), in whom the incidence of clinically evident SIADH is about 10%.
- Hyponatremia results from both **dilution** (water retention) *and* renal **sodium loss**.
- **Diagnostic criteria** for SIADH:

Diagnostic Criterion	Laboratory Equivalent
Hyponatremia	Serum Na$^+$ < 130 mEq/L
Persistent urinary Na$^+$ excretion, suggesting volume expansion	Urine Na$^+$ > 20-30 mEq/L
Serum hypotonicity	Serum osmolality < 270 mOsm/kg
Urine that is maximally dilute	Urine osmolality > 75-100 mOsm/kg (usually > 200)
Normal renal function	Serum creatinine < 1.4
Coexisting hypouricemia is highly suggestive	Serum uric acid < 3 mg/dl
Absence of edema, ascites	—

Symptoms and Signs of Hyponatremia

- It is often difficult to sort out the symptoms and signs due to hyponatremia from those due to underlying problems (the cancer itself, side effects of medications).

- *Mild hyponatremia* may cause
  - Fatigue and lethargy.
  - Myalgias or cramps.
  - Anorexia; nausea.
  - Headaches.
- When hyponatremia develops rapidly or *serum Na$^+$ < 115 mEq/L*:
  - Confusion, psychosis.
  - Seizures.
  - Coma.

Management of Hyponatremia

Management of hyponatremia in advanced cancer depends in part on the presumed cause.

Cause	Management Measures
SIADH	Whenever possible, **treat the underlying malignancy** (chemotherapy will correct most cases of SIADH due to SCLC). *Mild hyponatremia*: • Encourage moderate alcohol intake (e.g., a glass of sherry before meals). • Slightly increase dietary Na$^+$ intake. *Moderate hyponatremia*: • Moderate fluid restriction (< 1000 ml/day). • **Demeclocycline** (Declomycin), **300 mg PO bid**. *Severe, symptomatic* (coma, seizures) *hyponatremia*: • IV infusion of **0.9–3% saline** as required (see below*). • **Furosemide, 40–80 mg IV q8h**. • Discontinue saline infusion and furosemide when serum Na$^+$ ≥ 120 mEq/L.

*Data needed to calculate precise Na$^+$ requirements:
- Amount of Na$^+$ needed to increase the serum Na$^+$ to 125 mEq/L = (125 − serum Na$^+$) × 0.6 (body weight in kg).
- Normal saline contains 154 mEq of Na$^+$ per liter.
- 3% saline contains 514 mEq of Na$^+$ per liter.
- Aim of treatment is to increase serum Na$^+$ by no more than 0.5 to 1 mEq/L/hr.

EXAMPLE: A 60-kg patient has a serum Na$^+$ = 105 mEq/L.
- Amount of Na$^+$ required to correct his deficit = (125 − 105) × (0.6 × 60) = 720 mEq.
- That correction will require either
  - 4.7 L of normal saline, *or*
  - 1.5 L of 3% saline

Note: Check patient's clinical status frequently to make certain he is not developing signs of heart failure. → Be prepared to give diuretics if pulmonary crackles or dyspnea develops.

Cause	Management Measures
Edematous states	**Spironolactone**, 100 mg PO qam + **furosemide**, 40-80 mg PO qam. Moderate fluid restriction. Treat for underlying condition (e.g., heart failure) where appropriate and feasible.
Overuse of diuretics	Liberalize salt in diet. Oral fluids ad lib.
Hypovolemia	Normal saline to reexpand ECF volume.

Hypernatremia

Definition

Serum Na⁺ > 145 mEq/L (severe hypernatremia: serum Na⁺ > 160 mEq/L).

Incidence

Hypernatremia occurs in approximately 22% of patients during the last days of life.

Causes of Hypernatremia in Advanced Cancer

- **Decreased or absent fluid intake** accounts for most cases.
- Hypotonic fluid losses (sweating, vomiting, nasogastric suction).
- Osmotic diuresis (tube feeding, hyperglycemia).
- Diabetes insipidus (breast cancer with metastases to hypothalamus).

Signs and Symptoms of Hypernatremia

Signs and symptoms are nonspecific and are rarely distinguishable clinically from those produced by the illness.

Management of Hypernatremia in Advanced Cancer

- Moderate hypernatremia is common toward the end of life and does not require treatment.
- For *severe hypernatremia* in a patient whose life expectancy is more than a few days:

- If there is marked hypovolemia (oliguria, orthostatic hypotension, signs of dehydration), give normal **saline** as needed to cover salt and water deficits (1.5–2 L/24 hr IV).
- When hemodynamically stable, give 5% dextrose in water (**D5W**). Calculate the volume needed as follows:

$$\text{Liters of D5W/24 hr} = \frac{\text{serum Na}^+ - 140}{140} \times 0.6 \text{(body weight in kg)}$$

Hypokalemia

Definition

Serum K⁺ < 3.3 mEq/L.

Incidence

Relatively **rare** in advanced cancer (< 1% of patients).

Most Common Causes of Hypokalemia in Patients with Advanced Cancer

- **Iatrogenic:** loop diuretics given without potassium replacement; corticosteroids.
- Chronic diarrhea.
- **Vomiting** or nasogastric suction.
- **Fistulas.**
- Ectopic secretion of ACTH (SCLC, pancreatic cancer, malignant thymoma).

Symptoms and Signs of Hypokalemia

Symptoms and signs may be difficult to distinguish from those of the underlying condition.
- Symptoms usually do not become evident until serum K⁺ is < 2.5 mEq/L.
- Neuromuscular disturbances: paresthesias, cramps, ↓reflexes, restless legs.
- Constipation or ileus.
- Cardiac dysrythmias.

Management of Hypokalemia in the Patient with Advanced Cancer

- *Mild to moderate hypokalemia* (K^+ = 2.5–3.3):
  - Increase dietary potassium (citrus fruits, tomatoes, bananas, avocado).
  - Give oral potassium supplementation of 80 to 150 mEq/day.
  - In patients requiring diuretics, add a potassium-sparing diuretic (spironolactone) to the loop diuretic.
- *Severe, symptomatic hypokalemia* (K^+ < 2.5 mEq/L):
  - Give **intravenous KCl** in concentrations up to 60 mEq/L at a rate no faster than 30 mEq/hr.
  - If intravenous access is not feasible for any reason, KCl may be given by **subcutaneous infusion** by adding up to 34 mEq KCl to each liter of saline (see Appendix 2 for techniques of SQ infusion).

Hyperkalemia

Definition

Serum K^+ > 5.0 mEq/L.

Incidence

Relatively **common**, especially during the last days of life when the incidence approaches 40%.

Most Common Causes of Hyperkalemia in Patients with Advanced Cancer

- Renal insufficiency.
- Acidosis.
- Blood transfusions.
- Gastrointestinal bleeding.
- Rapid tumor lysis during chemotherapy (lymphomas and leukemias).

Symptoms and Signs of Hyperkalemia

Symptoms and signs usually do not occur until serum K^+ is > 6.5 mEq/L.
- Weakness, paresthesias.
- Areflexia.
- Ascending paralysis.
- Bradycardia.

Management of Hyperkalemia in Advanced Cancer

- Stop potassium supplements and potassium-sparing diuretics.
- Avoid high-potassium foods (citrus, bananas, avocados, tomatoes).
- Consider intravenous glucose.
- More aggressive treatments such as ion-exchange resins (Kayexalate, 20–30 gm PO q6h) should be reserved for patients with an otherwise reasonable life expectancy, for side effects may be very uncomfortable.

Hypocalcemia

Definition

Corrected serum Ca^{2+} < **8.9 mg/dl**

corrected $Ca^{2+} = Ca^{2+} \times 0.8$ (4 – serum albumin)

Causes of Hypocalcemia in Advanced Cancer

- Therapy for hypercalcemia, especially ongoing therapy with biphosphonate.
- Pancreatitis.
- Magnesium deficiency (most commonly with diuretic Rx, cisplatin, or prolonged nasogastric drainage).

Symptoms and Signs of Hypocalcemia

- Lethargy, confusion.
- **Tetany**, worsened by alkalosis (e.g., by hyperventilation):
  - Numbness and tingling of the face, hands, feet.
  - Muscle cramps.
- **Chvostek's sign**: Twitching of facial muscles after tapping on the facial nerve anterior to the ear.
- **Trousseau's sign**: Carpopedal spasm produced by occluding the brachial artery for 3 to 5 minutes (most easily done with a blood pressure cuff).

Management of Hypocalcemia in Advanced Cancer

- *Moderate hypocalcemia* (serum Ca^{2+} 7–8 mg/dl):
  - Oral calcium carbonate (e.g., Tums Extra Strength, Oscal), 1 to 2 gm PO tid taken with food, preferably supplemented with oral magnesium.

- *Severe, symptomatic hypocalcemia* (serum Ca^{2+} < 6 mg/dl):
  - Give **20 ml of 10% calcium gluconate IV over 10 minutes**, followed by an infusion of 60 ml in 500 ml of D5W over 6 to 8 hours.
  - For serum magnesium < 1.5 mg/dl or level not known, also give **magnesium sulfate, 1 gm IV**.
  - Switch to oral calcium supplementation after initial IV corrective dose.

Hypercalcemia

See Chapter 42.

References and Further Reading

Berl T. Treating hyponatremia: What is all the controversy about? *Ann Intern Med* 113:417, 1990.

Hainsworth JD, Workman R, Greco FA. Management of the syndrome of inappropriate antidiuretic hormone secretion in small cell lung cancer. *Cancer* 51:161, 1983.

Kruse JA, Carlson RW. Rapid correction of hypokalemia using concentrated intravenous potassium chloride infusions. *Arch Intern Med* 150:613, 1990.

Leaf A. The clinical and physiologic significance of the serum sodium concentration. *N Engl J Med* 267:25 & 267:77, 1962.

List AF, Hainsworth JD, Davis BW, et al. The syndrome of inappropriate secretion of antidiuretic hormone (SIADH) in small-cell lung cancer. *J Clin Oncol* 4:1191, 1986.

Lockton JA, Thatcher N. A retrospective study of thirty-two patients with small-cell bronchogenic carcinoma and inappropriate secretion of antidiuretic hormone. *Clin Radiol* 37:47, 1986.

Passamonte PM. Hypouricemia, inappropriate secretion of antidiuretic hormone, and small cell carcinoma of the lung. *Arch Intern Med* 144:1569, 1984.

Schen RJ, Arieli S. Administration of potassium by subcutaneous infusion in elderly patients. *Br Med J* 285:1167, 1982.

Silverman P, Distelhorst CWE. Metabolic emergencies in clinical oncology. *Semin Oncol* 16:504, 1989.

Trump DL. Serious hyponatremia in patients with cancer: Management with demeclocycline. *Cancer* 47:2908, 1981.

Fever and Infection

44 Fever and Infection

Incidence

Infection occurs commonly among patients with advanced cancer and is the proximate cause of death in 50% of all cancer patients.

Significance of Fever in Patients with Advanced Cancer

- **Fever may occur without infection** in advanced cancer. Other causes of fever include
  - **Tumor** (neoplastic fever), especially
    - Lymphoma.
    - Renal cell carcinoma.
    - Primary or metastatic tumor in the liver.
    - Atrial myxoma.
  - **Treatment side effects**:
    - Chemotherapy: Bleomycin, cisplatin, interferon, interleukin, colony-stimulating factors.
    - Radiation therapy → pneumonitis, pericarditis.
    - Pyrogenic reaction to blood transfusion.
    - Drug allergy.
  - **Central nervous system metastases** (e.g., meningeal carcinomatosis) or other intracranial processes (stroke).
  - **Dehydration**.
  - Adrenal insufficiency, usually induced by corticosteroid withdrawal.

- **Infection may occur without fever** in advanced cancer. Fever may be suppressed by
  - General debility.
  - Corticosteroids.
  - Nonsteroidal anti-inflammatory drugs.
- Give **symptomatic treatment** when fever causes distress.
  - In adults, fever below 103°F (39.4°C) usually does not cause discomfort.

Symptom	*Treatment*
Fever of unknown origin	**Acetaminophen,** 500-1000 mg PO q4-6h around the clock (not prn) to suppress temperature fluctuations that lead to chills and sweats.
Suspected neoplastic fever	**Naproxen,** 250 mg PO q12h.
Shaking chills (rigors)	**Promethazine,** 12.5-25 mg PO/IM/IV q6-8h prn. Some centers use **meperidine,** 25 mg slowly IV, followed by SQ infusion as needed to control rigors.

Significance of Infection in Patients with Advanced Cancer

- Many factors combine to make the patient with advanced cancer more susceptible to infection:

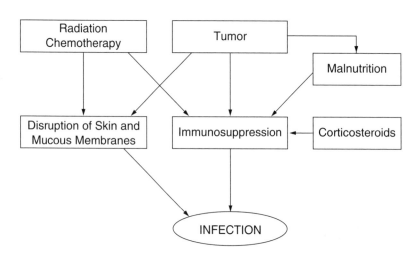

- In many cases, **infection is part of the natural dying process** in patients with cancer → aggressive treatment of infection does not alter the prognosis.

Principles of Managing Infections in the Terminally Ill Cancer Patient

- **Treat the patient, not the laboratory result.**
  - Bacteriuria is common in patients with advanced cancer and is universal in catheterized patients; it should not be treated if there are no symptoms of urinary tract infection (fever, dysuria).
  - Similarly, a marked left shift in the differential white blood cell count often signals **occult sepsis** but need not trigger aggressive workup and treatment for sepsis in the patient who is otherwise comfortable.
- **All patients** with infections **should receive comfort measures** to relieve distressing symptoms.
- *If it is possible to return the patient to good functional status* by definitive treatment for infection, carry out the appropriate workup (Gram's stains, cultures), and administer appropriate antibiotics.
- *If infection is part of the dying process*, treat only symptomatically, and do not subject the patient to diagnostic procedures.

Management of Specific Problems

Infection	Comfort Measures for All Patients	Indications for Workup and Antibiotic Rx	Workup and Treatment
Urinary tract infection	**Phenazopyridine** (Pyridium), 100–200 mg PO qid.	Dysuria. Fever, rigors.	Urine culture. Start **TMP/SMZ*** (160 mg/800 mg) PO tid–qid pending results of culture.
Pneumonia Bronchitis	Inhalations of neb-ulized **morphine**, 2.5 mg + **dexamethasone**, 2 mg + **saline**, 1.5 ml. Mucolytics for tenacious sputum.	Severe dyspnea. Fever, rigors. Cough with copious or purulent sputum.	Physical examination. Sputum Gram's stain, acid-fast stain, and culture.

*TMP/SMZ = trimethoprim-sulfamethoxazole (Septrin, Bactrim).   *continued*

Infection	Comfort Measures for All Patients	Indications for Workup and Antibiotic Rx	Workup and Treatment
Pneumonia Bronchitis *cont.*	Postural drainage.		Start **erythromycin**, 250 mg PO qid.
Candidal esophagitis	Lidocaine syrup. Analgesics as needed.	Dysphagia.	**Nystatin** oral suspension, 3–6 ml PO q6h ± **fluconazole**, 150 mg PO qam × 5 days.
Fungating tumors	Saline rinses. Charcoal pads. Topical application of Maalox.	Foul odor.	**Metronidazole 0.8% gel** topically. **Metronidazole**, 200–400 mg PO tid.
Enterocolitis	Rest the bowel. Oral rehydration. **Tincture of opium**, 15–20 gtt PO q4h, *or* **loperamide**, 2 mg PO × 2, then after each diarrheal stool.	Fever. Dysentery. Intractable symptoms.	Stool culture. **TMP/SMZ*** (160 mg/800 mg) PO tid.
Ulcerated tumors of the head and neck	Saline dressings. Analgesia.	Sudden increase in pain intensity.	**Cephalexin**, 500 mg PO qid.

References and Further Reading

Brown NK, Thompson DJ. Nontreatment of fever in extended care facilities. *N Engl J Med* 300:1246, 1979.

Bruera E, MacDonald N. Intractable pain in patients with advanced head and neck tumors: A possible role of local infection. *Br Med J* 70:691, 1986.

Carter Burks L, Aisner J, Fortner CLE. Meperidine for the treatment of shaking chills and fever. *Arch Intern Med* 140:483, 1980.

Chang JC. Naproxen test in the differential diagnosis of fever of undetermined origin in patients with cancer. *Cancer Ther Control* 1:64, 1989.

Chang JC. Neoplastic fever. *Arch Intern Med* 149:1728, 1989.

Coyle N, Portenoy R. Infection as a cause of rapidly increasing pain in cancer patients. *J Pain Symptom Manage* 6:266, 1991.

Johnson MJ. Pethidine for the treatment of disease related rigors. *Palliative Med* 8:339, 1994.

Terminal Care

45   The Final Hours

Aims of Care in the Terminal Phase

- To keep the patient as comfortable as possible.
- To maintain the patient's dignity.
- Neither to shorten nor to prolong the dying process.
- To prepare the patient's family for what is to come and to support them through the patient's final hours.

Symptoms and Signs of Approaching Death

A study of cancer patients during the last 48 hours of life showed the following frequencies of major symptoms and signs:

Symptom or Sign	% of Patients
Noisy and moist breathing	56
Urinary dysfunction	53
Incontinence	32
Retention	21

continued

Symptom or Sign	% of Patients
Pain	51
Restlessness and agitation	42
Dyspnea	22
Nausea and vomiting	14
Sweating	14
Jerking, twitching, plucking	12
Confusion	9

Based on Lichter & Hunt, 1990.

It is important to **prepare the family**, especially when the patient is being cared for at home, **for the changes they will see** as the patient nears death, so that those changes will not be unduly frightening:
- **State of consciousness**:
  - Usually becomes clouded in the hours before death, but the patient **may remain aware of the presence of family even when comatose**.
  - Speech becomes less frequent, more confused, then ceases altogether.
  - Senses are progressively dulled.
    - Hearing seems to be retained longest, even when the patient is apparently comatose →
    - It may comfort the patient if a family member speaks quietly to him or her.
  - The patient may become **restless or agitated** and may pick at the bedclothes or resist being covered with a sheet or blanket.
  - **Myoclonic jerks** are sometimes evident, especially in patients taking high doses of opioids.
- **Skin**:
  - Hands and feet become **cold and mottled**, often somewhat cyanotic.
  - The face takes on a gray cast; lips may be cyanosed.
  - The skin may feel cold and clammy.
- The **eyes** become **sunken** and glazed.
- **Respirations**:
  - Signs of **respiratory distress** occur relatively frequently.
  - Respirations usually become more rapid initially (Cheyne-Stokes or central neurogenic hyperventilation) → become irregular → gradually slow down → terminal gasps.

- Respirations may be vocalized (**grunting**).
- **Noisy tachypnea** or "**death rattle**" is common → families need to be reassured that grunting, snorting, gurgling, or rattling respirations do not signal distress.
- **Digestive tract**:
  - The patient's digestive system ceases to function.
  - **Swallowing** becomes progressively more **difficult** → the patient becomes less and less able to take foods, fluids, and medications by mouth.
- **Urinary tract**: The patient may become **incontinent** of urine or unable to pass urine.

Stopping Medications and Other Measures that Are No Longer Necessary

Medications

Most patients become unable to take medications by mouth during the last days and hours of life →
- Oral medications that are no longer necessary (e.g., laxatives, hypoglycemics) should be stopped.
- Medications that are needed to control ongoing symptoms (e.g., pain, nausea, seizures) should be given rectally or parenterally (usually continuous SQ infusion is most convenient and least intrusive).
- If a required medication is not available in parenteral form, a substitute medication that *can* be given parenterally should be found (see Table 45.1).
- As death approaches, the patient's medications can often be limited to the "**final four**":
  - Morphine (continuous SQ infusion).
  - Midazolam or methotrimeprazine (continuous SQ infusion).
  - Furosemide (IM/IV as needed).
  - Atropine (IM/IV as needed).

Nutrition and Hydration

- During the last days of life, patients tend naturally to take in less and less food and fluid.
  - Reduced intake of food and fluids preterminally is probably a **normal physiologic mechanism** that prepares the organism for death.

Table 45.1   Stopping Medications in the Last Hours of Life

Class	Drug	Stop or Continue?	Alternative Routes/Medications
Analgesics	Acetaminophen	Stop	
	NSAIDs	Stop oral dosing	If needed in patient with bone metastases to prevent pain on being turned, give indomethacin, naproxen, or diclofenac, ½ hour before activity.
	Weak opioids	Stop	Low doses of morphine by SQ infusion.
	Strong opioids	Continue morphine at ⅓ oral dose by SQ infusion.	
Antiemetics	Metoclopramide	Continue by SQ infusion	
	Haloperidol	Continue by SQ infusion	
	Methotrimeprazine	Continue by SQ infusion	
	Domperidone	Stop	Metoclopramide by SQ infusion.
	Ondansetron	Stop	Metoclopramide or haloperidol by SQ infusion.
Laxatives	All categories	Stop	
Sedative-hypnotics	Benzodiazepines (e.g., temazepam)	Stop oral forms	Midazolam IM hs or by SQ infusion.
Anticonvulsants	Phenytoin	Stop	Midazolam or phenobarbital by SQ infusion.
Corticosteroids	Dexamethasone	Stop oral dosing	If dosage ≥ 4 mg/day at the time oral dosing is stopped, give by SQ infusion, tapering gradually.
Diuretics	Spironolactone	Stop	

Category	Medication	Action	Comments
	Furosemide	Stop oral dosing	If given for overhydration (pleural effusion, ascites, severe edema, signs of heart failure) and if patient is catheterized, continue by IM or IV dosing qd–bid.
Peptic ulcer Rx/prophylaxis	Antacids Sulcralfate H_2 blockers	Stop Stop Stop oral dosing	If symptoms of peptic ulcer, reflux esophagitis, or upper GI bleeding are present, continue ranitidine, 50 mg IV qid or by continuous SQ infusion.
Bronchodilators	Theophylline, etc.	Stop	Albuterol by inhalation with dexamethasone, morphine, and atropine as required by the situation.
Urinary sedatives or antispasmodics	Phenazopyridine Oxybutynin	Stop Stop	If dysuria is a problem in the catheterized patient, irrigate the bladder with lidocaine in saline.
Antidepressants	Amitriptyline, etc.	Stop	None.
Anticoagulants	Warfarin sodium Aspirin	Stop Stop	None.
Antihypertensives and other cardiac medications	All categories	Stop	None.
Hypoglycemics	All categories	Stop	None.
Vitamins	All categories	Stop	None.
Antibiotics	All categories	Stop	None.
Hormonal agents	Thyroid hormone, Tamoxifen, etc.	Stop	None.

- **Hunger and thirst are rare** in the last days of life and can be controlled by simple measures (e.g., moistening the lips and mouth).
- **Enteral feeding should be stopped** when the patient can no longer swallow reliably.
- **Ideally, parenteral fluids should not be given.** Allowing the patient to become slightly dehydrated will prevent or ameliorate many otherwise distressing problems in the last hours:

Consequence of IV Hydration	Symptoms
↑ Respiratory secretions	Cough Pulmonary congestion Sensations of choking and drowning
↑ Urine output	Bedwetting, bedpans, catheters
↑ Gastrointestinal secretions	Vomiting
↑ Total body water	↑ Edema, ascites, pleural effusions
↓ Serum urea	↑ Awareness → ↑ distress, ↓ pain threshold

- **Management of terminal dehydration**:
  - **Explain** to the family that
    - The patient no longer needs significant amounts of food and fluids.
    - The patient does not feel hunger or thirst.
    - Intravenous fluids may increase the patient's discomfort.
  - If, despite explanations, the patient or family is still uncomfortable with a decision to withhold intravenous therapy, give **intravenous or subcutaneous fluids at a rate not exceeding 1 to 1.5 L/day**; use furosemide as needed to control symptoms of overhydration.
  - If parenteral fluids are *not* given, **prevent symptoms of thirst** by
    - Attention to oral hygiene (mouth care every hour by the family).
    - Small sips of fluids.
    - Giving small amounts of crushed ice to suck.

Pain Management During the Last Days and Hours of Life

- Adequate **pain control must be ensured so long as the patient remains alive.**

- Patients may experience pain even when unconscious.
- A patient who has required regular opioid analgesics in the preterminal period will continue to need opioids to remain relatively free of pain.
- In Lichter and Hunt's study (1990), 40% of hospice patients required an *increase* in analgesic dose during the last 48 hours of life; 12% required a decrease; and in 39%, the dosage of analgesics was unchanged.
- When the patient is no longer able to swallow, switch to **continuous SQ infusion** of opioids, starting with one-third to one-half the previous 24-hour oral dosage. (Example: A patient who was taking MS Contin, 150 mg PO bid, should be started on 100–150 mg/24 hr by SQ infusion.)
- In a patient with **new pain** who has not previously taken opioids, start with morphine, 30 mg/24 hr by continuous SQ infusion.
- Movement-related pain ("disturbance pain") during the last hours of life can be minimized by gentle, slow handling and avoiding unnecessary movement of the patient.

Terminal Restlessness

> *As to the motions of the arms...if they move before the face, hunt in the empty air, pluck nap from the bedclothes, pick up bits and snatch chaff from the walls—all these signs are bad, in fact deadly.*
>
> HIPPOCRATES, *PROGNOSTIC,* IV

Restlessness and agitation occur during the last days or hours of life in up to 40% of patients dying of cancer.

Clinical Findings

- Agitation.
- Tossing and turning.
- Moaning.
- Impaired consciousness.
- Myclonic twitching or spasms.
- Clinical picture of terminal restlessness may *overlap* with
  - Delirium (organic brain syndrome).
  - Terminal anguish (mental torment from "unfinished business").

Management of Terminal Restlessness

- Terminal restlessness can be very distressing to the patient and family.
- **Identify and treat reversible causes of restlessness:**
  - Full bladder.
  - Fecal impaction.
  - Pain.
  - Dyspnea (e.g., from hypoxemia, secretions, pulmonary edema).
  - Nausea.
  - Pruritus.
  - Drugs (corticosteroids, neuroleptics).
- Provide **verbal and tactile reassurance.** Instruct family members to
  - Hold the patient's hand or provide other physical contact.
  - Speak quietly to the patient, on the assumption that now and then the patient is conscious enough to hear and understand.
- Pharmacologic management:
  - **Midazolam:** Give a **SQ loading dose** of **5 mg,** and start a **continuous SQ infusion** (by syringe driver) at a rate of **30 mg/24 hr.**
    - If desired effect has not been achieved within an hour, give a second bolus of 3 mg, and increase the infusion rate by 0.5 to 1 mg/hr.
    - Larger dosage may be required when restlessness is accompanied by multifocal myoclonus.
    - Median dosage required is 35 mg/24 hr (range = 10–240 mg/24 hr).
    - Midazolam may be combined with other medications (morphine, metoclopramide) in the same syringe.
  - Some centers use **chlorpromazine** as an alternative to midazolam.
    - Chlorpromazine is equally effective for terminal restlessness and also relieves preterminal dyspnea.
    - The cost of midazolam is 30 to 100 times higher than that of chlorpromazine.
    - Dosage of chlorpromazine for terminal restlessness and dyspnea:
      - **12.5 mg IV q4–12h,** *or*
      - 25 mg PR q4–12h (useful for home care).

Death Rattle

Definition

Noisy terminal respirations caused by the presence of secretions in the airway (usually the upper airway) in patients who are too weak to cough effectively.

Management of the Death Rattle

- Treatment must involve both the patient and the family.
  - The **patient is usually unaware** of the noise and undisturbed by the secretions.
  - **Families**, however, **find the noise very disturbing**; they need to be prepared for the noise and reassured that it does not signal distress on the part of the patient.
- As a first step, **reposition the patient** (e.g., from supine to lateral recumbent).
- Noise can be further minimized by giving agents that dry respiratory secretions, if those agents are given *at the onset of symptoms*:
  - **Furosemide**, 20–40 mg IV +
  - **Atropine**, 1 to 2 mg IM, *or* scopolamine, 0.3 to 0.6 mg IM/SQ q4h.
  - By inhalation, **via nebulizer**: atropine, 2 mg + morphine, 2.5 mg + dexamethasone, 2 mg.
  - Another, less invasive approach, which may be particularly useful in patients being cared for at home, is to apply a **scopolamine patch** behind one ear. The patch usually takes effect within a few hours to dry secretions and minimize death rattle.
  - Since all these medications also cause dryness of the mouth, the patient's mouth should be wiped periodically with a moistened gauze pad.
- If secretions are persistent and copious, gentle **suctioning** may be used but should be kept to an absolute minimum, since suctioning disturbs the patient.

Control of Other Symptoms

- The control of most symptoms during the last hours of life is simply a continuation of the measures already taken, with changes from oral to parenteral drugs as required.

- Every effort should be made to **use multipurpose drugs** to minimize the total number of medications the patient must be given (e.g., hydroxyzine as an antiemetic, mild sedative, and analgesic).
- For information on control of specific symptoms, see relevant chapters (e.g., dyspnea, cough, nausea and vomiting, confusional states, seizures).

Support of the Patient's Family During the Agonal Period

- The impending death of a loved one is a **stressful event** and produces signs of stress.
  - Those close to the dying patient may not always behave rationally or decorously.
  - People under stress need
    - **Guidance** ("You can sit and stroke his arm like this, to let him know that you're nearby.").
    - **Information**, for example:
      ○ The patient can still hear from time to time and be aware of your presence even when he seems to be unconscious.
      ○ Noisy or grunting respirations do not mean that the patient is in distress.
      ○ The patient is not suffering from hunger or thirst.
    - **Support**:
      ○ Permission to have conflicting feelings ("Many people in circumstances like yours wish that death will come quickly to their loved one, to end his suffering, and then they feel guilty for wishing something like that. Maybe you've felt the same way.").
      ○ Encouragement to stay with the patient, but also
      ○ Permission to be absent if the death vigil becomes exhausting or overwhelming.
- When death occurs:
  - Be prepared to deal with the family's grief, which may express itself in various ways:
    - Sadness, weeping.
    - Anger, sometimes directed at the medical team.
    - Guilt.
    - Apathy.
    - Physical symptoms (e.g., fainting, hyperventilation syndrome, chest pain).

- Allow the family time alone with the body.
- Help the family to contact those most important to them and to make necessary arrangements.

References and Further Reading

Back IN. Terminal restlessness in patients with advanced malignant disease. *Palliative Med* 6:293, 1992.

Billings JA. Comfort measures for the terminally ill: Is dehydration painful? *Am Geriatr Soc* 33:808, 1985.

Bottomley DM, Hanks GW. Subcutaneous midazolam infusion in palliative care. *J Pain Symptom Manage* 7:94, 1990.

Burke AL, Diamond PL, Hulbert J, et al. Terminal restlessness—its management and the role of midazolam. *Med J Aust* 155:485, 1991.

Dawson HR. The use of transdermal scopolamine in the control of death rattle. *J Palliative Care* 5:31, 1989.

Fainsinger R, Bruera E. The management of dehydration in terminally ill patients. *J Palliative Care* 10(3):55, 1994.

Johanson GA. Midazolam in terminal care. *Am J Hospice Palliative Care* 10(1):13, 1993.

Lamerton R. Dehydration in dying patients. *Lancet* 337:981, 1991.

Lichter I, Hunt E. The last 48 hours of life. *J Palliative Care* 6:7, 1990.

Lombard DJ, Oliver DJ. The use of opioid analgesics in the last 24 hours of life in patients with advanced cancer. *Palliative Med* 3:27, 1989.

McCann RM, Hall WJ, Groth-Juncker A. Comfort care for terminally ill patients: The appropriate use of nutrition and hydration. *JAMA* 272:1263, 1994.

McNamara P, Minton M, Twycross RG. Use of midazolam in palliative care. *Palliative Med* 5:244, 1991.

Melver B, Walsh D, Nelson K. The use of chlorpromazine for symptom control in dying cancer patients. *J Pain Symptom Manage* 9:341, 1994.

Oliver D. Terminal dehydration. *Lancet* ii:631, 1984.

Terminal dehydration (editorial). *Lancet* i:301, 1986.

Ventafridda V, Ripamonti C, deConno F, et al. Symptom prevalence and control during cancer patients' last days of life. *J Palliative Care* 6:7, 1990.

Waller A, Hershkowitz M, Adunsky A. The effect of intravenous fluid infusion on blood and urine parameters of hydration and on the state of consciousness in terminal cancer patients. *Am J Hospice Palliative Care* 11(6):22, 1994.

Witzel L. Behaviour of the dying patient. *Br Med J* 2:81, 1975.

Appendices

Appendix 1.A

Drugs Used in Palliative Care: Generic and Trade Names of Commonly Used Drugs

There is considerable variation throughout the English-speaking world among the trade names (and even some generic names) of medications. In this table, we summarize generic and trade names in some English-speaking countries of medications commonly used in palliative care. Not all of the drugs listed are available in all countries.

Medications are listed alphabetically in the left-hand column. If the name is a GENERIC NAME, it is given in capital letters; if the name is a trade name, it is in lower case. In the middle column are listed the equivalent generic or trade names, as the case may be, for each citation. For each drug, an indication of its class or principal actions is listed in the right-hand column.

For drugs marketed outside the United States, the symbol (C) following a drug name indicates a Canadian trade name, the symbol (UK) indicates a British trade name, and the symbol (AU) indicates an Australian trade name. Where the symbol follows a *generic* name, it means that the drug is available in that country only and not in the United States.

Drug		Class or Principal Action
Abitren	DICLOFENAC	NSAID
Abrol	ACETAMINOPHEN (PARACETAMOL)	Analgesic, antipyretic
Acamol	ACETAMINOPHEN (PARACETAMOL)	Analgesic, antipyretic
ACETAMINOPHEN	Abrol, Acamol, Dexamol, Panadol, Tylenol	Analgesic, antipyretic
Acilac (C)	LACTULOSE	Osmotic cathartic
ACTIVATED CHARCOAL	Charcoal Plus, Carbosylane	Antiflatulent
Acupan	NEFOPAM	NSAID
ACYCLOVIR	Zovirax	Antiviral
Adolan	METHADONE	Opioid agonist
Advil	IBUPROFEN	NSAID
Aerolin (UK)	ALBUTEROL (SALBUTAMOL)	β_2-Adrenergic agonist
ALBUTEROL (SALBUTAMOL)	Aerolin (UK), Proventil, Salamol (UK), Ventolin	β_2-Adrenergic agonist
Aldactone	SPIRONOLACTONE	K+-sparing diuretic
Algolysin	PROPOXYPHENE HCL	Weak opioid agonist
Allegron (UK)	NORTRIPTYLINE	Tricyclic antidepressant
ALPRAZOLAM	Xanax	Benzodiazepine
Amersol (C)	IBUPROFEN	NSAID
Amitril (C)	AMITRIPTYLINE	Tricyclic antidepressant
Amitrip (AU)	AMITRIPTYLINE	Tricyclic antidepressant
AMITRIPTYLINE	Amitril (C), Amitrip (AU), Elatrol, Elavil, Eltrafon, Lentizol (UK), Levate (C), Novotriptyn (C), Saroten (AU), Triavil, Tryptanol (AU), Tryptizol (UK)	Tricyclic antidepressant
AMPHOTERICIN B lozenges	Fungilin (UK)	Antifungal lozenge for oral candidiasis
Anaprox	NAPROXEN SODIUM	NSAID
Ansaid	FLURBIPROFEN	NSAID

Drug		Class or Principal Action
Antenax (AU)	DIAZEPAM	Benzodiazepine
Antepsin (UK)	SUCRALFATE	Sulfated aluminum anti-peptic ulcer agent
Anti-naus (AU)	PROCHLORPERAZINE	Phenothiazine
Antivert	MECLIZINE	Antihistamine, anti-motion sickness
Anxanil	HYDROXYZINE	Antihistamine with analgesic properties
Apo-Diazepam (C)	DIAZEPAM	Benzodiazepine
Apo-Dimenhydrinate (C)	DIMENHYDRINATE	Antihistamine antiemetic
Apo-piroxicam (C)	PIROXICAM	NSAID
Apo-Sulfatrim (C)	TRIMETHOPRIM-SULFAMETHOXAZOLE	Antibiotic
Aquamide (AU)	FUROSEMIDE	Diuretic
Aredia	PAMIDRONATE	Biphosphonate
Arret	LOPERAMIDE	Antidiarrheal opioid
Assival	DIAZEPAM	Benzodiazepine
Astramorph	MORPHINE SULFATE injection	Opioid agonist
Atarax	HYDROXYZINE	Antihistamine
Ativan	LORAZEPAM	Benzodiazepine
Atrofen	BACLOFEN	Skeletal muscle relaxant
Atrovent	IPRATROPIUM BROMIDE	Anticholinergic bronchodilator
Aventyl	NORTRIPTYLINE	Tricyclic antidepressant
Avilac	LACTULOSE	Osmotic cathartic
B & O Supprettes	ATROPINE + OPIUM suppositories	Anticholinergic/opioid
BACLOFEN	Atrofen, Baclosal, Lioresal	Skeletal muscle relaxant
Baclosal	BACLOFEN	Skeletal muscle relaxant
Bactrim	TRIMETHOPRIM-SULFAMETHOXAZOLE	Antibiotic
Baridium	PHENAZOPYRIDINE	Bladder local anesthetic

Drug		Class or Principal Action
Benadryl	DIPHENHYDRAMINE	Antihistamine
BENZOCAINE oral pastes	Orajel, Orabase with Benzocaine	Local anesthetic for oral pain
BENZTROPINE MESYLATE	Cogentin	Antiparkinsonian
BENZYDAMINE (AU, C, UK)	Bioplex (UK), Bioral Gel (UK), Difflam (UK), Easy Gel (C), Tantum (AU)	NSAID with local anesthetic action
BETAMETHASONE DIPROPIONATE	Diprolene, Lotrisone	Corticosteroid cream
Bioplex (UK)	BENZYDAMINE (C, UK)	NSAID with local anesthetic action
Bioral Gel (UK)	BENZYDAMINE (C, UK)	NSAID with local anesthetic action
BISACODYL	Bisalax (AU), Contalax, Dulcolax, Dulco-Lax (UK), Durolax, Laxadin, Raykit, Toilex (AU)	Stimulant laxative
Bisalax (AU)	BISACODYL	Stimulant laxative
Bonamine (C)	MECLIZINE	Antihistamine antiemetic
Bonefos (UK)	CLODRONATE	Biphosphonate
Bonine	MECLIZINE	Antihistamine antiemetic
Brufen (UK)	IBUPROFEN	NSAID
Buccastem (AU, UK)	PROCHLORPERAZINE (buccal preparation)	Phenothiazine antiemetic
BUPIVACAINE HCL	Marcaine	Local anesthetic
Buprenex	BUPRENORPHINE	Opioid partial agonist
BUPRENORPHINE	Buprenex, Nopan, Temgesic (UK)	Opioid partial agonist
Buscopan (UK)	HYOSCINE BUTYL-BROMIDE (UK)	Anticholinergic antispasmodic
BUTORPHANOL	Stadol	Opioid agonist-antagonist
Caprin (UK)	ACETYLSALICYLIC ACID (ASPIRIN)	NSAID
CAPSAICIN	Zostrix	Irritant analgesic

Drug		Class or Principal Action
Carafate	SULCRALFATE	Sulfated aluminum anti–peptic ulcer agent
CARBAMAZEPINE	Epitol, Mazepime, Novo-Carbamaz (C),Tegretol	Anticonvulsant
Carbosylane	ACTIVATED CHARCOAL + SIMETHICONE	Antiflatulent
CARMELLOSE solutions	Glandosane, Luborant (UK), Salivace (UK)	Artificial saliva
CASANTHRANOL + DOCUSATE	Peri-Colace	Stimulant laxative + stool softener
Cephulac	LACTULOSE	Osmotic cathartic
Charcoal Plus	ACTIVATED CHARCOAL + SIMETHICONE	Antiflatulent
Chlorazine	PROCHLORPERAZINE	Phenothiazine
CHLORHEXIDINE mouthwash (UK)	Corsodyl (UK), Eludril (UK)	Antiplaque rinse for oral hygiene
Chlor-Promanyl (C)	CHLORPROMAZINE	Phenothiazine
CHLORPROMAZINE	Chlor-Promanyl (C), Largactil (C, UK), Ormazine, Procalm (AU), Promacid (AU), Promaz,Thorazine	Phenothiazine
CHOLINE MAGNESIUM TRISALICYLATE	Trilisate	NSAID
CHOLINE SALICYLATE (UK)	Teegel (UK)	Salicylate oral gel
Chronulac	LACTULOSE	Osmotic cathartic
CIMETIDINE	Dyspamet (UK),Tagamet	H_2 blocker
CISAPRIDE	Prepulsid (UK), Propulsid	Promoter of GI tract motility
Clinoril	SULINDAC	NSAID
CLODRONATE (UK)	Bonefos (UK), Loron (UK), Ostac	Biphosphonate
CLONAZEPAM	Clonex, Klonopin, Rivotril (C, UK)	Benzodiazepine anti-spasmodic
Clonex	CLONAZEPAM	Benzodiazepine anti-spasmodic

Drug		Class or Principal Action
CLOTRIMAZOLE lozenge	Mycelex	Antifungal lozenge for oral candidiasis
Codalax	CO-DANTHRAMER	Stimulant laxative
CO-DANTHRAMER	Codalax	Stimulant laxative
CO-DANTHRUSATE	Normax	Stimulant laxative
Cogentin	BENZTROPINE MESYLATE	Antiparkinsonian
Colace	DOCUSATE	Stool softener
Colax-C (C)	DOCUSATE	Stool softener
Coloxyl (AU)	DOCUSATE	Stool softener
Compazine	PROCHLORPERAZINE	Phenothiazine
Contalax	BISACODYL	Stimulant laxative
Convulex (UK)	VALPROIC ACID	Anticonvulsant
Cyclimorph (UK)	MORPHINE-CYCLIZINE injection	Opioid agonist + antihistamine antiemetic
CYCLIZINE	Marzine (C), Marezine (C), Mazerine, Valoid (UK)	Antihistamine antiemetic
CYCLOBENZAPRINE	Flexeril	Skeletal muscle relaxant
Cyklokapron	TRANEXAMIC ACID	Plasmin/plasminogen inhibitor
Cylert	PEMOLINE	Central nervous system stimulant
Cystrin (UK)	OXYBUTYNIN	Smooth muscle antispasmodic (bladder)
Cytotec	MISOPROSTOL	Synthetic prostaglandin E_1 analog
Daktarin (UK)	MICONAZOLE	Antifungal
Dantoin	DIPHENYLHYDANTOIN	Anticonvulsant
Dantrium	DANTROLENE	Skeletal muscle relaxant
DANTROLENE	Dantrium	Skeletal muscle relaxant
Darvon	PROPOXYPHENE HCL (DEXTROPROPOX-YPHENE)	Weak opioid agonist
Daypro	OXAPROZIN	NSAID
Decadron	DEXAMETHASONE	Corticosteroid

Drug		Class or Principal Action
Decasone	DEXAMETHASONE	Corticosteroid
Delaxin	METHOCARBAMOL	Skeletal muscle relaxant
Demerol	MEPERIDINE, PETHIDINE	Opioid agonist
Depakene	VALPROIC ACID	Anticonvulsant
Deprexan	DESIPRAMINE	Tricyclic antidepressant
Deronil (C)	DEXAMETHASONE	Corticosteroid
DESIPRAMINE	Deprexan, Norpramine, Pertofrane	Tricyclic antidepressant
Dexacort	DEXAMETHASONE	Corticosteroid
DEXAMETHASONE	Decadron, Decasone (C), Deronil (C), Dexacort, Hexadrol, Maridex (C), Oradexon (AU)	Corticosteroid
Dexamol	ACETAMINOPHEN (PARACETAMOL)	Analgesic, antipyretic
Dexasone (C)	DEXAMETHASONE	Corticosteroid
Dexedrine	DEXTROAMPHETAMINE SULFATE	Amphetamine
DEXTROAMPHETAMINE SULFATE	Dexedrine	Amphetamine
DEXTROPROPOXYPHENE	Algolysin, Darvon	Opioid agonist (weak)
DF 118 Forte (UK)	DIHYDROCODEINE (UK)	Opioid agonist
DHC Continus (UK)	DIHYDROCODEINE (UK)	Opioid agonist
Diagesil (UK)	HEROIN (DIAMORPHINE) (UK)	Opioid agonist
Dialar (UK)	DIAZEPAM	Benzodiazepine
Dialose	DOCUSATE	Stool softener
DIAMORPHINE HCL (HEROIN) (UK)	Diagesil (UK)	Opioid agonist
Diaphine (UK)	HEROIN (DIAMORPHINE) (UK)	Opioid agonist
Diastatin (AU)	NYSTATIN	Antifungal

Drug		Class or Principal Action
DIAZEPAM	Antenax (AU), Apo-Diazepam (C), Assival, Dialar (UK), Ducene (AU), Meval (C), Novodipam (C), Stesolid, Valium	Benzodiazepine
Di-Azo	PHENAZOPYRIDINE	Bladder local anesthetic
DIBUCAINE	Nupercainal	Local anesthetic ointment
DICLOFENAC	Abitren, Diclomax (UK), Motifene (UK), Voltarol, Volteran	NSAID
Diclomax Retard (UK)	DICLOFENAC	NSAID
Didronel	ETIDRONATE	Biphosphonate
Difflam (UK)	BENZYDAMINE (C, UK)	NSAID with local anesthetic action
Diflucan	FLUCONAZOLE	Antifungal
DIFLUNISAL	Dolobid	NSAID
DIHYDROCODEINE	DF 118 Forte (UK), DHC Continus (UK), Fortuss (AU), Paracodin (AU), Synalgos	Opioid agonist
Dilantin	PHENYTOIN	Anticonvulsant
Dilaudid	HYDROMORPHONE	Opioid agonist
DIMENHYDRINATE	Apo-Dimenhydrinate (C), Dramamine, Gravol (C), Travamine (C)	Antihistamine antiemetic
Dioctyl (UK)	DOCUSATE	Stool softener
DIPHENHYDRAMINE	Benadryl	Antihistamine
DIPHENOXYLATE	Lomotil	Antidiarrheal
Diprolene cream	BETAMETHASONE DIPROPIONATE cream	Corticosteroid cream
Ditropan	OXYBUTYNIN	Antispasmodic (bladder)
DOCUSATE	Colace, Colax (C), Coloxyl (AU), Dialose, Dioctyl (UK), Doxate (C), Norgalax Microenema (UK), Regulex (C)	Stool softener

Drug		Class or Principal Action
Dolobid	DIFLUNISAL	NSAID
Dolophine	METHADONE	Opioid agonist
Doloxene (C)	PROPOXYPHENE	Opioid agonist
DOMPERIDONE (AU, UK)	Evoxin (UK), Motilium (AU, UK)	Promoter of GI tract motility
Dormicum	MIDAZOLAM	Benzodiazepine
Doxate C (C)	DOCUSATE	Stool softener
Dozic	HALOPERIDOL	Neuroleptic, antiemetic
Dramamine	DIMENHYDRINATE	Antihistamine antiemetic
DRONABINOL	Marinol	Cannabinoid antiemetic-antianorectic
Dryptal	FRUSEMIDE (FUROSEMIDE)	Diuretic
Ducene (AU)	DIAZEPAM	Benzodiazepine
Dulco-Lax (UK)	BISACODYL	Stimulant laxative
Dulcolax	BISACODYL	Stimulant laxative
Duphalac	LACTULOSE	Osmotic cathartic
Duragesic	FENTANYL	Opioid agonist (transdermal)
Duramorph	MORPHINE SULFATE injection	Opioid agonist
Durolax (AU)	BISACODYL	Stimulant laxative
Dysman (UK)	MEFENAMIC ACID	NSAID
Dyspamet (UK)	CIMETIDINE	H_2 blocker
Easy Gel (C)	BENZYDAMINE	NSAID with local anesthetic action
Elatrol	AMITRIPTYLINE	Tricyclic antidepressant
Elavil	AMITRIPTYLINE	Tricyclic antidepressant
Emex (C)	METOCLOPRAMIDE	Antidopaminergic GI motility promoter
Encypalmed	PANCREATIN combination product	Pancreatic enzyme replacement
Endone (AU)	OXYCODONE	Opioid agonist

Drug		Class or Principal Action
Epanutin (UK)	PHENYTOIN	Anticonvulsant
Epilim (UK)	VALPROIC ACID	Anticonvulsant
Epimorph (C)	MORPHINE SULFATE	Opioid agonist
Epitol	CARBAMAZEPINE	Anticonvulsant
ETIDRONATE	Didronel	Biphosphonate
Etrafon	AMITRIPTYLINE	Tricyclic antidepressant
Euhypnos	TEMAZEPAM	Benzodiazepine
Evoxin (UK)	DOMPERIDONE (UK)	Promoter of GI tract motility
FAMOTIDINE	Gastro, Pepcid	H$_2$ blocker
Feldene	PIROXICAM	NSAID
Fenbid (UK)	IBUPROFEN	NSAID
FENBUFEN	Lederfen (UK)	NSAID
FENOPROFEN	Fenopron (UK), Nalfon, Progesic (UK)	NSAID
Fenopron (UK)	FENOPROFEN	NSAID
FENTANYL (transdermal)	Duragesic	Opioid agonist
FENTANYL (transmucosal)	Fentanyl Oralet	Opioid agonist for buccal administration
Flagyl	METRONIDAZOLE	Antibacterial, antiprotozoal
FLAVOXATE HCL	Urispas	Urinary tract spasmolytic
FLECAINIDE	Tambocor	Local anesthetic, antiarrhythmic
Fleet	PHOSPHOSODA	Enema
Flexeril	CYCLOBENZAPRINE	Skeletal muscle relaxant
FLUCONAZOLE	Diflucan	Antifungal
FLUNITRAZEPAM (UK)	Hypnodorm, Rohypnol (UK)	Benzodiazepine hypnotic
FLUOXETINE	Prozac	Antidepressant
FLUPHENAZINE	Prolixin, Fludecate	Phenothiazine
FLURBIPROFEN	Ansaid, Froben	NSAID

Drug		Class or Principal Action
Fortral	PENTAZOCINE	Opioid agonist-antagonist
Fortunan	HALOPERIDOL	Neuroleptic, antiemetic
Fortuss (AU)	DIHYDROCODEINE	Opioid agonist
Froben (UK)	FLURBIPROFEN	NSAID
FRUSEMIDE (FURO-SEMIDE)	Aquamide (AU), Dryptal, Frusid (AU, UK), Fusid, Lasix, Novosemide (C), Uremide, Uritol (C)	Diuretic
Frusid (AU, UK)	FRUSEMIDE (FURO-SEMIDE)	Diuretic
Fungilin (UK)	AMPHOTERICIN B	Antifungal lozenge for oral candidiasis
FUROSEMIDE (FRUSE-MIDE)	Aquamide (AU), Dryptal, Frusid (AU, UK), Fusid, Lasix, Novosemide (C), Uremide (AU), Uritol (C)	Diuretic
Fusid	FRUSEMIDE (FURO-SEMIDE)	Diuretic
Gastro	FAMOTIDINE	H_2 blocker
Gastrobid	METOCLOPRAMIDE	Antidopaminergic GI motility promoter
Glandosane	CARMELLOSE solution	Artificial saliva
GRANESITRON	Kytril	5-HT_3-blocking antiemetic
Gravol (C)	DIMENHYDRINATE	Antihistamine antiemetic
Halcion	TRIAZOLAM	Benzodiazepine hypnotic
Haldol	HALOPERIDOL	Neuroleptic, antiemetic
Haley's MO	MILK OF MAGNESIA + MINERAL OIL	Stimulant laxative
Halidol	HALOPERIDOL	Neuroleptic, antiemetic
HALOPERIDOL	Dozic, Fortunan, Haldol, Halidol, Novoperidol (C), Pacedol (AU), Peridol (C), Serenace (AU, UK)	Neuroleptic, antiemetic

Drug		Class or Principal Action
HEROIN (DIAMOR-PHINE HCL) (UK)	Diagesil (UK)	Opioid agonist
Hexadrol	DEXAMETHASONE	Corticosteroid
Hexakapron	TRANEXAMIC ACID	Plasmin/plasminogen inhibitor
Hyalase (UK)	HYALURONIDASE	Enzymatic diffusing substance (hypodermoclysis)
HYALURONIDASE	Wydase, Hyalase (UK)	Enzymatic diffusing substance (hypodermoclysis)
HYDROCODONE	Lortab, Vicodin (with acetaminophen)	Opioid agonist
HYDROMORPHONE	Dilaudid	Opioid agonist
HYDROXYZINE	Anxanil, Atarax, Marax, Ulcerax (UK), Vistaril	Antihistamine with analgesic properties
HYOSCINE BUTYL-BROMIDE (UK)	Buscopan (UK), Pamine	Anticholinergic antispasmodic
HYOSCINE (SCOPO-LAMINE) HYDRO-BROMIDE	Isopto Hyoscine, Triptone	Anticholinergic
HYOSCINE (SCOPO-LAMINE) HYDRO-BROMIDE transdermal	Scopoderm, Transderm Scop	Anticholinergic
Hypnodorm	FLUNITRAZEPAM (UK)	Benzodiazepine hypnotic
Hypnovel	MIDAZOLAM	Benzodiazepine
IBUPROFEN	Advil, Amersol (C), Brufen, Fenbid (UK), Motrin	NSAID
Imbrilon (UK)	INDOMETHACIN	NSAID
IMIPRAMINE	Impril (C), Novopramin (C), Tofranil	Tricyclic antidepressant
Imodium	LOPERAMIDE	Antidiarrheal opioid
Impril (C)	IMIPRAMINE	Tricyclic antidepressant
Indocin	INDOMETHACIN	NSAID
Indomax (UK)	INDOMETHACIN	NSAID

Drug		Class or Principal Action
INDOMETHACIN	Imbrilon (UK), Indocin, Indomax (UK), Indomed, Mobilan (UK)	NSAID
IPRATROPRIUM BROMIDE	Atrovent	Anticholinergic bronchodilator
Ketalar	KETAMINE	Dissociative anesthetic
KETAMINE	Ketalar	Dissociative anesthetic
KETOCONAZOLE	Nizoral	Antifungal
KETOPROFEN	Orudis (UK)	NSAID
KETOROLAC	Topadol, Toradol	NSAID
Klonopin	CLONAZEPAM	Benzodiazepine (antispasmodic, anticonvulsant)
Korostatin	NYSTATIN	Antifungal
Kytril	GRANISETRON	$5-HT_3$-blocking antiemetic
LACTULOSE	Acilac (C), Avilac, Cephalac, Chronulac, Duphalac	Osmotic cathartic
Laractone (UK)	SPIRONOLACTONE	K^+-sparing diuretic
Largactil (C, UK)	CHLORPROMAZINE	Phenothiazine
Lasilactone (UK)	FUROSEMIDE/ SPIRONOLACTONE	Loop diuretic + K^+-sparing diuretic
Lasix	FUROSEMIDE	Diuretic
Laxadin	BISACODYL	Stimulant laxative
Lederfen (UK)	FENBUFEN	NSAID
Lentizol (UK)	AMITRIPTYLINE	Tricyclic antidepressant
Levate (C)	AMITRIPTYLINE	Tricyclic antidepressant
Levo-Dromoran	LEVORPHANOL	Opioid agonist
LEVOMEPROMAZINE (METHOTRIMEPRAZINE)	Levoprome, Nozinan (C, UK)	Phenothiazine with antihistaminic and analgesic properties
LEVORPHANOL	Levo-Dromoran	Opioid agonist
LIDOCAINE	Xylocaine	Local anesthetic
LIGNOCAINE	Xylocaine	Local anesthetic

Drug		Class or Principal Action
Lioresal	BACLOFEN	Skeletal muscle relaxant
Lomotil	DIPHENOXYLATE + ATROPINE	Antidiarrheal
LOPERAMIDE	Arret, Imodium	Antidiarrheal opioid
LORAZEPAM	Ativan, Lorivan, Novo-lorazepam (C)	Benzodiazepine
Lorivan	LORAZEPAM	Benzodiazepine
Loron (UK)	CLODRONATE (UK)	Biphosphonate
Lortab	HYDROCODONE + ACETAMINOPHEN	Opioid/NSAID
Losec (UK)	OMEPRAZOLE	Benzimidazole gastric acid pump inhibitor
Lotrisone cream	BETAMETHASONE DI-PROPIONATE cream	Corticosteroid cream
Luminal	PHENOBARBITAL SODIUM	Barbiturate
Maalox	ALUMINUM HYDROX-IDE + MAGNESIUM HYDROXIDE	Antacid
Magel	ALUMINUM HYDROX-IDE + MAGNESIUM HYDROXIDE	Antacid
Marax	HYDROXYZINE	Antihistamine with analgesic properties
Marcaine	BUPIVACAINE HCL	Local anesthetic
Marezine	CYCLIZINE	Antihistamine anti-emetic
Marinol	DRONABINOL	Cannabinoid antiemetic-antianorectic
Marzine (C)	CYCLIZINE	Antihistamine anti-emetic
Maxeran (C)	METOCLOPRAMIDE	Antidopaminergic GI motility promoter
Maxidex (C)	DEXAMETHASONE	Corticosteroid
Maxolon (AU, C, UK)	METOCLOPRAMIDE	Antidopaminergic GI motility promoter
Mazepime	CARBAMAZEPINE	Anticonvulsant

Drug		Class or Principal Action
MCR	Controlled-release MORPHINE SULFATE	Opioid agonist
MECLIZINE	Antivert, Bonamine (C), Bonine, Sea Legs (UK)	Antihistamine
MECLOFENAMATE	Meclomen	NSAID
Meclomen	MECLOFENAMATE	NSAID
Medrol	METHYLPREDNISO-LONE	Corticosteroid
MEFENAMIC ACID	Dysman (UK), Ponstan (C), Ponstel	NSAID
Megace	MEGESTROL ACETATE	Progestational agent, antianorectic
MEGESTROL ACETATE	Megace, Pallace	Progestational agent, antianorectic
Mepergan	MEPERIDINE (PETHI-DINE)	Opioid agonist
MEPERIDINE (PETHI-DINE)	Demerol, Mepergan, Pamergan (UK)	Opioid agonist
Metamide (AU)	METOCLOPRAMIDE	Antidopaminergic GI motility promoter
Metamucil	PSYLLIUM	Bulk-forming stool softener
Metastron	STRONTIUM-89	Radioisotope for meta-static bone pain
METHADONE	Aldolan, Dolophine, Methadose, Physep-tone (C, UK)	Opioid agonist
Methadose	METHADONE	Opioid agonist
Methidate	METHYLPHENIDATE	CNS stimulant
METHOCARBAMOL	Delaxin, Robaxin	Centrally-acting muscle relaxant
METHOTRIMEPRAZINE (LEVOMEPROMA-ZINE)	Levoprome, Nozinan (C, UK)	Phenothiazine with antihistaminic and analgesic properties
METHSCOPOLAMINE BROMIDE	Pamine	Anticholinergic anti-spasmodic
METHYLPHENIDATE	Methidate, Ritalin	Central nervous sys-tem stimulant

Drug		Class or Principal Action
METHYLPREDNISO-LONE	Medrol	Corticosteroid
METOCLOPRAMIDE	Emex (C), Gastrobid (UK), Maxerin (C), Maxolon (AU, C, UK), Metamide (AU), Metramid, Parmid (UK), Pramin (AU), Primperan (AU, UK), Reglan	Antidopaminergic GI motility promoter
Metramid (UK)	METOCLOPRAMIDE	Antidopaminergic GI motility promoter
MetroGel	METRONIDAZOLE Gel	Antifungal
METRONIDAZOLE	Flagyl, MetroGel, Novonidazol (C), Rosex Gel	Antifungal
Meval (C)	DIAZEPAM	Benzodiazepine
MEXILETINE	Mexitil	Orally-active local anesthetic
Mexitil	MEXILETINE	Orally-active local anesthetic
MICONAZOLE	Daktarin (UK)	Antifungal
MIDAZOLAM	Dormicum, Hypnovel, Versed	Benzodiazepine
MIR	Immediate-release MORPHINE SULFATE	Opioid agonist
MISOPROSTOL	Cytotec	Synthetic prostaglandin E_1 analog
Mobilan (UK)	INDOMETHACIN	NSAID
MORPHINE HCL (C)	Morphitec (C), M.O.S. (C)	Opioid agonist
MORPHINE SULFATE, immediate release	Epimorph (C), MIR, MSIR, Sevredol (UK), Statex (C)	Opioid agonist
MORPHINE SULFATE, controlled release	MCR, MS Contin, MS Continus (UK), Roxanol	Opioid agonist
MORPHINE SULFATE suppository	MSP, RMS	Opioid agonist
Morphitec (C)	MORPHINE HCL (C)	Opioid agonist

Drug		Class or Principal Action
M.O.S. (C)	MORPHINE HCL (C)	Opioid agonist
Motifene (UK)	DICLOFENAC	NSAID
Motililum	DOMPERIDONE (AU, UK)	Dopamine antagonist that promotes GI motility
Motrin	IBUPROFEN	NSAID
MS Contin	Controlled-release MORPHINE SULFATE	Opioid agonist
MSIR	MORPHINE SULFATE	Opioid agonist
MSP	MORPHINE SULFATE suppository	Opioid agonist
MST Continus (UK)	Sustained-release MORPHINE SULFATE	Opioid agonist
Mycelex lozenge	CLOTRIMAZOLE	Antifungal lozenge for oral candidiasis
Mycolog	NYSTATIN	Antifungal
Mycostatin	NYSTATIN	Antifungal
Mylanta	MAGNESIUM HYDROXIDE + ALUMINUM HYDROXIDE	Antacid
NALBUPHINE	Nubain	Opioid agonist-antagonist
Nalfon	FENOPROFEN	NSAID
NALOXONE	Narcan	Opioid antagonist
Napratec (UK)	NAPROXEN	NSAID
Naprosyn	NAPROXEN	NSAID
NAPROXEN	Naxen (C), Naxyn, Napratec (UK), Naprosyn, Nycopren (UK)	NSAID
NAPROXEN SODIUM	Anaprox, Synflex (UK)	NSAID
Narcan	NALOXONE	Opioid antagonist
Navoban	TROPISETRON	5-HT$_3$-blocking anti-emetic
Naxen (C)	NAPROXEN	NSAID
Naxyn	NAPROXEN	NSAID
NEFOPAM	Acupan	NSAID

Drug		Class or Principal Action
Nembutal	PENTOBARBITAL	Barbiturate
Nilstat	NYSTATIN	Antifungal
Nizoral	KETOCONAZOLE	Antifungal
Nopan	BUPRENORPHINE	Opioid partial agonist
Norgalax Micro-enema (UK)	DOCUSATE	Stool softener
Normax	CO-DANTHRUSATE	Stimulant laxative
Normison	TEMAZEPAM	Benzodiazepine
Norpramine	DESIPRAMINE	Tricyclic antidepressant
NORTRIPTYLINE	Allegron (UK), Aventyl, Pamelor	Tricyclic antidepressant
Novatrimel (C)	TRIMETHOPRIM–SULFAMETHOXA-ZOLE	Antibiotic
Novitropan	OXYBUTYNIN	Smooth muscle anti-spasmodic
Novo-Carbamaz (C)	CARBAMAZEPINE	Anticonvulsant
Novodipam (C)	DIAZEPAM	Benzodiazepine
Novolorazepam	LORAZEPAM	Benzodiazepine
Novonidazol (C)	METRONIDAZOLE	Antifungal
Novoperidol (C)	HALOPERIDOL	Neuroleptic, antiemetic
Novopirocam (C)	PIROXICAM	NSAID
Novopramine (C)	IMIPRAMINE	Tricyclic antidepressant
Novosemide (C)	FUROSEMIDE	Diuretic
Novo-Spiroton (C)	SPIRONOLACTONE	K⁺-sparing diuretic
Novotriptyn (C)	AMITRIPTYLINE	Tricyclic antidepressant
Novoxapam (C)	OXAZEPAM	Benzodiazepine
Nozinan (C, UK)	METHOTRIMEPRAZINE (LEVOMEPROMA-ZINE)	Phenothiazine with antihistaminic and analgesic properties
Nubain	NALBUPHINE	Opioid agonist-antagonist
Numorphan	OYXMORPHONE	Opioid agonist
Nupercainal	DIBUCAINE	Local anesthetic ointment

Drug		Class or Principal Action
Nutrizym (UK)	PANCREATIN	Pancreatic enzymes
Nycopren (UK)	NAPROXEN	NSAID
Nystan	NYSTATIN	Antifungal
NYSTATIN	Diastatin (AU), Korostatin, Mycolog, Mycostatin, Nilstat, Nystan	Antifungal
OCTREOTIDE	Sandostatin	Somatostatin analog
OMEPRAZOLE	Losec (UK), Prilosec	Benzimidazole gastric acid pump inhibitor
ONDANSETRON	Zofran	$5\text{-}HT_3$-blocking antiemetic
Orabase with benzocaine	BENZOCAINE	Local anesthetic for oral pain
Oradexon (AU)	DEXAMETHASONE	Corticosteroid
Orajel	BENZOCAINE	Local anesthetic for oral pain
Oramorph SR	Sustained-release MORPHINE SULPHATE	Opioid agonist
Ormazine	CHLORPROMAZINE	Phenothiazine
Orudis (UK)	KETOPROFEN	NSAID
Ostac	CLODRONATE	Biphosphonate
OXAPROZIN	Daypro	NSAID
OXAZEPAM	Novoxapam (C), Oxpam (C), Serax, Vaben, Zapex (C)	Benzodiazepine
Oxpam (C)	OXAZEPAM	Benzodiazepine
OXYBUTYNIN	Cystrin (UK), Ditropan, Novitropan	Smooth muscle antispasmodic (bladder)
OXYCODONE	Endone (AU), Proladone (AU, UK), Supeudol (C), Roxicodone; with acetaminophen: Percocet, Tylox; with aspirin: Percodan	Opioid agonist
OXYMORPHONE	Numorphan	Opioid agonist
Pacedol (AU)	HALOPERIDOL	Neuroleptic, antiemetic

Drug		Class or Principal Action
Pallace	MEGESTROL ACETATE	Progestational agent; antianorectic
Pamelor	NORTRIPTYLINE	Tricyclic antidepressant
Pamergan (UK)	PETHIDINE (MEPERIDINE)	Opioid agonist
PAMIDRONATE	Aredia	Biphosphonate
Pamine (UK)	HYOSCINE BUTYL-BROMIDE	Anticholinergic
Panadol	ACETAMINOPHEN (PARACETAMOL)	Analgesic, antipyretic
Pancrease	PANCREATIN combination product	Pancreatic enzyme replacement
PANCREATIN products	Encypalmed, Nutrizym (UK), Pancrease, Viokase	Pancreatic enzyme replacement
PAPAVERINE	Pavabid	Antispasmodic opioid derivative
PARACETAMOL	Abrol, Acamol, Dexamol, Panadol, Tylenol	Analgesic, antipyretic
Paracodin (AU)	DIHYDROCODEINE	Opioid agonist
Parmid (UK)	METOCLOPRAMIDE	Antidopaminergic GI motility promoter
Pavabid	PAPAVERINE	Antispasmodic opioid derivative
PEMOLINE	Cylert, Volital (UK)	Central nervous system stimulant
PENTAZOCINE	Fortral, Talwin	Opioid agonist-antagonist
PENTOBARBITAL	Nembutal	Barbiturate
Pentothal	THIOPENTAL	Barbiturate
Pepcid	FAMOTIDINE	H_2 blocker
Percocet	OXYCODONE + ACETAMINOPHEN	Opioid/NSAID
Percodan	OXYCODONE + ASPIRIN	Opioid/NSAID
Peri-Colace	CASANTHRANOL + DOCUSATE	Stimulant laxative + stool softener
Peridol (C)	HALOPERIDOL	Neuroleptic, antiemetic

Drug		Class or Principal Action
Pertofran (UK)	DESIPRAMINE	Tricyclic antidepressant
PETHIDINE (MEPERI-DINE)	Demerol, Mepergan	Opioid agonist
Phenazo (C)	PHENAZOPYRIDINE	Bladder local anesthetic
PHENAZOPYRIDINE	Baridium, Di-Azo, Phenazo (C), Pyridium, Pyronium (C), Sedural (UK)	Bladder local anesthetic
Phenergan	PROMETHAZINE	Antihistamine
PHENOBARBITAL SODIUM	Luminal	Barbiturate
PHENYTOIN	Epanutin (UK), Dilantin	Anticonvulsant
Physeptone (C, UK)	METHADONE	Opioid agonist
PIROXICAM	Apo-piroxicam (C), Feldene, Novopriocam (C)	NSAID
Ponstan (C)	MEFENAMIC ACID	NSAID
Ponstel	MEFENAMIC ACID	NSAID
Pramin (AU)	METOCLOPRAMIDE	Dopamine antagonist, promoter of GI motility
Prepulsid (UK)	CISAPRIDE	Promoter of gastric/gut motility
Prilosec	OMEPRAZOLE	Benzimidazole gastric acid pump inhibitor
Primperan (AU, UK)	METOCLOPRAMIDE	Antidopaminergic GI motility promoter
Procalm (AU)	CHLORPROMAZINE	Phenothiazine
PROCHLORPERAZINE	Anti-naus (AU), Buccastem (AU, UK), Chlorazine, Compazine, Stemetil	Phenothiazine
Progesic (UK)	FENOPROFEN	NSAID
Proladone (AU, UK)	OXYCODONE	Opioid agonist
Prolixin	FLUPHENAZINE	Phenothiazine
Promacid (AU)	CHLORPROMAZINE	Phenothiazine
Promaz	CHLORPROMAZINE	Phenothiazine

Drug		Class or Principal Action
PROMETHAZINE	Phenergan	Antihistamine
PROPOXYPHENE HCL	Algolysin, Darvon, Doloxene (C)	Opioid agonist (weak)
Propulsid	CISAPRIDE	Promoter of gastric/ gut motility
Proventil	ALBUTEROL	β_2-Adrenergic agonist
Prozac	FLUOXETINE	Antidepressant
PSYLLIUM	Metamucil	Bulk-forming stool softener
Pyridium	PHENAZOPYRIDINE	Bladder local anesthetic
Pyronium (C)	PHENAZOPYRIDINE	Bladder local anesthetic
Quinamm	QUININE SULFATE	Alkaloid muscle relaxant
QUININE SULFATE	Quinamm	Alkaloid muscle relaxant
RANITIDINE	Zantac	H_2 blocker
Raykit	BISACODYL	Stimulant laxative
Reglan	METOCLOPRAMIDE	Antidopaminergic GI motility promoter
Regulex (C)	DOCUSATE	Stool softener
Rescudose	MORPHINE SULFATE oral solution	Opioid agonist
Restoril	TEMAZEPAM	Benzodiazepine
Ritalin	METHYLPHENIDATE	Central nervous system stimulant
Rivotril (C, UK)	CLONAZEPAM	Benzodiazepine anticonvulsant
RMS	Rectal MORPHINE SULFATE	Opioid agonist
Robaxin	METHOCARBAMOL	Centrally-acting muscle relaxant
Rohypnol (UK)	FLUNITRAZEPAM	Benzodiazepine hypnotic
Rosex Gel	METRONIDAZOLE Gel	Antifungal
Roxanol	MORPHINE SULFATE controlled oral solution	Opioid agonist

Drug		Class or Principal Action
Roxicodone	OXYCODONE	Opioid agonist
Salamol (UK)	ALBUTEROL (SALBU-TAMOL)	β_2-Adrenergic agonist
SALBUTAMOL	Aerolin (UK), Proventil, Salamol (UK), Ventolin	β_2-Adrenergic agonist
Sandostatin	OCTREOTIDE	Somatostatin analog
Saroten (AU)	AMITRIPTYLINE	Tricyclic antidepressant
Scopoderm	SCOPOLAMINE	Anticholinergic (transdermal)
SCOPOLAMINE (HYOSCINE) HYDROBROMIDE	Isopto Hyoscine, Triptone	Anticholinergic
SCOPOLAMINE transdermal	Scopoderm, Transderm Scop, Transderm V (C)	Anticholinergic
Sea Legs (UK)	MECLIZINE	Antihistaminic antiemetic
Sedural	PHENAZOPYRIDINE	Bladder anesthetic
Senokot S	SENNA + DOCUSATE	Stimulant laxative
Septra	TRIMETHOPRIM–SULFAMETHOXA-ZOLE	Antibiotic
Septrin	TRIMETHOPRIM–SULFAMETHOXA-ZOLE	Antibiotic
Serax	OXAZEPAM	Benzodiazepine
Serenace (AU)	HALOPERIDOL	Neuroleptic, antiemetic
Sevredol (UK)	Immediate-release MORPHINE SULFATE	Opioid agonist
Spiroctan (UK)	SPIRONOLACTONE	K$^+$-sparing diuretic
Spirolone (UK)	SPIRONOLACTONE	K$^+$-sparing diuretic
SPIRONOLACTONE	Aldactone, Laratone (UK), Novo-Spiriton (C), Spiroctan (UK), Spirolone (UK), Spirotone (AU)	K$^+$-sparing diuretic
Spirotone (AU)	SPIRONOLACTONE	K$^+$-sparing diuretic

Drug		Class or Principal Action
Stadol	BUTORPHANOL	Opioid agonist-antagonist
Statex (C)	MORPHINE SULFATE	Opioid agonist
Stemetil	PROCHLORPERAZINE	Phenothiazine
Stesolid	DIAZEPAM	Benzodiazepine
STRONTIUM-89	Metastron	Radioisotope for metastatic bone pain
Sucralat	SUCRALFATE	Sulfated aluminum anti-peptic ulcer agent
SUCRALFATE	Antepsin (UK), Carafate, Sucralat, Sulcrate (C), Ulsanic	Sulfated aluminum anti-peptic ulcer agent
Sulcrate (C)	SUCRALFATE	Sulfated aluminum anti-peptic ulcer agent
SULINDAC	Clinoril	NSAID
Supeudol (C)	OXYCODONE	Opioid agonist
Synalgos	DIHYDROCODEINE combination	Opioid agonist
Synflex (UK)	NAPROXEN SODIUM	NSAID
Tagamet	CIMETIDINE	H_2 blocker
Talwin	PENTAZOCINE	Opioid agonist-antagonist
Tambocor	FLECAINIDE	Local anesthetic, anti-arrhythmic
Tantum (AU)	BENZYDAMINE	NSAID with local anesthetic action
Tegretol	CARBAMAZEPINE	Anticonvulsant
Temaril	TRIMEPRAZINE	Phenothiazine anti-pruritic
TEMAZEPAM	Euhypnos, Normison, Restoril	Benzodiazepine
Temgesic (UK)	BUPRENORPHINE	Opioid agonist
THIOPENTAL	Pentothal	Barbiturate
Thorazine	CHLORPROMAZINE	Phenothiazine
Tofranil	IMIPRAMINE	Tricyclic antidepressant
Toilex (AU)	BISACODYL	Stimulant laxative
Tolectin	TOLMETIN	NSAID

Drug		Class or Principal Action
TOLMETIN	Tolectin	NSAID
Topadol	KETOROLAC	NSAID
Toradol	KETOROLAC	NSAID
TRANEXAMIC ACID	Cyklokapron, Hexakapron	Plasmin/plasminogen inhibitor
Transderm Scop	SCOPOLAMINE transdermal	Anticholinergic
Transderm V (C)	SCOPOLAMINE transdermal	Anticholinergic
Travamine (C)	DIMENHYDRINATE	Antihistamine antiemetic
Triavil	AMITRIPTYLINE	Tricyclic antidepressant
TRIAZOLAM	Halcion	Benzodiazepine hypnotic
Trilisate	CHOLINE MAGNESIUM TRISALICYLATE	NSAID
TRIMEPRAZINE	Temaril	Phenothiazine antipruritic
TRIMETHOPRIM–SULFAMETHOXAZOLE	Apo-Sulfatrim (C), Bactrim, Novatrimel (C), Septra, Septrin	Antibiotic
Trisilate	CHOLINE MAGNESIUM TRISALICYLATE	NSAID
TROPISETRON	Navoban	5-HT$_3$-blocking antiemetic
Tryptanol (AU)	AMITRIPTYLINE	Tricyclic antidepressant
Tryptizol (UK)	AMITRIPTYLINE	Tricyclic antidepressant
Tylenol	ACETAMINOPHEN (PARACETAMOL)	Analgesic, antipyretic
Tylenol #3	ACETAMINOPHEN + CODEINE	Opioid/antipyretic
Tylox	OXYCODONE + ACETAMINOPHEN	Opioid/antipyretic
Ulcerax (UK)	HYDROXYZINE	Antihistamine with analgesic properties
Ulsanic	SUCRALFATE	Sulfated aluminum antipeptic ulcer agent
Uremide (AU)	FUROSEMIDE (FRUSEMIDE)	Diuretic

Drug		Class or Principal Action
Urispas	FLAVOXATE HCL	Urinary tract spasmolytic
Uritol	FUROSEMIDE	Diuretic
Vaben	OXAZEPAM	Benzodiazepine
Valium	DIAZEPAM	Benzodiazepine
Valoid (UK)	CYCLIZINE	Antihistamine, antiemetic
VALPROIC ACID	Convulex (UK), Depakene, Depolept, Epilim (UK)	Anticonvulsant
Ventolin	SALBUTAMOL (ALBUTEROL)	β_2-Adrenergic agonist
Versed	MIDAZOLAM	Benzodiazepine
Vicodin	HYDROCODONE + ACETAMINOPHEN	Opioid/antipyretic
Viokase	PANCREATIN combination product	Pancreatic enzyme replacement
Vistaril	HYDROXYZINE	Antihistamine with analgesic properties
Volital (UK)	PEMOLINE	Central nervous system stimulant
Voltarol	DICLOFENAC	NSAID
Volteran	DICLOFENAC	NSAID
Wydase	HYALURONIDASE	Enzymatic diffusing substance (hypodermoclysis)
Xanax	ALPRAZOLAM	Benzodiazepine
Xylocaine	LIDOCAINE (LIGNOCAINE)	Local anesthetic
Zantac	RANITIDINE	H_2 blocker
Zapex (C)	OXAZEPAM	Benzodiazepine
Zofran	ONDANSETRON	5-HT_3–blocking antiemetic
Zostrix	CAPSAICIN	Irritant analgesic
Zovirax	ACYCLOVIR	Antiviral

Appendix 1.B

Drugs Used in Palliative Care: Drug Profiles

Keep well in your memory drugs and their properties, both simple and compound....Remember their modes and their number and variety in the several cases. This in medicine is the beginning, middle, and end.

HIPPOCRATES, *DECORUM*, IX

Acetaminophen (Paracetamol)

Trade Names:	Acephen, Datril, Feverall, Tylenol, Valadol.
Mechanism of Action:	*Analgesic and antipyretic* but only very weakly anti-inflammatory (it may be inactivated by the peroxides found in peripheral inflammatory lesions). Acts centrally, inhibiting cerebral cyclooxygenase. No adverse effects on gastric mucosa, platelets, bleeding time, or uric acid excretion. Analgesic potency identical to aspirin.
Pharmacology:	Major active metabolite of phenacetin, without its major toxicity. Rapidly and almost completely absorbed from the GI tract. Peak plasma concentrations in 30–60 minutes; half-life in plasma about 2 hours. The onset of action of an oral dose occurs in 5–30 minutes and peaks in ½–2 hours. A single dose is effective for 4–6 hours. Readily crosses the blood-brain barrier. Metabolized primarily by hepatic microsomal enzymes.
Indications in Palliative Care:	Mild pain. Drug of choice for **headache** in cancer patients.
Contraindications:	Known hypersensitivity.
Adverse Side Effects:	Occasional erythematous or urticarial rash. Excessive dose (>10 gm) may cause potentially fatal hepatic necrosis. Chronic overuse may lead to nephrotoxicity.
Incompatibility:	Enhances hypoglycemic effects of sulfonylureas. Absorption of acetaminophen is *decreased* by concomitant anticholinergics, activated charcoal, or opioids.
How Supplied:	Tablets: 160 mg, 325 mg, 500 mg, and 650 mg. Capsules: 325 mg and 500 mg. Suppositories: 120 and 325 mg Elixir: 120 mg/5 ml, 160 mg/5 ml, and 325 mg/5 ml.
Dosage and Administration:	**500–1000 mg PO q4–6h.**

Acetylsalicylic Acid (Aspirin)

Trade Names:	Sold generically and under various trade names. A component of Alka-Seltzer, Ascriptin, Bufferin, Darvon compound, Ecotrin, Empirin, Excedrin, Norgesic, Percodan.
Mechanism of Action:	As an analgesic, acts peripherally by inhibiting the synthesis of the prostaglandins that sensitize pain receptors to mechanical and chemical stimulation. Exerts its anti-inflammatory and antipyretic effects through a similar mechanism, i.e., inhibiting PGE_2 synthesis.
Pharmacology:	Absorbed rapidly after oral administration, partly from the stomach but mostly from the upper small intestine. Peak serum levels are reached within 2 hours of an oral dose, then gradually decline. The onset of action occurs within 5–30 minutes of an oral dose and peaks in ½–2 hours. **A single oral dose is effective for 4–6 hours.** The rate of absorption is affected by the rate of disintegration of the tablet, gastric emptying time, and the pH of the mucosal surface (rise in pH facilitates absorption). Food in the stomach delays absorption. Rectal absorption is slower, less complete, and unpredictable and therefore not recommended. Biotransformed in the liver and excreted in the urine mostly as salicyluric acid. Urinary excretion is extremely variable and pH dependent (alkaline urine favors excretion). Renal disease and agents that compete for tubular transport (e.g., probenecid) reduce aspirin excretion and may lead to elevated serum levels.
Indications in Palliative Care:	**Mild** to moderate **pain** (prototype drug for step I of the WHO ladder). Pain from **pancreatic** and **head and neck cancers**.
Contraindications:	Peptic **ulcer** disease. **Bleeding** dyscrasias. **Urticaria** (aspirin can markedly worsen an allergic reaction to another allergen). Asthma with nasal polyps. Use with *caution* in multiple myeloma and in renal failure.
Adverse Side Effects:	Gastritis and upper GI bleeding. Decreased platelet function → prolonged bleeding time.
Incompatibility:	Interferes with diuretic action of spironolactone (reduces diuretic effect by up to 70%). Additive effects with anticoagulants.
How Supplied:	Tablets: 325 mg, 500 mg, 600 mg, and 625 mg. Enteric-coated tablets (Ecotrin): 325 mg and 500 mg. Suppositories: 200 mg, 300 mg, 325 mg, 600 mg, 650 mg, and 1200 mg. Chewing gum (Aspergum): 227.5 mg/stick.
Dosage and Administration:	**650–1000 mg PO q6h.**

Activated Charcoal–Simethicone

Trade Name:	Charcoal Plus (= activated charcoal, 400 mg; simethicone, 80 mg).
Mechanism of Action:	Simethicone is a surface-active agent that reduces the surface tension of gas bubbles in the stomach, thereby destroying mucosal pockets of gas that cause distress. Activated charcoal is a high-capacity gas absorbent active in the intestine; its highly porous surface absorbs and adsorbs gases, poorly soluble substances, and toxins. It reduces the volume of intestinal gas and thereby decreases flatulence. It also absorbs microbial metabolites in the gut that may generate gas (e.g., hydrogen and methane).
Pharmacology:	Not absorbed into the bloodstream.
Indications in Palliative Care:	For relief of **stomach gas**, **intestinal gas**, and **flatulence**. For relief of **hiccups** when associated with gastric stasis and distention (very commonly in advanced cancer).
Contraindications:	None known.
Adverse Side Effects:	None reported.
Incompatibility:	May adsorb other medications in the digestive tract → give other medications 1 hour before or 2 hours after activated charcoal. May cause temporary blackening of the stool.
How Supplied:	Two-phase tablets.
Dosage and Administration:	**2 tablets PO qid** (pc & hs).

Albuterol (Salbutamol)

Trade Names:	Aerolin (UK), Proventil, Salamol (UK), Ventolin
Mechanism of Action:	β₂-*Adrenergic agonist* drug with preferential affinity for β-receptors of bronchial smooth muscle. Acts by stimulating the conversion of ATP to cyclic AMP, whose presence leads to *relaxation of bronchial smooth muscle* and inhibits release of mediators of immediate hypersensitivity.
Pharmacology:	Systemic levels of albuterol are low after inhalation of recommended dosage (< 20% reaches the systemic circulation). Onset of improvement of pulmonary function (as measured by FEV_1 and MMEF) occurs within 15 minutes of inhaling a therapeutic dose; peak improvement occurs within 60–90 minutes, and duration of effect is 3–4 hours.
Indications in Palliative Care:	Relief of respiratory distress caused by **bronchospasm** when inhaled corticosteroids fail to relieve wheezing.
Contraindications:	Known hypersensitivity to the drug.
Adverse Side Effects:	**Tremor** (11%). **Nausea** (3%), heartburn. **Headache** (3%). Paradoxical **bronchospasm** (15%). Muscle cramps.
Incompatibility:	Do not use with other sympathomimetic agents. Use with extreme caution in patients taking MAO inhibitor or tricyclic **antidepressant** drugs, which may potentiate the actions of albuterol on the vascular system. β-Blocking agents and albuterol are mutually inhibitory.
How Supplied:	Solution for nebulizer in a concentration of 5 mg/ml. Metered-dose inhalers.
Dosage and Administration:	**0.5 ml (2.5 mg) diluted in 2.5 ml of normal saline** and **nebulized over 5–15 minutes, tid–qid.** May be combined in nebulizer with dexamethasone and/or morphine.

Amitriptyline

Trade Names:	Amitril (C), Amitrip (AU), Elavil, Endep, Enovil, Levate (C), Lentizol (UK), Mevaril (C), Tryptizol (UK).
Mechanism of Action:	**Tricyclic antidepressant** with **sedative** effects. Mechanism of action not known. *Not* a MAO inhibitor, and it does not act primarily by stimulation of the CNS. Inhibits the membrane pump mechanism responsible for uptake of norepinephrine and serotonin in adrenergic and serotonergic neurons. This action may potentiate or prolong neuronal activity, since reuptake of these amines is important in terminating transmitting activity. **Analgesic** that potentiates the effect of opioids and, on its own, relieves some neuropathic pain (superficial dysesthesias). Mechanism not known.
Pharmacology:	Quite lipid soluble and therefore well absorbed from the GI tract and has a high volume of distribution. Highly protein-bound in plasma and tissues; extensive biotransformation in the liver; slowly eliminated. Mean half-lives in serum for amitriptyline and its metabolite nortriptyline are 15 hours and 27 hours. Half-life prolonged in the elderly. The onset of action for an analgesic effect takes up to 5 days, for antidepressant effect up to 2 weeks. Enterohepatic recirculation occurs. About ⅔ eventually excreted in urine.
Indications in Palliative Care:	For relief of symptoms of **depression** (endogenous). For **neuropathic pain** (superficial dysesthesias). As a **co-analgesic** with opioids when there are additional reasons for prescribing amitriptyline (for its sedative or antidepressant effects). For control of **bladder spasms**.
Contraindications:	Not recommended in recovery phase of AMI, and should be used with *caution* in patients with known cardiac disease. Because of atropine-like actions, use with *caution* in patients with h/o seizures, urinary retention, angle-closure glaucoma. Contraindicated in patients taking MAO inhibitors.
Adverse Side Effects:	**Sedation.** Peripheral **anticholinergic** effects: dry mouth, tachycardia, blurred vision, urinary retention; **constipation** in up to 50% (in the elderly may progress to paralytic ileus); CNS effects: difficulty concentrating, psychomotor slowing. Cardiac effects: **orthostatic hypotension** in 20%; **tachycardia** and **palpitations** are common; aggravation of heart block; rarely AMI.
Incompatibility:	MAO inhibitors → hyperpyretic crises, severe convulsions, death. Quinidine, procainamide → worsen impaired conduction. Antihistamines → toxic confusional and delirious state in elderly. Anticholinergics → paralytic ileus, hyperpyrexia.

Incompatibility *cont.*	Cimetidine → ↓hepatic metabolism of tricyclics → ↑serum levels → toxicity.
How Supplied:	Tablets: 10 mg, 25 mg, 50 mg, 75 mg, 100 mg, 150 mg. Injection: 10 mg/ml.
Dosage and Administration:	▪ For *depression in terminal illness*: Start with **10–25 mg PO hs** (use the lower dosage in elderly or very debilitated patients); every 3-7 days thereafter, **increase dosage by 10–25 mg** (whichever was used as the starting dose) until maximum dose of 75-100 mg has been reached. The occurrence of dry mouth is a good indication that therapeutic plasma levels have been achieved. Therapeutic effects take >14 days to become manifest for depression. Therefore, maintain total dose for 2-3 weeks before concluding that the drug is ineffective. ▪ As a *co-analgesic with opioids* or for *neuropathic pain*: Dosage regimen is the same as for depression, but *effects are more rapid in onset and may be achieved at lower dosages*. ▪ For *bladder spasms*: **25–50 mg PO hs**. Amitriptyline should not be withdrawn abruptly but rather tapered over a period of 2 weeks.

Antacids: Aluminum Hydroxide/ Magnesium Hydroxide

Trade Name:	Maalox.
Mechanism of Action:	*Buffers* gastric acid to raise the pH of gastric contents and thereby provides pain relief in peptic ulcer disease and other states of hyperacidity. Magnesium hydroxide is a potent antacid, but frequent doses can cause severe osmotic diarrhea. Therefore magnesium hydroxide is combined with aluminum hydroxide, which has a constipating effect.
Pharmacology:	Minimal absorption when used over the short term.
Indications in Palliative Care:	Preferred antacid formulation for relief of • Symptomatic **gastric hyperacidity**. • Reflux **esophagitis**. Calcium carbonate antacids should be avoided. By topical application, for **fungating or malodorous cutaneous tumors**, to relieve burning and reduce odor.
Contraindications:	Use magnesium-containing compounds with caution in patients with renal failure.
Adverse Side Effects:	Occasional diarrhea (usually not a problem in patients taking opioids).
Incompatibility:	Do not administer to patient taking any tetracycline preparation (may prevent absorption of the antibiotic). The aluminum hydroxide also binds thyroxine and chlorpromazine and may reduce absorption of those agents.
How Supplied:	Maalox: 12-ounce bottles of suspension (shake before using).
Dosage and Administration:	For gastric hyperacidity or reflux esophagitis: **30 ml PO** **½ hour pc and hs**. For fungating cutaneous tumors: Apply topically after bathing and as needed.

Atropine Sulfate

Trade Name:	Atropine sulfate.
Mechanism of Action:	Anticholinergic, competitive antagonist at muscarinic sites both peripherally and in the ganglion. Inhibits salivary and gastric secretion, slows peristalsis throughout the GI tract, opposes vagally-induced bronchoconstriction; inhibits secretions of the nose, mouth, pharynx, and bronchi and thus dries the mucous membranes of the respiratory tract.
Pharmacology:	Belladonna alkaloid that readily enters the circulation from the GI tract or when applied to mucosal surfaces. Peak inhibitory effects on salivation occur within 30 minutes of an oral or IM dose. Half-life is approximately 4 hours; about half of the drug is metabolized in the liver, and the remainder is excreted unchanged in the urine.
Indications in Palliative Care:	By nebulizer, to alleviate respiratory distress in patients who are too weak to cough up copious secretions. To dry **excess respiratory secretions** (death rattle) in the immediate preterminal phase.
Contraindications:	None when given preterminally.
Adverse Side Effects:	Tachycardia and tachydysrhythmias (bradycardia with low doses). Drowsiness. Midriasis. Dry mouth. Decreased sweating, sometimes leading to elevations of body temperature.
Incompatibility:	Additive anticholinergic effects with tricyclic antidepressants, phenothiazines.
How Supplied:	Ampules: 1 mg in 1 ml.
Dosage and Administration:	For excessive secretions, **0.5–1 mg by nebulizer** in 2.5 ml of normal saline delivered over 5–15 minutes (may be combined with morphine and/or dexamethasone). For terminal secretions (death rattle), **1 mg IM or slowly IV**.

Baclofen

Trade Names:	Atrofen, Lioresal
Mechanism of Action:	*Muscle relaxant and antispastic.* Precise mechanism of action unknown. Baclofen can inhibit both monosynaptic and polysynaptic reflexes at the spinal level and has general CNS depressant properties.
Pharmacology:	Rapidly absorbed and eliminated; excreted primarily by the kidney in unchanged form. Onset of therapeutic action varies from hours to weeks. About 15% is metabolized in the liver; the rest is excreted unchanged by the kidneys.
Indications in Palliative Care:	**Muscle spasm**, especially caused by spinal cord compression.
Contraindications:	Use with caution in seizure-prone patients, especially those on antiepileptic medications.
Adverse Side Effects:	Transient **drowsiness**. Dizziness, weakness, confusion, headache, insomnia. **Nausea**. **Constipation**. Urinary frequency.
Incompatibility:	Sedative effects may be additive to those of other CNS depressants.
How Supplied:	Tablets: 10 mg and 20 mg.
Dosage and Administration:	5 mg PO tid × 3 days, then 10 mg PO tid × 3 days, then 15 mg PO tid × 3 days, then 20 mg PO tid × 3 days. Additional increments may be necessary, but final total dose should not exceed 80 mg/day (i.e., 20 mg qid). If benefits are not evident after trial period, slowly withdraw the drug.

Bisacodyl

Trade Names:	Bisalax (AU), Biscolax, Contalax, Dulcolax, Theralax.
Mechanism of Action:	**Contact stimulant laxative** that acts directly on the colonic mucosa to produce normal peristalsis throughout the large bowel. On contact with colonic mucosa, stimulates sensory nerve endings → parasympathetic reflexes → increased peristalsis. Also promotes fluid/electrolyte accumulation in colon → increased laxative effect. Bowel movement usually produced within 6 hours after oral administration and 15–60 minutes after rectal administration.
Pharmacology:	Very poorly absorbed, if at all, in the small bowel following oral administration or in the large bowel following rectal administration.
Indications:	For treatment of **mild constipation**. Used together with an osmotic cathartic to prevent constipation in patients on chronic opioid therapy.
Contraindications:	Rectal **bleeding**. Gastroenteritis. Bowel **obstruction** or signs suggestive of obstruction (nausea, vomiting, colicky abdominal pain).
Adverse Side Effects:	Occasional abdominal discomfort, especially if taken with milk or antacids.
Incompatibility:	None reported.
How Supplied:	Tablets: 5 mg. Rectal suppositories: 5 mg and 10 mg. Enema: 0.33 mg/100 ml.
Dosage and Administration:	Tabs: **1–2 tabs qhs–bid**. Suppositories: **1 suppository qd**. Enema: 1 prn.

Carbamazepine

Trade Names:	Epitol, Mazepine, Tegretol.
Mechanism of Action:	Anticonvulsant: Acts by reducing polysynaptic responses and blocking the post-tetanic potentiation. As an analgesic, depresses thalamic potential and bulbar and polysynaptic reflexes. Mechanism of action unknown.
Pharmacology:	Both suspension and tablet forms deliver equivalent amounts of drug to the systemic circulation (suspension absorbed faster). Thrice-daily dosage schedule of suspension gives comparable steady-state plasma levels to twice-daily dosage of tablets. Onset of analgesic action takes 3–4 days. Plasma levels are variable and may range from 0.5–25 µg/ml without apparent relation to daily intake of the drug. Usual adult therapeutic levels are between 4 and 12 µg/ml. Following chronic oral administration of tablets, plasma levels peak at 4–5 hours. Because carbamazepine may induce its own metabolism, the half-life is variable (25–65 hours). Metabolized by the liver → 75% excreted in feces, 25% in urine.
Indications in Palliative Care:	Stabbing **neuropathic pain**. (Usually added after a trial of a tricyclic antidepressant has not sufficiently relieved pain.) Psychomotor and **temporal lobe seizures** from brain metastases. **Trigeminal neuralgia** and glossopharyngeal neuralgia.
Contraindications:	History of bone marrow depression (obtain CBC before treatment). Known sensitivity to tricyclic compounds. Patient taking MAO inhibitors.
Adverse Side Effects:	Possible **aplastic anemia** and **agranulocytosis** (rare, but the most serious potential side effect). **Nausea and vomiting*** are the most frequent adverse effects, especially during initial phases of therapy. Dizziness, drowsiness, unsteadiness and ataxia, nystagmus.* Severe dermatologic reactions including toxic epidermal necrolysis (**Lyell's syndrome**) and Stevens-Johnson syndrome. Possible liver toxicity (follow **LFTs**).
Incompatibility:	Concurrent MAO inhibitors → hypertensive crisis. Concurrent phenobarbital, phenytoin, or primodone→ ↓ serum carbamazepine. Carbamazepine → ↓serum haloperidol. Concurrent **erythromycin, cimetidine, propoxyphene, fluoxetine**, or **calcium channel blockers** → ↑carbamazepine levels→ possible toxicity. Concurrent lithium → ↑risk of neurotoxic side effects.

*Incidence of nausea, ataxia, and nystagmus can be decreased by starting with 100 mg bid and increasing the daily dosage no more than 200 mg/wk.

How Supplied:	Chewable tablets: 100 mg. Tablets: 200 mg. Suspension: 100 mg/5 ml.		
Dosage and Administration:	*Form*	*Starting Dose*	*Titration*	*Maximum Dose*
	Tabs	**200 mg hs** on the first day	After 3 days,* ↑ to **200 mg bid**; after 3 more days ↑ to **200 mg tid**; after 3 more days ↑ to **200 mg qid**	1200 mg/ 24 hr
	Suspension	**2 tsp (10 ml) hs** on the first day	After 3 days,* ↑ to **2 tsp bid**; after 3 more days, **2 tsp tid**; after 3 more days, **2 tsp qid**	1200 mg/ 24 hr

Cisapride

Trade Names:	Prepulsid (UK), Propulsid.
Mechanism of Action:	Mechanism not well understood; probably facilitates release of acetylcholine in the myenteric plexus of the gut. Cisapride increases esophageal sphincter tone and esophageal motility. The effects of cisapride in enhancing gastric emptying and small bowel motility are similar to those of metoclopramide and domperidone; however, cisapride—unlike those drugs—has additional activity on the colon, where it *increases colonic motility*. Thus it increases the frequency of bowel movements. It is not a dopaminergic blocker, and its actions are blocked by atropine. It does not cause extrapyramidal symptoms.
Pharmacology:	Maximum plasma concentrations occur 1–2 hours after an oral dose. The presence of food enhances absorption of the drug. Bioavailability is 40–50%, indicating first-pass metabolism in the liver or gut. Cisapride is 98% bound to plasma proteins. It is metabolized in the liver. The elimination half-life is about 10 hours but may be longer in the elderly or in the presence of liver disease. Elimination is *not* significantly altered in renal insufficiency.
Indications in Palliative Care:	Reflux **esophagitis**. Nonulcer **dyspepsia**. Symptoms caused by **gastric hypomotility**, especially when an additional, mild laxative effect is desired.
Contraindications:	No absolute contraindications in advanced cancer.
Adverse Side Effects:	Generally well tolerated, and the few side effects are related to its pharmacologic action: Transient abdominal cramping and borborygmi. Diarrhea or loose stools (4%).
Incompatibility:	May enhance the depressant effects of ethanol and benzodiazepines by increasing their absorption. Anticholinergics may decrease cisapride's therapeutic effects. Concurrent administration of cimetidine → ↑cisapride plasma concentration.
How Supplied:	Tablets: 5 mg and 10 mg.
Dosage and Administration:	For *dyspepsia*: Start with **5 mg PO tid**; dose may be doubled if necessary. For *esophagitis*: **10 mg PO tid and hs**. Cisapride should be taken **15 minutes before meals**. In the elderly and in hepatic insufficiency, start with half the recommended dosage.

Clodronate

Trade Names:	**Ostac, Bonefos.**
Mechanism of Action:	Anti-osteolytic activity → ↓bone resorption → ↓serum calcium; at the same time there is ↓calcuria, ↑PTH. Diminishes bone pain. With chronic therapy, also decreases the occurrence of fractures and the appearance of new osteolytic foci in both myeloma and metastatic disease (soft tissue metastases not affected).
Pharmacology:	Not metabolized: absorbed, excreted, and stored unchanged. Intestinal absorption is poor (only 1–10%) and is reduced by food intake, especially calcium products. Rapidly cleared from the serum and taken up into the skeleton, where it has a very long (perhaps lifetime) half-life.
Indications in Palliative Care:	Treatment of **bone pain** from bony metastases. Treatment of **hypercalcemia of malignancy.**
Contraindications:	Renal failure.
Adverse Side Effects:	When given orally: • **Nausea, abdominal pain, flatulence, diarrhea**, especially at the start of treatment. • Dizziness, fatigue (less common). By infusion: • **Renal insufficiency** when large doses are given very rapidly. • Hypocalcemia. • Alterations in liver function tests (↑LDH).
Incompatibility:	Food high in **calcium** (e.g., milk products) or medications high in **bivalent cations** (e.g., antacids, iron) reduce absorption of clodronate when taken orally.
How Supplied:	Not currently available in the United States. Elsewhere: Capsules: 400 mg. Infusion concentrate: 60 mg/ml in 5 ml (Bonefos). Infusion concentrate: 30 mg/ml in 10 ml (Ostac).
Dosage and Administration:	Orally: **1600–2400 mg PO qd** (may be taken as a single dose at night or, to improve GI tolerance, may be divided into two daily doses). Should be taken with sufficient fluid, but *not with milk*! Nothing should be eaten 1 hour before and 1 hour after clodronate ingestion. Treatment may be continued up to 6 months. Infusion: **300 mg in 500 ml of normal saline infused over 3 hours daily for 3–5 consecutive days.** (If given for hypercalcemia, rehydration must precede biphosphonate treatment.) For bone pain, continue with oral clodronate after the initiation of therapy by infusion.

Clonazepam

Trade Names:	Klonopin, Rivotril (C, UK).
Mechanism of Action:	Benzodiazepine tranquilizer. Suppresses spike-and-wave discharge in petit mal seizures and decreases frequency, duration, and spread of discharge in minor motor seizures. Thought to act by modulating the effect of the inhibitory neurotransmitter χ-amino butyric acid in the brain.
Pharmacology:	After a single oral dose, maximum blood levels are achieved in 1-2 hours; half-life varies from 18-50 hours. Its action begins in 20-60 minutes, peaks in 1-2 hours, and persists 6-8 hours. The drug is mostly excreted in the urine.
Indications in Palliative Care:	**Neuropathic pain.**
Contraindications:	Acute narrow-angle glaucoma. Significant hepatic disease.
Adverse Side Effects:	Drowsiness (50%). Ataxia (30%). Behavioral disturbances (25%). Increased salivation and hypersecretion in upper respiratory passages. Possible respiratory depression. When given to patients with underlying seizure disorders of different types, may precipitate grand mal seizures.
Incompatibility:	CNS-depressant effects may be potentiated by alcohol, narcotics, barbiturates, nonbarbiturate hypnotics, phenothiazines, butyrophenones, MAO inhibitors, and tricyclic antidepressants.
How Supplied:	Tablets: 0.5 mg (orange), 1 mg (blue), and 2 mg (white).
Dosage and Administration:	Start with **0.5 mg PO tid**; increase by **0.5 mg every 3 days** until symptoms are controlled or signs of toxicity appear. Do not exceed a daily dosage of 20 mg. Abrupt withdrawal of clonazepam after long-term use may precipitate status epilepticus. Taper dosage over several days when stopping the drug.

Dexamethasone

Trade Names:	Decadron, Decasone (C), Oradexon (AU).
Mechanism of Action:	Known anti-inflammatory effects do not account for most of the therapeutic effects of dexamethasone in advanced cancer.
Pharmacology:	Readily absorbed orally and parenterally.
Indications in Palliative Care:	Nausea and **vomiting**. **Anorexia**. As an **adjuvant analgesic**, especially for bone pain. To **improve sense of well-being**. **Dyspnea** due to lymphangitic spread of cancer in the lung. By inhalation, for **bronchospasm** induced by tumor or (combined with inhaled morphine) for **uncontrollable coughing**. Symptoms produced by **inflammatory edema** surrounding a tumor. **Superior vena cava syndrome**. Pain due to **stretching of liver capsule**. Symptomatic **cerebral metastases**. Acute **spinal cord compression** by tumor or metastases. Morphine-induced **sweating**.
Contraindications:	Active **upper GI bleeding**. Systemic **fungal infection**. Active **tuberculosis**.
Adverse Side Effects:	Activation of latent **diabetes**. **Psychiatric** disturbance. Headache. Oral **candidiasis**. Peptic **ulcer**, with possible perforation or hemorrhage, if given with NSAIDs. Impaired wound healing. ↑ Protein catabolism.
Incompatibility:	Phenytoin, phenobarbital, ephedrine, and rifampin enhance clearance of corticosteroids → ↓blood levels. Therefore, especially in patients taking phenytoin or phenobarbitone, it is necessary to *double the anticipated dose of dexamethasone*. May cause hypokalemia when given together with potassium-depleting diuretics or β_2 sympathomimetics.
How Supplied:	Elixir: 0.5 mg/5 ml. Tablets: 0.25 mg (orange), 0.5 mg (yellow), 0.75 mg (bluish-green), 1.5 mg (pink), 4 mg (white), and 6 mg (green). Oral solution: 0.5 mg/5 ml and 0.5 mg/0.5 ml. Injection (IV/IM): In vials of 4 mg/ml, 10 mg/ml, 20 mg/ml, and 24 mg/ml (IV use only). Inhaler (Decadron Respihaler) supplying 0.084 mg of dexamethasone with each activation.

continued

Dexamethasone *continued*

Dosage and Administration:	For *most indications* (e.g., nausea, anorexia, bone pain, dyspnea, sense of well-being): **4 mg PO qam**. Taper dose by ⅓ every 3 days until minimal effective dose is reached. (*Note*: Because of its long half-life, dexamethasone may be given only once daily, in the morning, thereby avoiding the evening overstimulation and insomnia that occur with twice-daily dosing.) For *dyspnea* or *uncontrollable coughing*: Given by inhalation: **2 mg in 2.5 ml of saline qid** (with other agents according to pathophysiology of the dyspnea (see Chapter 24). For *symptomatic cerebral metastases*: **16–36 mg PO qam**, then decrease dose by 2 mg every 3 days. For *acute spinal cord compression*: **100 mg IV stat**, then 4-24 mg q6h; follow with radiation therapy if prognosis >3-4 weeks.

Diclofenac Sodium

Trade Names:	Diclomax (UK), Voltaren.
Mechanism of Action:	Nonsteroidal anti-inflammatory drug (NSAID) with analgesic and antipyretic properties, which may derive from its ability to inhibit prostaglandin synthesis.
Pharmacology:	When taken on an empty stomach, diclofenac is completely absorbed from the GI tract, with peak plasma levels in 2-3 hours. If taken with food, there is a delay in absorption of 1-5 hours. Due to first-pass metabolism, though, only about half the absorbed dose is systemically available. The analgesic action has its onset at 15-30 minutes after an oral dose, peaks at 1-3 hours, and lasts 4-6 hours. Eliminated through metabolism and subsequent urinary and biliary excretion of the glucuronide.
Indications in Palliative Care:	**Bone pain** due to metastatic disease in bone. Mild to moderate visceral pain.
Contraindications:	Use with caution in **multiple myeloma**. Known allergy to aspirin or other NSAIDs.
Adverse Side Effects:	**Dyspepsia** or nausea (20%). **GI bleeding**, ulceration, perforation (in 1% of patients treated for 3-6 months). May aggravate **renal failure**. **Headache**, dizziness. Confusion. Abnormal LFTs. Fluid retention and **edema**.
Incompatibility:	May lead to elevated serum levels of digoxin, lithium, methotrexate. May inhibit the activity of diuretics.
How Supplied:	Tablets: 25 mg, 50 mg, and 75 mg.
Dosage and Administration:	Tabs: **50 mg PO bid**.

Diphenhydramine

Trade Name:	Benadryl.
Mechanism of Action:	H$_1$ blocking agent (*antihistamine*) in the ethanolamine family. Competes with histamine for H$_1$ receptor sites on smooth muscle of the bronchi, GI tract, and arteries, thereby blocking histamine-induced changes at those sites. Also has significant antimuscarinic and central sedative properties. Diphenhydramine suppresses the cough reflex by a direct action on the cough center. Because of its structural relationship to local anesthetics, it has anesthetic effects when applied topically.
Pharmacology:	Single oral dose of diphenhydramine HCl is quickly absorbed and widely distributed throughout the body, including the CNS. Onset of action is within 15–30 minutes. Maximum activity occurs in approximately 1 hour. The duration of activity following oral administration is 4–6 hours. Degraded in the liver and nearly completely excreted within 24 hours.
Indications in Palliative Care:	For **reversal of extrapyramidal reactions** to phenothiazine and other psychotropics. Also useful to control symptoms of **allergic reactions** (urticaria, pruritus). For **vomiting** of vestibular origin.
Contraindications:	Use with caution in patients with bladder neck obstruction.
Adverse Side Effects:	Sedation (may be a useful effect in patients with pruritus). Epigastric distress. Thickening of bronchial secretions.
Incompatibility:	Additive effects with other CNS depressants (e.g., hypnotics, sedatives, tranquilizers). Should not be given to patients taking MAO inhibitor antidepressants (which will intensify the anticholinergic effects of antihistamines).
How Supplied:	Tablets: 25 mg and 50 mg. Capsules: 25 mg and 50 mg. Elixir: 12.5 mg/5 ml (14% alcohol). Syrup: 12.5 mg/5 ml and 13.3 mg/5 ml (5% alcohol). Vials (for injection): 10 mg/ml. Disposable syringe: 50 mg in 1 ml. Ampules: 50 mg in 1 ml.
Dosage and Administration:	For *extrapyramidal reactions*: **50 mg PO/IM stat**, and repeat in 6 hours. For *allergic reactions*: **25–50 mg PO tid–qid**. As a *sedating antipruritic*: **50 mg PO hs**. For *vomiting* from vestibular or vomiting center origin: **50 mg PO/IM q4h**.

Docusate Sodium

Trade Names:	Colace, Colax (C), Dialose, Dioctyl (UK).
Mechanism of Action:	Surface-active agent that helps to **keep the stool soft** by facilitating the absorption of water by the stool. Latency of about 3 days. Does not interfere with normal peristalsis.
Pharmacology	At least partially absorbed, since docusate appears in the bile in significant concentrations.
Indications in Palliative Care:	As part of a regimen to prevent or treat **constipation** (usually given together with a bowel stimulant ± an osmotic laxative). To prevent painful defecation in patients with anorectal lesions.
Contraindications:	Contraindicated in patients receiving mineral oil (may increase absorption of mineral oil to dangerous levels).
Adverse Side Effects:	May cause slight nausea or throat irritation (syrup).
Incompatibility:	Tends to increase the intestinal absorption of other drugs given at the same time and may therefore increase their toxicity. Coadministration with aspirin may increase damage to intestinal mucosa.
How Supplied:	Colace capsules: 50 mg and 100 mg. Colace 1% liquid solution: 10 mg/ml. Colace syrup: 20 mg/5 ml. Pericolace capsules: docusate, 100 mg + casanthranol, 30 mg. Pericolace syrup: docusate, 60 mg + casanthranol, 30 mg/15 ml. Dialose tablets: 100 mg. Dialose Plus tablets: docusate, 100 mg + phenolphthalein, 65 mg. Senokot-S tablets: docusate, 50 mg + standardized senna, 8.6 mg.
Dosage and Administration:	**100 mg qd–tid** prn. The liquid forms should be taken in juice to mask the bitter taste.

Etidronate Disodium

Trade Name:	Didronel.
Mechanism of Action:	Acts mainly on bone, to inhibit the formation, growth, and dissolution of hydroxyapatite crystals and their precursors. The number of osteoclasts is reduced. The result is a *reduction of normal and abnormal bone resorption* (responsible for its therapeutic benefit in hypercalcemia); secondarily, etidronate reduces bone formation.
Pharmacology:	Not metabolized. Absorption after *oral administration* = 1% of a 5-mg/kg dose → 6% of a 20-mg/kg dose. Absorption is decreased if taken with meals. Most of the absorbed drug is cleared from the blood in 6 hours and excreted in the urine within 24–36 hours; the remainder is adsorbed to bone, especially in areas of ↑osteogenesis. After *IV administration*, a large fraction of the infused dose is excreted rapidly and unchanged in the urine; the remainder is eliminated slowly through bone turnover (half-life = 90 days).
Indications in Palliative Care:	**Hypercalcemia** of malignancy that has not responded adequately to hydration. Intractable **bone pain** due to bone metastases (etidronate is not officially approved for this indication). To retard osteoclastic activity and bone destruction in metastatic bone disease (etidronate is not officially approved for this indication).
Contraindications:	Impaired renal function (serum **creatinine > 5.0**; use reduced dosage in patients with creatinine 2.5–4.9).
Adverse Side Effects:	Metallic or altered taste (effect disappears after infusion). Asymptomatic hyperphosphatemia after oral doses of 10–20 mg/kg/day. Occasional diarrhea.
Incompatibility:	None known.
How Supplied:	Tablets: 200 mg and 400 mg. Ampules: 300 mg in 6 ml.
Dosage and Administration:	For *bone pain*: **200 mg PO bid** × 1–2 months. Should be taken on an empty stomach 2 hours or more before eating. For *hypercalcemia*, after establishing hydration and diuresis, give **7.5 mg/kg diluted in >250 ml of normal saline and infused over at least 2 hours qd × 3.**

Famotidine

Trade Name:	Pepcid.
Mechanism of Action:	H_2 receptor blocker. *Inhibits gastric secretion*—basal, nocturnal, and that stimulated by food (both volume and acid concentration).
Pharmacology:	After oral administration, onset of antisecretory effect occurs within 1 hour; maximum effect is dose-dependent and occurs within 1–3 hours; duration of inhibition of secretion is 10–12 hours. Eliminated by renal (70%) and metabolic (30%) routes. No clinically significant age-related changes in pharmacokinetics in the elderly.
Indications in Palliative Care:	Symptoms of **peptic ulcer disease**. Prophylaxis of peptic ulcer disease in vulnerable patients taking corticosteroids or NSAIDs (controversial). *Note*: Famotidine is the preferred H_2 blocker in palliative care because of the small size of the tablet, which makes it easier to swallow, and the absence of interference with other commonly used medications. Ranitidine is second choice. Cimetidine should be avoided because of its interactions with many agents used in oncology and palliative care.
Contraindications:	Known hypersensitivity to the drug.
Adverse Side Effects:	Headache (5%). Dizziness (1%).
Incompatibility:	Like other H_2 blockers, may cause the enteric coating of some pills to dissolve too rapidly. May decrease the absorption of ketoconazole.
How Supplied:	Tablets: 20 mg (beige) and 40 mg (orange). Flavored oral suspension: 40 mg/5 ml. Vials for intravenous injection: 10 mg/1 ml.
Dosage and Administration:	**40 mg PO hs × 4–6 weeks**, then maintenance dose of 20 mg PO hs.

Fentanyl

Trade Name:	Duragesic.
Mechanism of Action:	Synthetic **opioid** analgesic. Activates (supraspinal) μ- and (intraspinal) κ-receptors to produce analgesia, particularly to nociceptive (as opposed to neuropathic) pain. Inhibits interneurons and output neurons of the spinothalamic tract that would otherwise convey nociceptive messages to higher cortical centers. Fentanyl also acts directly on smooth muscle of the GI tract to increase tone and decrease propulsive contractions.
Pharmacology:	Used in palliative medicine in the form of a **transdermal patch** that provides continuous systemic delivery of the drug for **72 hours**—the amount of drug released per hour being proportional to the surface area of the patch. Onset of action is gradual, requiring 12-24 hours before plasma levels reach a steady state. Peak serum levels occur 24-72 hours after a single application. After the patch is removed, fentanyl levels decline gradually (falling 50% in 13-22 hours) because of continued absorption of fentanyl from skin depots. Clearance of fentanyl may be reduced in geriatric patients. Fentanyl is metabolized chiefly in the liver, and the metabolites are mostly excreted in the urine.
Indications in Palliative Care:	For patients whose opioid requirements are stable and who are unable to take oral medication or to follow a regular oral dosing schedule.
Contraindications:	Consider a different opioid alternative in patients who • Require very high dosage of morphine (which would entail using a large number of patches). • Have varying opioid requirements (rapid dose titration is not possible with fentanyl because of slow onset of action). Known sensitivity to fentanyl or adhesives.
Adverse Side Effects:	As for other opioids: Nausea and vomiting.* Respiratory depression.* Drowsiness.* Miosis. Constipation. Myoclonus. Acute urinary retention. Pruritus.
Incompatibility:	Other CNS depressants (phenothiazines, tranquilizers, skeletal muscle relaxants, sedating antihistamines, alcoholic beverages) may produce additive depressive effects.
How Supplied:	Duragesic 25: 10 cm² patch containing 2.5 mg; releases 25 μg/hr. Duragesic 50: 20 cm² patch containing 5 mg; releases 50 μg/hr.

*Denotes side effects that tend to remit after several days of treatment.

How Supplied *cont.*	Duragesic 75: 30 cm² patch containing 7.5 mg; releases 75 µg/hr. Duragesic 100: 40 cm² patch containing 10 mg; releases 100 µg/hr
Dosage and Administration:	To convert patients from oral or IM morphine: • **Calculate the previous 24-hour morphine require ment,** then use table below to find fentanyl dosage. • Start fentanyl with the recommended dosage, and **titrate** upward, starting every 3 days after the first fentanyl dose and no more often than every 6 days thereafter. • **Apply the patch to nonirritated, nonirradiated skin on a flat surface** of the **upper torso.** Clip (do *not* shave) hair at the site. Use only clear water to cleanse the skin prior to application of the patch; do not use soaps, oils, lotions, alcohol, or other potentially irritating agents. Allow the skin to dry thoroughly before applying the patch. • *For the first 24 hours of treatment,* analgesia should be provided with a **short-acting morphine** preparation. Thereafter, rescue doses of morphine may occasionally be required for breakthrough pain. • Some patients will require a new fentanyl patch every 48 hours rather than every 72 hours. To discontinue transdermal fentanyl and switch to another opioid: • Remove the patch. • Start treatment with half the equianalgesic dose of the new opioid 12-18 hours after patch removal. • Thereafter, titrate the dosage of the new opioid upward as required.

Morphine: Fentanyl Conversion Table

Oral 24-hour morphine (mg/day)	IM 24-hour morphine (mg/day)	Duragesic dose (µg/hr)
45-134	8-22	25
135-224	23-37	50
225-314	38-52	75
315-404	53-67	100
405-494	68-82	125
495-584	83-97	150
585-674	98-112	175
675-764	113-127	200
765-854	128-142	225
855-944	143-157	250
945-1034	158-172	275
1035-1124	173-187	300

Furosemide (Frusemide)

Trade Names:	Frusid (AU, UK), Lasix, Novosemide (C), Uremide (C).
Mechanism of Action:	**Diuretic.** Inhibits primarily the absorption of Na$^+$ and Cl not only in the proximal and distal tubules but also in the loop of Henle, independent of inhibitory effects of aldosterone. The result is to promote the excretion of Na$^+$, Cl, K$^+$, and water.
Pharmacology:	*Oral administration*: About 60% of a dose of furosemide is absorbed from the GI tract. Absorption is delayed by food. Onset of diuresis is within 1 hour; peak effect within the first or second hour; duration of diuretic effect is 6–8 hours. *IV administration*: Onset of diuresis is within 5 minutes; peak effect within the first half hour; duration of effect about 2 hours.
Indications in Palliative Care:	Peripheral **edema**. **Ascites.** Acute **pulmonary edema**. For amelioration of **pleural effusions**, together with spironolactone, when thoracentesis is not feasible. To reduce respiratory secretions **preterminally**.
Contraindications:	Anuria or worsening azotemia. Allergy to sulfonamides.
Adverse Side Effects:	**Tinnitus** and hearing impairment (if given by rapid IV injection, in very high doses, or in patients with severe renal impairment). **Hypokalemia** and hypomagnesemia. Hyperuricemia.
Incompatibility:	*Aminoglycoside* antibiotics (furosemide may increase their ototoxicity). *Salicylates* (furosemide increases their toxicity by limiting their excretion). *Lithium* (furosemide limits lithium excretion → toxicity). *Indomethacin* interferes with furosemide's diuretic action.
How Supplied:	Tablets: 20 mg, 40 mg, and 80 mg. Oral solution: 10 mg/ml and 40 mg/5 ml. Ampules and single-use vials: 10 mg/ml (for IV or IM use). Prefilled syringes: 10 mg/ml.
Dosage and Administration:	For *edema or ascites* in patients able to swallow: Start with **40 mg PO qam**, increase to 80 mg PO qam if no response. Give together **with spironolactone** to avoid hypokalemia and, in ascites or edema, to counter secondary hyperaldosteronism. *Note*: In patients who do not have an indwelling urinary catheter, it is best to give diuretic medications as a single dose in the morning, so that their sleep is not disturbed by the necessity to void. In catheterized patients, diuretics may be given in divided doses two or three times daily. For treatment of *pulmonary edema* or *excessive respiratory secretions* preterminally, start with **40 mg slowly IV**. In renal impairment or shutdown, if the first dose does not produce diuresis, try 240 mg slowly IV.

Haloperidol

Trade Names:	Haldol, Novoperidol (C), Peridol (C), Serenace (AU, UK).
Mechanism of Action:	Butyrophenone tranquilizer. Reduces dopaminergic neurotransmission in the CNS. Its dopamine-blocking effects on the CTZ probably account for haloperidol's antiemetic action. Haloperidol also has weak anticholinergic, α-adrenergic, and ganglionic blocking activity.
Pharmacology:	Onset of action of antiemetic effects occurs within 1–2 hours of an oral dose and 10–30 minutes of an IM dose. The peak antiemetic effect occurs 2–4 hours after an oral dose and 30–45 minutes after an IM dose. The half-life is 12–38 hours. Haloperidol is metabolized extensively by the liver.
Indications in Palliative Care:	**Nausea and vomiting** (in low doses). **Psychotic disturbances** (higher doses).
Contraindications:	Comatose states. Parkinson's disease.
Adverse Side Effects:	**Extrapyramidal symptoms** (Parkinson-like, akathisia, or dystonia, including opisthotonos and oculogyric crisis) reported frequently, often during the first few days of treatment; extrapyramidal symptoms are dose-related and can be controlled by lowering the dosage or giving an antiparkinsonian drug such as trihexyphenidyl (Artane), benztropine (Cogentin), or diphenhydramine (Benadryl). **Tardive dyskinesias**, potentially irreversible, especially in elderly women. Consists of rhythmic, involuntary movements of the tongue, face, mouth, or jaw, accompanied by involuntary movements of the extremities. Risk increases with increasing dosage and duration of treatment, but dyskinesias may develop even at low doses after brief treatment period. There is no known treatment, although the syndrome may remit if haloperidol is withdrawn. **Neuroleptic malignant syndrome** (hyperpyrexia, rigidity, catatonia, dysrhythmias, diaphoresis, myoglobinuria, acute renal failure). Transient **hypotension** and precipitation of angina. May precipitate **seizures** in patients with a seizure history.
Incompatibility:	Can potentiate other CNS depressants (e.g., opiates). Interferes with the metabolism of phenytoin → phenytoin toxicity.
How Supplied:	Tablets: 0.5 mg (white), 1 mg (yellow), 2 mg (pink), 5 mg (green), 10 mg (aqua), and 20 mg (salmon). Drops: solution of 2 mg/ml. Ampules: 5 mg/ml.
Dosage and Administration:	For *nausea and vomiting*: • **0.5 mg PO tid** *or* **1.5 mg PO hs**. • By continuous **infusion, 1.5 mg/24 hr**. For *psychotic episodes*: • Start with 3–5 mg PO/IM tid + 3–5 mg prn → titrate upward according to previous day's total dosage.

Hydromorphone

Trade Name:	Dilaudid.
Mechanism of Action:	Semisynthetic **opioid** analgesic, **5–6 times more potent than morphine** (1.5 mg IM hydromorphone = 10 mg IM morphine). Activates (supraspinal) µ- and (intraspinal) κ-receptors to produce analgesia, particularly to nociceptive (as opposed to neuropathic) pain. Inhibits interneurons and output neurons of the spinothalamic tract that would otherwise convey nociceptive messages to higher cortical centers. Hydromorphone's antitussive effect is due to direct action on the medullary cough center; its peripheral effects are due to direct action on smooth muscle.
Pharmacology:	Hydrogenated ketone of morphine. The analgesic effect of parenterally administered hydromorphone is apparent within 15 minutes and usually lasts more than 5 hours. Onset of action of oral hydromorphone is slower, with analgesia occurring within 30 minutes, peaking within 1 hour, and lasting 4–6 hours. Oral bioavailability is 37–62%, somewhat better than that of morphine. Given rectally, hydromorphone's onset of action is in 10–15 minutes, peak effect in ½ hour, and duration of action is 6–8 hours. By the spinal route, hydromorphone causes less pruritus than morphine.
Indications in Palliative Care:	Because of its potency, hydromorphone is the opioid of choice for **continuous SQ infusion by syringe driver** in patients requiring **high opioid dosage**. As an alternative to morphine in patients who seem to be developing **morphine unresponsiveness** (i.e., increasing doses of morphine do not achieve better control of nociceptive pain) or morphine intolerance.
Contraindications:	Known hypersensitivity to hydromorphone.
Adverse Side Effects:	As for other opioids: Nausea and vomiting.* Respiratory depression.* Drowsiness.* Miosis. Constipation. Myoclonus. Acute urinary retention. Pruritus.
Incompatibility:	Additive CNS depression may occur with patients who are also receiving phenothiazines, tranquilizers, sedative-hypnotics, antidepressants, or alcohol.
How Supplied:	Ampules: 1 mg/ml, 2 mg/ml, 4 mg/ml, and 10 mg/ml. Multidose vials: 2 mg/ml in 20 ml.

*Denotes side effects that tend to remit after several days of treatment.

How Supplied: *cont.*	Color-coded tablets: 1 mg (green), 2 mg (orange), 3 mg (pink), and 4 mg (yellow). Rectal suppositories: 3 mg. Nonsterile powder for prescription compounding: 15-grain vial. Cough syrup: 1 mg/5 ml.
Dosage and Administration:	Calculate the patient's morphine requirement over the previous 24 hours. Start with ⅛ to ⅙ **the patient's 24-hour morphine dosage**: • If the patient was taking oral morphine, give hydromorphone orally, in six divided doses per day. • If the patient was receiving parenteral morphine, give hydromorphone by syringe driver, over 24 hours.

Hydroxyzine HCl

Trade Names:	Atarax, Ulcerax (UK), Vistaril.
Mechanism of Action:	H_1 blocking agent (antihistamine) in the piperazine family (which includes also cyclizine, meclizine). Its antipruritic action is due to direct competition with histamine at cellular binding sites. Some of its other actions may be due to suppression of activity in key regions of the subcortical area of the CNS. Has known *bronchodilator, antihistaminic, antiemetic, antispasmodic, anticholinergic, local anesthetic,* and *analgesic* effects. Potentiates sedative and analgesic effects of opioids (opioid-sparing effect).
Pharmacology:	Rapidly absorbed from the GI tract. Antiemetic and sedative effects usually noted within 15-30 minutes after oral administration, peak in 2-3 hours, and last 4-6 hours. Hydroxyzine is metabolized almost completely by the liver, and the metabolites are excreted primarily in the urine.
Indications in Palliative Care:	**Pruritus.** Nausea and vomiting. Anxiety states. Nighttime sedation (in combination with hypnotic).
Contraindications:	None in terminal illness.
Adverse Side Effects:	**Dry mouth.** **Drowsiness.** Involuntary motor activity.
Incompatibility:	May potentiate the effects of other CNS depressants, such as narcotics or barbiturates. May block the vasopressor action of epinephrine.
How Supplied:	Tablets (Atarax): 10 mg, 25 mg, 50 mg, and 100 mg. Capsules (Vistaril): 25 mg, 50 mg, and 100 mg. Oral suspension (Vistaril): 25 mg/tsp (5 ml). Syrup (Atarax): 10 mg/tsp (5 ml). IM injection solution (Vistaril): 25 mg/ml and 50 mg/ml.
Dosage and Administration:	For pruritus: **25 mg PO hs**. For antiemetic, sedative, or bronchodilator effect: **6.25–25 mg PO hs** *or* **25 mg/24 hr** by continuous SQ infusion.

Lactulose

Trade Names:	Acilac (C), Chronulac.
Mechanism of Action:	By acidification and increasing the osmotic pressure of colon contents, lactulose increases stool water → **softens the stool**. Since lactulose does not exert its effect until it reaches the colon, it may take 24–48 hours to work. In higher doses, lactulose also enables "ion trapping" of ammonia by acidifying the colonic contents (thus facilitating the conversion of NH_3 → nonabsorbable NH_4).
Pharmacology:	Synthetic disaccharide that cannot be hydrolyzed in the human GI tract and therefore reaches the colon unchanged. In the colon, it is broken down by colonic bacteria to lactic acid and smaller amounts of acetic and formic acid. Only small amounts of an orally administered dose reach the blood (urinary excretion < 3%).
Indications in Palliative Care:	For the treatment of **constipation** or the prevention of constipation in patients on chronic opioid therapy.
Contraindications:	Since lactulose also contains galactose, it is contraindicated in patients who require a low galactose diet. Use lactulose with caution in unstable diabetics because of galactose and lactose content.
Adverse Side Effects:	Initial dosing may produce **flatulence** and intestinal **cramps**, which are usually transient. Occasional **nausea** and vomiting. Excessive dose can lead to diarrhea, with hypokalemia and hyponatremia.
Incompatibility:	Concomitant administration of **nonabsorbable antacids** may inhibit the drop in colonic pH necessary for lactulose's action.
How Supplied:	As a syrup in 8-ounce and 1-quart bottles, containing 10 gm/15 ml.
Dosage and Administration:	**15–30 ml PO qd–bid.** Some patients find the syrup easier to tolerate if mixed with fruit juice, water, or milk.

Loperamide

Trade Name:	Imodium.
Mechanism of Action:	Peripherally-acting opioid agonist without central opioid activity. Slows intestinal motility, and affects water and electrolyte movement through the bowel. Also has a specific antisecretory effect on the bowel wall mediated by an active transport mechanism. The net effect is to reduce the daily fecal volume, increase fecal viscosity and bulk density, and diminish the loss of fluid and electrolytes via the gut.
Pharmacology:	Peak plasma levels are obtained 5 hours after administration of capsules and 2.5 hours after administration of liquid form. Most is excreted in the feces.
Indications in Palliative Care:	Symptomatic relief of persistent **diarrhea**. *NOTE:* APPARENT DIARRHEA IN A TERMINALLY ILL PATIENT MAY IN FACT BE THE RESULT OF LEAKAGE AROUND A FECAL IMPACTION. RULE OUT FECAL IMPACTION BEFORE PRESCRIBING ANTIDIARRHEALS.
Contraindications:	Acute dysentery (with melena and fever). Use with caution in patients with ulcerative colitis and in pseudomembranous colitis associated with antibiotic agents.
Adverse Side Effects:	Hypersensitivity reactions (including rash). Abdominal pain and distention. Dry mouth.
Incompatibility:	None reported.
How Supplied:	Capsules: 2 mg. Flavored solution: 1 mg/5 ml.
Dosage and Administration:	**2 capsules (4 mg) PO initially** followed by **1 capsule (2 mg) after each subsequent loose stool** (total dose not to exceed 16 mg in 24 hours).

Megestrol Acetate

Trade Names:	Megace, Pallace.
Mechanism of Action:	Progestational agent that stimulates appetite and exerts an anabolic effect, producing weight gain through an increase in both fat and lean body mass. Its antineoplastic effect occurs through inhibition of progestin-sensitive breast and endometrial cancers.
Pharmacology:	Oral absorption variable. Peak plasma levels occur at 2 hours after an oral dose, and the plasma elimination half-life ranges from 13–105 hours.
Indications in Palliative Care:	To improve appetite in patients with **anorexia** and life expectancy > 1 month.
Contraindications:	Thrombophlebitis.
Adverse Side Effects:	Menstrual irregularities. Mild fluid retention. Occasional hypercalcemia after initial therapy. Tumor flare (breast cancer).
Incompatibility:	None reported.
How Supplied:	Tablets: 20 mg and 40 mg.
Dosage and Administration:	**40–120 mg PO qid.**

Methadone

Trade Names:	Aldolan, Dolophine HCl, Methadone HCl, Methadose, Physeptone (C, UK).
Mechanism of Action:	Synthetic **opioid** analgesic. Activates (supraspinal) μ- and (intraspinal) κ-receptors to produce analgesia, particularly to nociceptive (as opposed to neuropathic) pain. Inhibits interneurons and output neurons of the spinothalamic tract that would otherwise convey nociceptive messages to higher cortical centers. Methadone's peripheral effects are due to direct action on smooth muscle.
Pharmacology:	Racemic mixture of L-methadone, responsible for analgesic effect, and D-methadone, which has antitussive properties. A dose of 8–10 mg methadone is approximately equivalent in analgesic effect to 10 mg of morphine. With single-dose administration, the onset and duration of analgesic action of the two drugs are similar. Because of a high volume of distribution and 60–90% protein binding, methadone accumulates in tissues, more than morphine, resulting in a longer plasma half-life (especially in older patients), and cumulative toxicity is thus more of a problem than with morphine. Furthermore, changes in dosage may take several days to reach a steady state. Analgesia from methadone lasts 6–12 hours. Methadone is well absorbed by all routes. Oral bioavailability is about 80%. When given orally, methadone is half as potent as when given parenterally; with oral administration, onset of action is slower, peak action less, and duration of analgesia longer. Methadone is metabolized by the liver and excreted through the gut and kidneys. Its clearance is not affected by either liver or kidney disease, however.
Indications in Palliative Care:	As an alternative to morphine in patients who seem to be developing **morphine unresponsiveness** (i.e., increasing doses of morphine do not achieve better control of nociceptive pain) or morphine intolerance, when close supervision is possible.
Contraindications:	Use with caution in patients at risk of cumulative toxicity: ▪ Elderly patients. ▪ Demented or delirious patients.
Adverse Side Effects:	As for other opioids: Nausea and vomiting.* Respiratory depression.* Drowsiness.* Miosis. Constipation. Myoclonus. Acute urinary retention. Pruritus.

*Denotes side effects that tend to remit after several days of treatment.

Incompatibility:	**Rifampicin** speeds methadone metabolism → may lead to symptoms of withdrawal. **Cimetidine** inhibits methadone metabolism → may lead to drowsiness or coma. Additive sedative and respiratory depressive effects when given with phenothiazines.
How Supplied:	Dolophine HCl supplied as ▪ Ampules: 10 mg in 1 ml; 10-ml and 20-ml multidose vials of 1 mg/ml. ▪ Tablets: 5 mg and 10 mg. Methadone HCl supplied as ▪ Oral solution: 5 mg/5 ml and 10 mg/5 ml in bottles of 500 ml. ▪ Tablets: 5 mg and 10 mg.
Dosage and Administration:	For patients who have become relatively unresponsive to morphine, *start* with ½ to ⅔ **the patient's current 24-hour morphine dosage,** divided into 4 daily doses. After 3 days, eliminate one dose (i.e., reduce the 24-hour dosage by 25%), and go to tid dosing.

Methotrimeprazine (Levomepromazine)

Trade Names:	**Levoprome, Nozinan** (C, UK).
Mechanism of Action:	Phenothiazine with pharmacologic activity similar to that of chlorpromazine and promethazine, but with much stronger sedative and antiemetic activity; CNS effects like those of chlorpromazine; antihistaminic; anticholinergic; marked analgesic properties in addition.
Pharmacology:	Peak plasma concentrations in 1–4 hours after oral administration and 30–90 minutes after IM administration. Maximum analgesic effects occur in 20–40 minutes. Duration of sedation or analgesia is up to 4 hours. About 50% of orally absorbed drug reaches the systemic circulation. It is metabolized in the liver.
Indications in Palliative Care:	For **restlessness** when the objective is to sedate the patient. Strongest **antiemetic** acting on the CTZ; useful when sedation is also desirable. As an adjunct to analgesics for severe **pain**. For **terminal restlessness**. Together with opioid, corticosteroid, and papaverine in the treatment of **intestinal obstruction** without nasogastric intubation. Together with dexamethasone for symptomatic **brain metastases** when the objective is sedation. For intractable **hiccups**.
Contraindications:	In patients in whom sedation is not a desired effect.
Adverse Side Effects:	May cause severe **postural hypotension**. Pain at injection site. Extrapyramidal reactions. Anticholinergic effects (dry mouth).
Incompatibility:	Potentiates effects of antihypertensive drugs. Additive effects with benzodiazepines. Additive anticholinergic effects with atropine, scopolamine (hyoscine).
How Supplied:	Tablets: 2 mg, 5 mg, 25 mg, and 50 mg. Drops: 4% solution. Solution for IM injection: 20 mg/ml and 25 mg/ml. (*Note:* In the United States, methotrimeprazine is available only for injection.)
Dosage and Administration:	*For prevention of nausea & vomiting:* **2–6.25 mg PO tid** or **6.25–25 mg PO hs**. *For treatment of nausea & vomiting:* ▪ **IM: 2–6.25 mg tid**. ▪ SQ by syringe driver: **6–25 mg/24 hr.** * *For bowel obstruction:* SQ by syringe driver, **25–75 mg/24 hr**.

*Can be combined with morphine, metoclopramide, and/or promethazine in same syringe.

Dosage and Administration: *cont.*	*For restlessness:* Dose **titrated** according to effect, or until there is a fall in blood pressure. Start with 6.25 mg PO/IM tid; double the dosage if effect not adequate. *For pain associated with restlessness or nausea/vomiting* (combined with opioids): 15 mg of methotrimeprazine = 10 mg of morphine; choose dosage accordingly. *For hiccups:* **25–50 mg PO/IM tid** (strong sedative effect).

Methylphenidate HCl

Trade Names:	Methidate, Ritalin.
Mechanism of Action:	Mild *CNS stimulant* that is thought to work by activating the brainstem arousal system and cortex through release of norepinephrine from nerve endings (→ ↑nerve transmission). At high doses, dopamine stores are also activated.
Pharmacology:	Extensively absorbed after oral administration. Peak serum levels in 2 hours after oral administration. Duration of action is usually 4–6 hours (up to 8 hours with sustained-release tablets). Well tolerated in the elderly.
Indications in Palliative Care:	To **counteract excess sedation** in cancer patients taking opioids for pain. To treat **depression** in withdrawn, apathetic, elderly patients. To **enhance the analgesic effect of opioids** when a stimulatory effect is also desirable.
Contraindications:	Anxiety, tension, agitation. Glaucoma. Motor tics. Seizures.
Adverse Side Effects:	**Nervousness** and insomnia (controlled by reducing dosage). Headache. Palpitations. Hypersensitivity reactions (rash).
Incompatibility:	Use with caution in patients taking MAO inhibitor antidepressants. May inhibit metabolism of coumarin, anticonvulsant drugs, phenylbutazone, and tricyclic antidepressants to produce toxic effects of those drugs (dosages of those drugs should be lowered when given with methylphenidate). Stimulant action of methylphenidate is increased by caffeine.
How Supplied:	Tablets: 5 mg, 10 mg, and 20 mg. Sustained-release tablets: 20 mg. Ampules: 20 mg.
Dosage and Administration:	**10 mg PO at 0800** and **5 mg PO at 1200** for routine use. For special occasions, **10 mg PO 4 hours before and ½ hour before** the occasion in question.

Metoclopramide

Trade Names:	Gastrobid (UK), Maxerin (C), Maxalon (AU, C, UK), Pramin (AU), Reglan.
Mechanism of Action:	Stimulates motility of upper GI tract without stimulating gastric, biliary, or pancreatic secretions. Increases tone and amplitude of antral contractions; relaxes pyloric sphincter and duodenal bulb; increases peristalsis of duodenum and jejunum → **faster gastric emptying** and intestinal transit. Increases resting tone of lower esophageal sphincter. Antiemetic properties result from its **antagonism of** central and peripheral **dopamine receptors** (hence works both at **CTZ** and at stomach). Effect of metoclopramide on motility is not dependent on intact vagal innervation, but it can be abolished by anticholinergics.
Pharmacology:	**Onset of action** is 1–3 minutes following IV dose, 10–15 minutes following IM dose, and **30–60 minutes following oral dose. Effects persist 1–2 hours.** Rapidly and well absorbed; peak plasma concentrations 1–2 hours after a single oral dose. Eighty-five percent appears in urine within 72 hours. About 30% bound to protein; extensive body distribution. Excretion impaired when creatinine clearance ↓ → start with ½ dosage when creatinine clearance<40.
Indications in Palliative Care:	First-line drug for the **treatment of nausea and vomiting** in cancer patients. **Prevention of nausea and vomiting** associated with cancer chemotherapy or postoperatively. **Gastroesophageal reflux** with heartburn. To **improve appetite** when anorexia is due to gastric stasis.
Contraindications:	When stimulation of GI motility might be dangerous, as in **GI bleeding, high mechanical obstruction** (i.e., above the ligament of Treitz) or **perforation**. **Epilepsy.** Use with caution in patients receiving **other drugs likely to cause extrapyramidal reactions**.
Adverse Side Effects:	**Drowsiness.** **Depression.** **Extrapyramidal reactions**, mostly acute dystonic reactions, in 1 in 500 patients treated with 30–40 mg/day; usually seen within first 24–48 hours of treatment, more often in children/young adults (especially in higher doses used to prevent vomiting from chemotherapy). Treat with **diphenhydramine** (Benadryl), **50 mg PO/IM**, or **benztropine** (Cogentin), **0.5–4 mg PO bid**. Parkinson-like symptoms may occur within first 6 months of starting treatment. **Tardive dyskinesias** (with involuntary movements of tongue, face, mouth, or jaw) most likely in the elderly (especially women) may be irreversible; no known treatment. Restlessness, fatigue, lassitude in 10%.

continued

Metoclopramide *continued*

Incompatibility:	Effects on GI motility are antagonized by anticholinergics and narcotics. Additive sedative effects can occur when given with alcohol, sedatives, hypnotics, or tranquilizers. Increases absorption of aspirin, acetaminophen, diazepam, L-dopa, and lithium. Concomitant use with phenothiazines or butyrophenones more likely to produce extrapyramidal reactions. Use with caution (if at all) in patients on MAO inhibitors.
How Supplied:	Tablets: 5 mg and 10 mg. Syrup: 5 mg/5 ml. Vials and ampules: 5 mg/ml. Suppositories: 5 mg and 20 mg (not available in the United States).
Dosage and Administration:	For treatment of *nausea and vomiting:* **10 mg PO tid** *OR* **30–60 mg/24 hr SQ** via syringe driver. For *symptomatic gastroesophageal reflux:* **10–15 mg PO qid** ½ **hour ac and hs** (5 mg/dose in elderly). For *prevention of nausea/vomiting from chemotherapy:* Initial dosage: **1–2 mg/kg IV** diluted in not less than 50 ml of normal saline given slowly (over at least 15–30 minutes) 30 minutes before beginning chemotherapy, then q2h × 2, then q3h × 2.

Metronidazole

Trade Names:	Flagyl, MetroGel, Novonidazole (C), Protostat.
Mechanism of Action:	Antiprotozoal and antibacterial agent with particular activity against *anaerobic bacteria*, including *Bacteroides* and *Clostridium* species.
Pharmacology:	Well absorbed following oral administration, with peak plasma concentrations 1–2 hours after administration and an average elimination half-life of 8 hours. Plasma clearance is decreased in patients with decreased liver function.
Indications in Palliative Care:	Anaerobic bacterial infections causing distress to the patient, such as **fungating cutaneous metastases**.
Contraindications:	Known hypersensitivity. Severe hepatic impairment.
Adverse Side Effects:	To *oral* and *parenteral* forms: **Nausea** (12%) and vomiting. **Headache.** Diarrhea. Epigastric distress. Abdominal **cramping**. Seizures and peripheral neuropathy. Activation of latent candidiasis. *Topical* metronidazole has minimal adverse side effects (transient stinging or redness).
Incompatibility:	**Alcoholic beverages** should not be taken for the duration of treatment with metronidazole, for the combination will provoke abdominal cramps, nausea, vomiting, headaches, and flushing. Should not be given with disulfuram. Potentiates anticoagulant effect of **coumarin** anticoagulants → ↑prothrombin time. **Cimetidine** may prolong the half-life of metronidazole. Metronidazole may elevate serum **lithium** to toxic levels. Reduce dosage in patients with **hepatic disease**. Metronidazole interferes with laboratory determination of SGOT, SGPT, and LDH.
How Supplied:	Tablets: 250 mg and 500 mg. As an 0.75% gel for topical application (MetroGel). In vials for IV infusion of 500 mg for reconstitution in 4.4 ml of sterile water or normal saline for injection.
Dosage and Administration:	For *smelly tumors*: Apply **gel** to wound tid; if necessary, add **250 mg PO tid with meals** × **7–10 days.** (Warn patient that drug may cause a metallic taste and may turn the urine reddish-brown.) For *severe anaerobic infections* during active cancer treatment, IV infusion of 7.5 mg/kg q6h (not to exceed 4 gm/24 hr).

Mexiletine HCl

Trade Name:	Mexitil.
Mechanism of Action:	Local anesthetic, antiarrhythmic, structurally similar to lidocaine but active when taken orally. Developed as an antiarrhythmic drug to suppress ventricular dysrhythmias through its inhibitory effect on the sodium current (membrane-stabilizing effect).
Pharmacology:	Ninety percent absorbed from the GI tract, with a low first-pass metabolism. Peak blood levels are reached in 2–3 hours. The onset of analgesic effect takes up to 5 days and reaches a maximum within 2 weeks. The half-life of a single dose is 10–12 hours. Metabolized in the liver, with 10% excreted unchanged in the urine. Hepatic impairment prolongs the elimination half-life.
Indications in Palliative Care:	**Neuropathic pain,** especially sharp, lancinating, or electric shock–like pain when tricyclic antidepressant and/or anticonvulsant therapy has failed.
Contraindications:	Second- or third-degree AV block. *Caution* in patients with impaired renal function (more likely to suffer toxicity).
Adverse Side Effects:	Nausea, anorexia. Dizziness, light-headedness. Tremor.
Incompatibility:	Narcotics, atropine, and aluminum hydroxide/magnesium hydroxide slow the absorption of mexiletine. Metoclopramide accelerates absorption of mexiletine. Cimetidine may increase or decrease blood levels of mexiletine. Mexiletine may increase blood levels of theophylline. Discontinue treatment with tricyclic antidepressants for at least 3 days before starting mexiletine to avoid additive dysrhythmic effects.
How Supplied:	Capsules: 150 mg, 200 mg, and 250 mg.
Dosage and Administration:	Start with **150 mg bid** × 3 days, then 150 mg tid × 2 weeks, then, if the patient is still in pain, increase to 150 mg qid × 1 week; if still in pain, increase once more to a maximum of 750 mg/day in divided doses. Administration with food is recommended to decrease incidence of nausea and vomiting from the drug.

Midazolam

Trade Names:	Hypnovel (UK),Versed.
Mechanism of Action:	**CNS depressant** with sedative, antianxiety, anticonvulsant, and skeletal muscle relaxant activity.
Pharmacology:	Short-acting **benzodiazepine**. Onset of sedative effect after IM administration is 15 minutes and peaks in 30-60 minutes; onset of amnesic effect is 30-60 minutes after IM injection. Sedation after IV administration occurs in 3-5 minutes. Elimination half-life = 1.2-12.3 hours (clinical effects do not directly correlate with blood levels); about half is excreted in the urine in conjugated form; elimination half-life ↑ in patients with CHF and chronic renal failure.
Indications in Palliative Care:	**Terminal restlessness.** Short-term sedation for uncomfortable procedures. Sedation for managing catastrophic terminal events.
Contraindications:	Acute narrow-angle glaucoma.
Adverse Side Effects:	Adverse effects are most commonly observed after *IV* administration and include respiratory depression and respiratory arrest. Adverse effects seen principally after IM administration include **headache** (1.3%) and **pain at the injection site** (3.7%).
Incompatibility:	Clearance of midazolam may be delayed by concomitant administration of **cimetidine** (but not ranitidine). CNS depressant effects potentiated by opioids, barbiturates, antihistamines, and antidepressants.
How Supplied:	Vials: 1 mg/ml and 5 mg/ml. Prefilled 2-ml syringes: 5 mg/ml.
Dosage and Administration:	Initial dose in patients not receiving narcotics: • 0.07-0.08 mg/kg (≈ **5 mg) IM** in patients < **60** years old. • 0.02-0.05 mg/kg (≈ **2-3 mg) IM** in patients > **60** years old. May be given by **continuous SQ infusion**: Start at **5 mg/ 24 hr** and titrate upward (may be mixed with other agents, such as morphine, in the same infusion). For emergency sedation in terminal catastrophic events (e.g., exsanguination): 2.5 mg IV given over at least 2 minutes.

Misoprostol

Trade Name:	Cytotec.
Mechanism of Action:	Synthetic **prostaglandin E$_1$ analog** that both **inhibits secretion of gastric acid** and protects gastric mucosa. Opposes the ulcerogenic action of NSAIDs on the gastric mucosa (NSAIDs inhibit prostaglandin synthesis → ↓bicarbonate and mucus secretion → mucosal damage). Misoprostol inhibits basal and nocturnal gastric acid secretion. It increases gastric mucus secretion and mucosal blood flow as well as increasing duodenal bicarbonate secretion. It may also protect renal blood flow in patients with cirrhosis and ascites taking NSAIDs. May reverse nephrotoxicity caused by cyclosporine. Because of abortifacient properties, misoprostol is not given to women who might be pregnant.
Pharmacology:	Rapidly absorbed after oral administration, peaking in the serum at 12 minutes, with a half-life of 20–40 minutes. Inhibition of gastric acid secretion occurs within 30 minutes, peaks at 60–90 minutes, and lasts at least 3 hours after a given dose. Concentrations are diminished when the drug is taken with food or antacids, but the effect does not appear to interfere with clinical effectiveness of the drug.
Indications in Palliative Care:	Drug of choice to **prevent gastric ulcers caused by NSAIDs**, including aspirin. (Has not been shown to prevent *duodenal* ulcers.)
Contraindications:	Allergy to prostaglandins. Use with *caution* in patients with inflammatory bowel disease. No other absolute contraindications in palliative care.
Adverse Side Effects:	Diarrhea (13%), developing within first 2 weeks of therapy, usually self-limited; can be minimized by taking the medication with food. Crampy abdominal pain (7%). Flatulence.
Incompatibility:	None reported.
How Supplied:	Tablets: 100 µg and 200 µg.
Dosage and Administration:	**100–200 µg PO qid** (with meals and hs), for the duration of NSAID therapy.

Morphine Preparations

Trade Names:	Astramorph, Duramorph, Epimorph (C), Infumorph, M.O.S. (C), Morphitec (C), MS Contin, MST Continus (UK), MSIR, MS/S, Oramorph (UK), Rescudose, RMS Uniserts, Roxanol, Sevredol (UK), Statex (C).
Mechanism of Action:	Activates (supraspinal) μ- and (intraspinal) κ-receptors to produce analgesia, particularly to nociceptive (as opposed to neuropathic) pain. Morphine inhibits interneurons and output neurons of the spinothalamic tract that would otherwise convey nociceptive messages to higher cortical centers. Morphine given by inhalation is thought to act locally on specific endorphin receptors in the lung, since < 5% of an inhaled dose reaches the circulation.
Pharmacology:	Readily absorbed from the GI tract, rectal mucosa, and after SQ or IM injection. (Morphine given by inhalation is not significantly absorbed and acts locally on bronchial mucosa.) The bioavailability of oral morphine preparations is about 25%. The onset of action after oral administration is 15–60 minutes for immediate-release (MSIR) and 60–90 minutes for slow-release forms (MS Contin). Peak effect is at 30–60 minutes (immediate-release) and 1–4 hours (slow-release). Duration of action is 2–7 hours (immediate release) or 6–12 hours (slow-release). Given SQ, the onset of action of morphine is 15–30 minutes, the peak effect is in 50–90 minutes, and the duration of action is 2–7 hours. Only small quantities pass the blood-brain barrier. Morphine is metabolized by conjugation with glucuronic acid to form a more potent compound, morphine-6-glucuronide and an inactive, probably antagonistic compound, morphine-3-glucuronide. Morphine in its conjugated forms is eliminated by glomerular filtration.
Indications in Palliative Care:	Relief of moderate to severe **pain** (see Chapters 1 and 2). Given by nebulizer, to relieve **persistent cough or dyspnea**. Given IV to relieve **acute pulmonary edema**, especially that due to left heart failure.
Contraindications:	None, but use caution in Severe renal insufficiency (morphine-6-glucuronide may accumulate to toxic levels). Hepatic failure (morphine may not be conjugated and may accumulate to toxic levels).
Adverse Side Effects:	**Nausea** and vomiting.* **Respiratory depression.*** **Drowsiness.*** Miosis. **Constipation.** Myoclonus. Acute urinary retention. Pruritus. Bronchospasm.

*Denotes side effects that tend to remit after several days of treatment.   *continued*

Morphine Preparations   *continued*

Incompatibility:	Elimination of morphine is impaired by **cimetidine** → morphine toxicity. Additive sedative and respiratory depressive effects when given with phenothiazines.
How Supplied:	*Short-acting* (immediate-release) *tablets* (**MSIR**): 10 mg, 15 mg, and 30 mg given q3-4h. Flavored *oral solution*: **MSIR**:10 mg/5 ml and 20 mg/5 ml. **Roxanol**: 20 mg/ml, 30 mg/1.5 ml, and 10 mg/2.5 ml. **Rescudose**: 10 mg/2.5 ml. Unflavored, *concentrated oral solution* (**MSIR**): 20 mg/ml. *Long-acting* (sustained-release) *tablets*: **MS Contin**: 15 mg (blue), 30 mg (lavender), 60 mg (orange), and 100 mg (gray) given bid-tid. **Oramorph**: 30 mg, 60 mg, and 100 mg (all white) given bid-tid. Rectal *suppositories* (**MS/S**): 5 mg, 10 mg, 20 mg, and 30 mg given q4h. *Ampules* for continuous epidural or intrathecal infusion (**Infumorph**): 200 mg/20 ml and 500 mg/20 ml. *Ampules* for IV, epidural, or intrathecal use (**Astromorph**, **Duramorph**): 0.5 mg/ml and 1 mg/ml.
Dosage and Administration:	See Chapter 2. In general, initial **dosage titration** is carried out with **MSIR** **q4h + prn** until a satisfactory level of pain control is achieved. The total morphine requirement of the previous 24 hours is then toted up and divided by 2 to arrive at a twice-daily dosage for MS Contin. Subsequently, MSIR is used only in rescue doses to supplement MS Contin for incident or breakthrough pain. Maintenance doses in cancer patients are highly individual and may range from 60 mg/day to 2000 mg/day or higher. A **laxative regimen** should be started concurrently. For cancer pain, opioids are given **by the clock** and not on a prn basis. *By nebulizer, for cough or dyspnea*: Start with **2.5 mg** of morphine sulfate parenteral solution. Give together with dexamethasone 2 mg and 2.5 ml of normal saline q4-6h and prn. The dosage of nebulized morphine may be titrated upward as needed, but there is usually little additional benefit in exceeding a dosage of 100 mg by nebulizer. Most patients can be managed on doses under 20 mg per treatment.

Naproxen
Naproxen Sodium

Trade Names:	Naproxen: Naprotec (UK), Naprosyn, Naxen (C). Naproxen sodium: Aleve, Anaprox, Synflex (UK).
Mechanism of Action:	NSAID with analgesic, antipyretic, and anti-inflammatory actions thought to be mediated by inhibition of prostaglandin and leukotriene synthesis. The analgesic potency is about three times that of aspirin or ibuprofen but with slightly less GI toxicity than aspirin. Like aspirin, naproxen inhibits platelet aggregation and prolongs bleeding time. Naproxen does *not* have the uricosuric activity associated with aspirin.
Pharmacology:	Absorbed rapidly and completely from the GI tract; the sodium salt is more rapidly absorbed and achieves higher peak plasma levels. GI absorption is delayed by food and milk. The plasma half-life of naproxen is about 14 hours. Naproxen is metabolized in the liver, and its metabolic degradation products are excreted in the urine. The onset of analgesic action after an oral dose occurs in 30–60 minutes (onset of anti-inflammatory action may take up to 2 weeks); the peak analgesic effect occurs in 1–2 hours and lasts 7–12 hours. Naproxen is the NSAID of choice in palliative care because its longer half-life makes twice-daily dosing effective.
Indications in Palliative Care:	**Bone pain** in patients with metastases to bone. Mild to moderate visceral pain.
Contraindications:	Active **peptic ulcer** or recent history of GI bleeding. Use with caution in **multiple myeloma** because of the danger of precipitating renal failure. Patients in whom aspirin or other NSAIDs have induced wheezing, urticaria, or rhinitis. Patients with the triad of asthma, nasal polyps, and aspirin hypersensitivity. Renal impairment or prerenal failure. **Heart failure**.
Adverse Side Effects:	Peripheral **edema**, fluid retention, hypertension. Dyspepsia, nausea, **epigastric pain**, GI bleeding or perforation, constipation. Prolongation of bleeding time. Pruritus, rash. Tinnitus. May precipitate acute renal failure in patients with prerenal azotemia.
Incompatibility:	Bleeding may occur if used with **anticoagulants** (coumarin, heparin) or with other drugs that inhibit platelet aggregation (carbenicillin, piperacillin, valproic acid, other NSAIDs).

continued

Naproxen
Naproxen Sodium   *continued*

Incompatibility: *cont.*	May potentiate the hypoglycemic effects of **hypoglycemic agents** such as insulin or oral agents. Naproxen may displace protein-bound drugs from their receptors, leading to toxicity from drugs such as phenytoin, verapamil, or nifedipine. Naproxen may decrease the clinical effectiveness of diuretics and β-blocking antihypertensive agents.
How Supplied:	*Naproxen*: Tablets: 250 mg, 375 mg, and 500 mg. Oral suspension: 125 mg/5 ml. *Naproxen sodium*: Film-coated tablets: 275 mg and 550 mg. *Note*: 275 mg of naproxen sodium = 250 mg of naproxen.
Dosage and Administration:	**250–500 mg PO bid.** *Note*: Because of the high degree of plasma binding and the rapid urinary clearance of the drug, plasma concentrations of naproxen do not increase at doses higher than 500 mg bid, so there is little to be gained in exceeding that dosage.

Nystatin

Trade Names:	**Mycostatin, Nystatin.**
Mechanism of Action:	Macrolide antibiotic produced by *Streptomyces noursei*, structurally similar to amphotericin B but more toxic and therefore not used systemically. Antifungal activity results from binding to a sterol moiety present in the membrane of sensitive fungi. This produces increased permeability of the fungal membrane, allowing leakage of small molecules.
Pharmacology:	Not absorbed systemically from the GI tract, skin, or vaginal mucosa. When taken orally, nystatin is excreted unchanged in the feces.
Indications in Palliative Care:	Oral **candidiasis**.
Contraindications:	Known hypersensitivity.
Adverse Side Effects:	Bitter taste. Nausea when taken in high doses.
Incompatibility:	None known.
How Supplied:	Oral tablets: 500,000 U (Mycostatin). Oral suspension: 100,000 U/ml. Pastilles: 200,000 U (Mycostatin). Powder for oral administration: ⅛ tsp = 500,000 U, for reconstitution in water.
Dosage and Administration:	Oral suspension: **4–6 ml PO tid** after mouth care (swish in mouth and swallow). Pastilles: 1–2 PO qid. Allow to dissolve slowly in the mouth; do not chew or swallow whole.

Octreotide

Trade Name:	Sandostatin.
Mechanism of Action:	Synthetic analog of somatostatin that (1) decreases secretion of salt and water into the bowel lumen, while increasing intestinal absorption of water and electrolytes → decreases the volume of fluids within intestinal lumen and directly opposes pathogenic mechanisms in bowel obstruction; (2) slows gastric emptying and small-intestinal transit time; (3) decreases bile flow by inhibiting smooth muscle activity of gallbladder; (4) decreases abnormally raised lower esophageal sphincter pressure; and (5) may have a direct analgesic effect (binds to opioid receptors in the brain; central effects opposed by naloxone).
Pharmacology:	Octreotide is absorbed rapidly after SQ injection with peak serum concentrations in 25 minutes. Half-life is 100 minutes, peak of action is at 2 hours, and duration of action is 12 hours, although the half-life may be increased by up to 50% in the elderly, necessitating dosage adjustment. One third of the drug is excreted unchanged in the urine. In severe renal failure, clearance of the drug is reduced to 50% of normal.
Indications in Palliative Care:	For nonsurgical management of **malignant bowel obstruction** (not yet an FDA-approved indication). For control of intractable **diarrhea**, especially when caused by chemotherapy or the malignancy itself (not yet an FDA-approved indication). To decrease drainage from **cutaneous fistulas** (not yet an FDA-approved indication). Metastatic **carcinoid tumors**, to suppress the severe diarrhea and flushing associated with the disease. May have a role as an analgesic by intrathecal administration (not FDA approved for this use).
Contraindications:	Sensitivity to the drug.
Adverse Side Effects:	Dry mouth due to inhibition of salivary flow (usually abates after 24 hours). Increased flatulence (responds to ↓octreotide dosage). Pain on injection (can be minimized by warming the drug vial with the hands after removal from the refrigerator or by giving as a continuous SQ infusion). May cause hypo- or hyperglycemia. Rebound hyperglycemia may occur on discontinuation of the drug. Long-term use → >20% incidence of cholelithiasis.
Incompatibility:	Adjustment of dosage of oral hypoglycemics or insulin may be necessary after starting octreotide. May affect absorption of *any* orally administered drug.
How Supplied:	Ampules: 50 µg/ml, 100 µg/ml, and 500 µg/ml. Multidose vials: 20 µg/ml and 1000 µg/ml.

Dosage and Administration:	For *malignant bowel obstruction or cutaneous fistula*, start with

- 150 µg by SQ injection bid, *or*
- **300 µg/24 hr** by **continuous SQ infusion** (may be mixed with morphine and haloperidol in the same infusion).
- May increase to a total dosage of 600 µg/24 hr.

For *carcinoid tumors*, start with 150 µg SQ bid.

Omeprazole

Trade Names:	Losec (UK), Prilosec.
Mechanism of Action:	Benzimidazole drug that **inhibits gastric acid secretion** by specific inhibition of the K^+/H^+ ATPase enzyme system (proton pump) at the secretory surface of the parietal cell. *Not* an anticholinergic or H_2 receptor antagonist. Instead, omeprazole acts as a **gastric acid pump inhibitor** to block the final step of acid production.
Pharmacology:	Omeprazole is supplied in enteric-coated form to protect it from being inactivated in the acidic stomach contents; it is absorbed in the proximal small intestine. The onset of anti-secretory action of omeprazole occurs within 1 hour after oral administration; maximum effect is within 2 hours, and inhibitory effect is still 50% of maximum at 24 hours (lasts up to 72 hours)—this apparently because of prolonged binding of the drug to the parietal ATPase enzyme. After discontinuing the drug, gastric secretory activity gradually returns over 3–5 days. Omeprazole is mostly metabolized by the liver, and metabolites are excreted in the urine. The elimination rate is decreased in the elderly.
Indications in Palliative Care:	Short-term (4 weeks) treatment of **active duodenal ulcer**. Should *not* be used as maintenance therapy. Short-term treatment of **gastroesophageal reflux disease** that has not responded to H_2 receptor antagonists.
Contraindications:	None in palliative care.
Adverse Side Effects:	Headache (2.4%). Diarrhea (2%).
Incompatibility:	Can prolong the elimination of **diazepam, warfarin**, and **phenytoin** drugs → dosage adjustments may be necessary. *May* interfere with absorption of drugs that require low gastric pH (e.g., ampicillin).
How Supplied:	Delayed-release capsules: 20 mg.
Dosage and Administration:	**20 mg PO qam before eating.** Capsule should not be opened, chewed, or crushed but must be swallowed whole because of enteric coating that protects the drug from gastric acidity.

Ondansetron

Trade Name:	Zofran.
Mechanism of Action:	Selective antagonist of 5-HT$_3$ (serotonin) receptors, which are present centrally in the CTZ of the brain and peripherally on vagal nerve terminals; the antiemetic effect of ondansetron may be mediated at either or both sites. Ondansetron has no effect on GI motility, nor does it act at dopamine receptor sites.
Pharmacology:	The onset of action after an IV dose is within 30 minutes. Peak plasma concentrations occur within 1½ hours. The duration of action is 12–24 hours. When taken orally, ondansetron has a bioavailability of about 50% and reaches peak concentrations within 2 hours. Ondansetron is extensively metabolized, and its metabolic products are excreted in the urine. A reduction in renal clearance is seen in patients over 75 years old, but this has not necessitated any alteration in dosage.
Indications in Palliative Care:	Chemotherapy-induced nausea and vomiting (especially that caused by cisplatin-based regimens). Severe **nausea and vomiting** in terminal illness that has not responded to prokinetic and antidopaminergic agents. May be useful in cholestatic pruritus.
Contraindications:	Use with caution in patients with hepatic failure.
Adverse Side Effects:	Constipation (11%). Rash. Transient blurred vision.
Incompatibility:	None of clinical significance.
How Supplied:	IV injection: 2 mg/ml in 20-ml multidose vials. Tablets: 4 mg and 8 mg (not available for clinical use in the United States).
Dosage and Administration:	*Intravenous*: **0.15 mg/kg** diluted in 50 ml of normal saline or 5% dextrose and **infused over 15 minutes** (if given to prevent vomiting from chemotherapy, should be infused 30 minutes before the first dose of the emetogenic agent). Should not be mixed with other solutions, especially alkaline solutions. *Oral* (where available): **8 mg PO bid**.

Opium, tincture of

Trade Names:	No proprietary preparations; order generically.
Mechanism of Action:	As for morphine, but acts less rapidly than morphine, since opium is more slowly absorbed; the relaxing action of the *papaverine* and noscapine components on the intestine makes opium *more constipating than morphine* and accounts for its effectiveness in diarrhea.
Pharmacology:	Contains variable mixture of 25 alkaloids, including morphine (9-17%), noscapine (2-9%), thebaine, narceine, papaverine, and hydrocotarnine. The opium alkaloids act primarily in the GI tract and are metabolized by the liver.
Indications in Palliative Care:	Persistent **diarrhea**.
Contraindications:	Overflow diarrhea in fecal impaction. Diarrhea from pseudomembranous enterocolitis or ulcerative colitis (opium may precipitate toxic megacolon).
Adverse Side Effects:	As for morphine, but less frequent and less pronounced: sedation, nausea, vomiting.
Incompatibility:	None reported.
How Supplied:	Specially prepared by local pharmacies, in a concentration equivalent to 10 mg of morphine per milliliter.
Dosage and Administration:	**15–20 gtt PO tid prn.** Mix with sufficient water to ensure that all the opium reaches the stomach.

Oxybutynin Chloride

Trade Names:	Cystrin (UK), Ditropan.
Mechanism of Action:	Exerts a direct antispasmodic effect on smooth muscle and inhibits the muscarinic action of acetylcholine on smooth muscle. No antinicotinic effects. Clinically, relaxes bladder smooth muscle. The net effect is to reduce the urge to void, increase bladder capacity, and diminish bladder spasm.
Pharmacology:	Absorbed rapidly after oral administration. Therapeutic action has its onset within 30-60 minutes, peaks in 3-6 hours, and persists 6-10 hours. The drug is metabolized by the liver and excreted mainly in the urine.
Indications in Palliative Care:	**Bladder spasm.** Reflex neurogenic bladder (urgency, frequency, urge incontinence).
Contraindications:	Ileus or bowel obstruction. Obstructive uropathy. Extreme caution in patients with ulcerative colitis (may induce toxic megacolon) and reflux esophagitis.
Adverse Side Effects:	Dry mouth. **Constipation.** Drowsiness. Blurred vision. May produce heat stroke when administered in the presence of high environmental temperature because it interferes with sweating.
Incompatibility:	Additive effects when given with other anticholinergics. May induce tardive dyskinesia when given with haloperidol.
How Supplied:	Tablets: 5 mg. Syrup: 5 mg/ml.
Dosage and Administration:	**5 mg PO bid–tid.**

Oxycodone

Trade Names:	Roxicodone; Percodan (oxycodone + aspirin); Percocet (oxycodone + acetaminophen); Proladone (AU, UK); Supeudol (C).
Mechanism of Action:	*Semisynthetic narcotic analgesic* twice as potent as morphine. Like other narcotics, occupies μ_1-receptors to produce analgesic effect. No antitussive activity.
Pharmacology:	Onset of action after oral dosage occurs within 15–30 minutes, with peak effect within 1 hour. Duration of analgesia is 3–6 hours. The drug is metabolized in the liver and excreted mainly by the kidneys. Plasma half-life is about 5 hours. In the event of overdose, the actions of oxycodone can be antagonized by naloxone (Narcan).
Indications in Palliative Care:	Moderate **pain**. Bone pain (Percodan, because of the aspirin moiety).
Contraindications:	Percodan contraindicated in patients who cannot take aspirin for any reason (allergy, GI bleeding).
Adverse Side Effects:	Drowsiness. Constipation. Nausea and vomiting.
Incompatibility:	The use of MAO inhibitors or tricyclic **antidepressants** with oxycodone preparations may increase the effect of either the antidepressant or the oxycodone. Concurrent use of anticholinergics may produce paralytic ileus. Additive effects with other CNS depressants.
How Supplied:	Roxicodone tablets: oxycodone, 5 mg. Roxicodone oral solution: 5 mg/5 ml. Intensol concentrated oral solution: 20 mg/ml. Percodan tablets: Oxycodone HCl, 4.5 mg + oxycodone terephthalate, 0.38 mg + aspirin, 325 mg. Percocet tablets: oxycodone, 5 mg + paracetamol, 325 mg.
Dosage and Administration:	Roxicodone: Start with **5 mg PO q4–6h**, and titrate upward as needed. Percodan/Percocet: **1 tab PO q4–6h**. If this dosage does not produce adequate pain relief, switch to pure oxycodone to titrate upward or switch to a morphine preparation.

Pamidronate Disodium

Trade Name:	Aredia.
Mechanism of Action:	**Inhibits bone resorption** without inhibiting bone formation and mineralization, apparently by (1) adsorbing to calcium phosphate crystals in bone and (2) inhibiting osteoclast activity. Since osteoclastic hyperactivity and the resultant excessive bone resorption are the underlying derangements in metastatic bone disease and hypercalcemia of malignancy, pamidronate directly opposes those effects.
Pharmacology:	After IV infusion over 4–24 hours, about half is rapidly absorbed by bone; the rest is excreted unchanged in the urine within 72 hours. Biphasic excretion curve. Rate of elimination from bone unknown. Serum phosphate levels fall after pamidronate administration; usually return to normal within 7–10 days; urinary Ca^{2+}/Cr falls after treatment. Maximum calcium-lowering effect is usually seen 4–5 days after infusion.
Indications in Palliative Care:	Treatment of moderate to severe **hypercalcemia** associated with malignancy, with or without bone metastases. Treatment of **bone pain** secondary to metastases (not an officially approved use and effectiveness not fully established).
Contraindications:	Clinically significant hypersensitivity to biphosphonates.
Adverse Side Effects:	Transient mild temperature elevations (27%) and myalgias. Local soft-tissue symptoms (redness, swelling, induration) at the site of the IV catheter. Uveitis. Hypophosphatemia, hypokalemia, hypomagnesemia.
Incompatibility:	Concomitant administration of a loop diuretic did *not* improve calcium-lowering action of pamidronate.
How Supplied:	Ampules: 15 mg of pamidronate dissolved in 5 ml water, to be stored in refrigerator. Vials: 30 mg/ml for reconstitution with 10 ml of sterile water. Must be administered immediately after dilution in infusion solution.
Dosage and Administration:	Mild hypercalcemia (Ca^{2+} <12): Try hydration alone. Moderate hypercalcemia (Ca^{2+} = 12–13.5 mg/dl, corrected*): **60–90 mg**. Severe hypercalcemia (Ca^{2+} = >13.5, corrected*): **90 mg** The dosage is given as a **single-dose IV infusion over 4–6 hours**. NEVER give as a bolus injection. Pamidronate is best given with **acetaminophen, 500 mg PO/PR**, to prevent pamidronate fever.

continued

---

*To correct serum calcium for hypoalbuminemia:

Corrected $Ca^{2+} = Ca^{2+} + 0.8(4.0 - $ serum albumin$)$.

Pamidronate Disodium   *continued*

Dosage and Administration: *cont.*	Pamidronate should be **diluted in a calcium-free infusion solution** (e.g., normal saline, *not* Ringer's).
	In hypercalcemia associated with hematologic malignancies, may add a glucocorticoid.
	Serum calcium, phosphorus, and magnesium should be monitored when giving biphosphonates.
	Wait at least 7 days before repeating treatment, if needed.
	Dosage and administration for retreatment are the same as for initial treatment.

Pancreatin Preparations

Trade Names:	Creon, Donnazyme, Entozyme, Nutrizym (UK).
Mechanism of Action:	Pancreatin catalyzes the hydrolysis of fats to glycerol and fatty acids; starch to dextrins and short-chain sugars; and protein to proteoses. It substitutes for the endogenous lipases, proteases, and amylase that are insufficient or missing altogether in pancreatic disorders.
Pharmacology:	Most pancreatin preparations are formulated to resist gastric degradation and to deliver pancreatic enzymes to the duodenum, where they function in lieu of endogenous pancreatic enzymes. They are not absorbed but act locally in the GI tract.
Indications in Palliative Care:	For symptomatic conditions resulting from **exocrine pancreatic insufficiency** (usually in patients after GI bypass surgery, pancreatic surgery, etc.).
Contraindications:	Known hypersensitivity to pork protein. Acute pancreatitis.
Adverse Side Effects:	Rash. Nausea, cramping, diarrhea.
Incompatibility:	Not known.
How Supplied:	Enteric-coated or double-layer tablets or gelatin capsules containing variable amounts of lipase, protease, and amylase.
Dosage and Administration:	**2 tablets with each meal and with food taken between meals**, as needed. Tablets should not be chewed, but should be swallowed rapidly to minimize irritation of the mouth.

Papaverine

Trade Names:	Cerebid, Delapav, Papaverine, Pavabid, Pavadur, and others.
Mechanism of Action:	Smooth muscle relaxant, especially when muscle is spasmodically contracted. Acts directly on the muscle itself in the vascular system, bronchial musculature, and GI, biliary, and urinary tracts. Relaxes smooth muscles, especially those of larger arteries in spasm, unrelated to muscle innervation. Minimal actions on CNS, although very large doses cause sedation. Effect on the heart: relaxes coronary arteries → ↑coronary blood flow; mild inotropic effect; depresses conduction and prolongs the refractory period. Direct vasodilating action on cerebral arteries → ↑cerebral blood flow.
Pharmacology:	Hydrochloride of an alkaloid obtained from opium. Effective by all routes of administration. Peak plasma levels occur 1-2 hours after an oral dose; effects usually persist at least 6 hours. A considerable fraction of the drug localizes in fat depots and in the liver; the rest is distributed throughout the body. Metabolized by the liver; 90% bound to plasma protein. Plasma levels can be maintained by oral administration q6h.
Indications in Palliative Care:	Visceral spasm (ureteral, biliary, GI).
Contraindications:	IV administration contraindicated in the presence of **complete heart block**. Caution in patients with glaucoma. Discontinue if eosinophilia or abnormal LFTs develop.
Adverse Side Effects:	GI discomfort. Rash, flushing. Tachycardia. Sedation. Rare hepatitis.
Incompatibility:	Should not be added to lactated Ringer's (will precipitate). May decrease antiparkinsonian action of L-dopa. Effects may be potentiated by CNS depressants.
How Supplied:	Tablets: 30 mg, 60 mg, 100 mg, 200 mg, and 300 mg. Sustained-release tablets: 200 mg. Sustained-release capsules: 150 mg. Multidose vials: 30 mg/ml. Ampules: 60 mg in 2 ml.
Dosage and Administration:	**40–80 mg** PO/IM **qd–tid** or prn.

Promethazine

Trade Names:	Anergan, Phenergan, Phenazine, and others.
Mechanism of Action:	Phenothiazine derivative with **antihistaminic, sedative, antiemetic**, anti-motion sickness, and **anticholinergic** effects. As an antiemetic, it works mainly as an H$_1$ receptor blocking agent but is probably active as well at the CTZ.
Pharmacology:	Well absorbed from the GI tract; clinical effects apparent within 20 minutes after oral, rectal, or IM administration and last 4-6 hours (may persist up to 12 hours). Metabolized by liver.
Indications in Palliative Care:	Prevention and control of **nausea and vomiting** in situations where mild sedation is also desirable. To palliate **rigors**. Amelioration of allergic reactions to blood or plasma. Mild, uncomplicated allergic skin manifestations of urticaria, angioedema.
Contraindications:	**Asthma**. Use with *caution* in patients with narrow-angle glaucoma, stenosing peptic ulcer, pyloroduodenal obstruction, and obstructive uropathy (BPH).
Adverse Side Effects:	Possible oversedation if given with other CNS depressants (alcohol, narcotics, barbiturates). Has been associated with cholestatic jaundice. May lower the seizure threshold. Rare extrapyramidal symptoms (usually from parenteral high dose).
Incompatibility:	Do not give with MAO inhibitors, which intensify and prolong the action of phenothiazines. Additive sedative effects with other CNS depressants.
How Supplied:	Ampules: 25 mg/ml and 50 mg/ml. Tubex syringes: 25 mg/ml and 50 mg/ml. Tablets: 12.5 mg (orange), 25 mg (white), and 50 mg (pink). Syrup: 6.25 mg/5 ml and 25 mg/5 ml. Suppositories: 12.5 mg, 25 mg, and 50 mg.
Dosage and Administration:	For *nausea & vomiting*: 6.25 mg PO or 12.5 mg PR bid and 6.25-25 mg PO/IM prn. For *rigors*: 25 mg PO/IM. For *pruritus* of any cause: 6.25-25 mg PO hs. For *allergic reactions*: 25 mg PO hs or 6.25-12.5 mg tid. For *sedation*: 25 PO hs.

Ranitidine

Trade Name:	Zantac.
Mechanism of Action:	H_2 receptor blocker. *Inhibits* daytime and nocturnal *basal gastric acid secretion* as well as that stimulated by food.
Pharmacology:	Fifty percent absorbed after oral administration; absorption not affected by food or antacids. The onset of action is within 30 minutes of an oral dose and 15 minutes of a parenteral dose. Peak effect occurs 2–3 hours after an oral dose and 1–2 hours after parenteral administration. Duration of action is 8–12 hours for an oral dose and 6–8 hours for a parenteral dose. Elimination half-life is 2.5–3 hours. Excreted principally through the urine by active tubular clearance ($\rightarrow$ reduce dosage in renal insufficiency).
Indications in Palliative Care:	Symptoms of **peptic ulcer disease**. **Gastroesophageal reflux** disease. Erosive **esophagitis**. Prevention of peptic ulcer in vulnerable patients taking corticosteroids or NSAIDs (controversial; misoprostol is probably a better choice for this indication). *Note*: In palliative care, famotidine is the oral H_2 blocker of choice because of ease in swallowing and absence of interactions with other drugs.
Contraindications:	Known hypersensitivity to the drug. *Caution* in patients with impaired renal function.
Adverse Side Effects:	Headache, sometimes severe. Abnormal LFTs.
Incompatibility:	False-positive test for urine protein with MultiStix. May affect metabolism of warfarin.
How Supplied:	Tablets: 150 mg and 300 mg. Syrup: 16.8 mg/ml. Vials: 25 mg/ml.
Dosage and Administration:	**150 mg PO bid** *or* 300 mg PO hs (equally effective). May be given **IV: 50 mg** diluted in **100 ml of D5/W** and infused over 15–20 minutes **tid**. IV formulation can also be given by **continuous SQ infusion** (100–150 mg/24 hr).

Scopolamine (Hyoscine)

Trade Names:	Scopoderm TTS (UK), Transderm Scōp, Transderm V(C), Triptone.
Mechanism of Action:	Central *anticholinergic* activity. Inhibits vestibular input to the CNS, which inhibits the vomiting reflex. In addition, scopolamine may have a direct action on the vomiting center within the reticular formation of the brain stem. Its antimuscarinic properties decrease secretions and GI motility.
Pharmacology:	Belladonna alkaloid, sharing many pharmacologic properties with atropine. Available in *transdermal* form, which is programmed to deliver 0.5 mg of scopolamine via controlled release over 3 days. Antiemetic effect begins within 3–4 hours following application of the disk behind the ear. When given SQ or IM, effects are seen within 15–30 minutes.
Indications in Palliative Care:	**Nausea and vomiting,** especially that **due to bowel obstruction.** Also effective against chemotherapy-induced nausea and vomiting, when used together with metoclopramide. May be useful in **opioid-induced nausea** in ambulatory patients. In the patient's last hours, to dry secretions and thereby **prevent death rattle.**
Contraindications:	**Glaucoma.** Use with caution in known pyloric obstruction or bladder neck obstruction.
Adverse Side Effects:	**Dryness of the mouth** in 65% of patients. Drowsiness. Transient blurring of vision. Confusion, excitement, delirium may occur in the elderly.
Incompatibility:	Use with caution in patients receiving other belladonna alkaloids, antihistamines (including meclizine), and antidepressants.
How Supplied:	Transdermal patches: 1.5 mg. Vials and ampules for injection: 0.3 mg/ml, 0.4 mg/ml, 0.5 mg/ml, 0.86 mg/ml, and 1 mg/ml.
Dosage and Administration:	*Transdermal:* Apply **1 patch to dry skin in the hairless area behind one ear every 3 days.** Wash hands thoroughly with soap and water, and dry thoroughly, after applying the patch, to avoid scopolamine coming in contact with the patient's or caregiver's eyes. When removing the patch, discard the patch, and wash hands and the application site thoroughly with soap and water. If a new patch is applied after 3 days, place it behind the *other* ear. *By injection:* **0.3–0.6 mg IM/SQ** *or* **0.3–0.6 mg** by **continuous SQ infusion.**

Spironolactone

Trade Name:	Aldactone.
Mechanism of Action:	**Diuretic.** Specific antagonist of aldosterone. Acts mainly by competitive binding of receptors at the aldosterone-dependent Na^+/K^+ exchange sites in the *distal* renal tubule. Causes $\uparrow Na^+$ and water excretion while K^+ is retained, and therefore has both diuretic and antihypertensive actions. May be given alone or with diuretics that act on the proximal tubule or loop of Henle.
Pharmacology:	Rapidly metabolized to sulfur-containing products that are pharmacologically active. Peak serum concentrations occur at 3–5 hours after oral ingestion, but the onset of action is gradual, and peak effects are not seen until the third to fourth day of treatment. Its metabolites are excreted mainly in the urine. Taking spironolactone with food increases its bioavailability by 100%.
Indications in Palliative Care:	Given together with a proximal or loop diuretic (e.g., furosemide) for • Peripheral **edema** and lymphedema. • **Ascites.** • **Pleural effusions.** Can be given as a single drug for the treatment of **hypokalemia**.
Contraindications:	Anuria or acute renal failure. Hyperkalemia.
Adverse Side Effects:	Gynecomastia (dose and duration related). Cramping and diarrhea.
Incompatibility:	Do not give together with **potassium** supplements or potassium-rich foods (e.g., avocado). Do not give together with antihypertensives of the **ACE inhibitor** family (e.g., enalapril, captopril). Spironolactone increases the serum half-life of **digitalis** → may lead to digitalis toxicity if dosage is not adjusted. Concomitant administration of **aspirin** may reduce the effectiveness of spironolactone up to 70%.
How Supplied:	Tablets: 25 mg, 50 mg, and 100 mg.
Dosage and Administration:	For *peripheral edema*: **100–200 mg PO qam** with breakfast (usually given together with furosemide, 40–80 mg PO qam). For ascites: **200–800 mg PO qam** or in divided doses, with furosemide, 40–80 mg qam. *Note:* In patients who do not have an indwelling urinary catheter, it is best to give diuretic medications as a single dose in the morning, so that their sleep is not disturbed by the necessity to void. In catheterized patients, diuretics may be given in divided doses bid-tid.

Sucralfate

Trade Name:	Carafate.
Mechanism of Action:	Acts by a variety of mechanisms whose net effect is to protect the gastroduodenal mucosa against injury through local rather than systemic actions: (1) forms an ulcer-adherent complex with proteinaceous exudate at the site of peptic ulcer and may provide a barrier to diffusion of H^+ ions; (2) inhibits pepsin activity in gastric juice and adsorbs bile acids; (3) stimulates the gastric mucosa to synthesize and release prostaglandin E_2, which plays a major role in protection of the gastric mucosa; (4) stimulates the secretion of both mucus and bicarbonate in the stomach; (5) binds epidermal growth factor and causes it to accumulate in ulcerated areas; and (6) promotes epithelial restitution.
Pharmacology:	Sucrose backbone to which multiple sulfated aluminum salts are attached. Sucralfate is relatively insoluble and is minimally absorbed from the GI tract. Sucralfate is effective for 5 hours after oral administration. About 90% is excreted in the feces; the absorbed drug is excreted unchanged in the urine.
Indications in Palliative Care:	Symptoms of **peptic ulcer disease** or **reflux esophagitis**. **Mucositis**. Rectal bleeding from rectal tumor. Oozing cutaneous metastases.
Contraindications:	None known.
Adverse Side Effects:	Constipation in 2% of patients.
Incompatibility:	When given together with other aluminum-containing products (e.g., aluminum-based antacids) in patients with renal insufficiency, may lead to aluminum accumulation and toxicity. Reduces absorption of cimetidine, ciprofloxacin, digoxin, norfloxacin, phenytoin, ranitidine, tetracycline, and theophylline. If the patient is taking any of these drugs, they should be given *2 hours before sucralfate*.
How Supplied:	Tablets: 1 gm.
Dosage and Administration:	For *peptic ulcer disease* or *esophagitis*: **1 gm PO qid**. To administer through a nasogastric tube, place the sucralfate tablet in a 50-ml syringe, add 20–30 ml water, and allow the tablet to dissolve. Then inject the solution down the NG tube, and flush the tube 2–3 times with water.

continued

Sucralfate *continued*

Dosage and Administration: *cont.*	For *mucositis*: • 1-gm tablet crushed and spread through the mouth qid, *or* • Suspension[a]: Swish in mouth for 2 minutes, then swallow, pc and hs. For *oozing cutaneous metastases* or *rectal bleeding from tumor*: Apply **sucralfate paste**.[b]

[a]To make a **sucralfate suspension**: Dissolve eight 1-gm tablets in 40 ml of sterile water; add 40 ml of 70% sorbitol, and shake. In a separate container, dissolve 3 Ensure flavor packs in 10 ml of water; add to drug mixture; add water qs to 120 ml.

[b]To make up **sucralfate paste**, crush a 1-gm sucralfate tablet in 2–3 ml of water-soluble gel, such as K-Y Jelly.

Appendix 2

Subcutaneous (SQ) Infusions

Indications for the Subcutaneous Route

Patient unable to take oral medications or fluids:
- Intractable nausea and **vomiting** (e.g., bowel obstruction).
- **Dysphagia.**
- Vacillating level of consciousness.
- The **last** days or **hours of life.**

Advantages of SQ Infusions	*Disadvantages of SQ Infusions*
- Obviate need for frequent injections. - Maintain relatively constant plasma drug levels, without peaks and troughs of intermittent dosing. - Can be used comfortably at home. - Allow patient more freedom and control. - As opposed to *IV* infusion, less danger of inadvertent overhydration.	- May cause inflammation at the infusion site. - Dosage can be reassessed and changed only every 24 hours—rapid dose adjustments not possible. - May require expensive equipment (syringe driver) or costly disposables. - For home use, requires nursing and pharmacy backup.

Contraindications to Subcutaneous Drug Infusions

- Severe thrombocytopenia.
- Anasarca.
- Patient unwillingness.

Drugs that May Be Given by Subcutaneous Infusion

- Preferred drugs:

Class	Preferred SQ Drugs
Opioids	Morphine Hydromorphone Methadone
Antiemetics	Haloperidol Metoclopramide Methotrimeprazine
Somatostatin analog	Octreotide
Sedatives	Midazolam Phenobarbital
Antihistamines	Promethazine Dimenhydrinate Hydroxyzine
Anticholinergic	Atropine Scopolamine
Corticosteroid	Dexamethasone
H_2 blockers	Ranitidine Famotidine
NSAIDs	Ketorolac

- The following cause subcutaneous inflammation and should *not* be given by SQ infusion:
  - Diazepam.
  - Chlorpromazine.
- It is possible to combine several drugs together in the same syringe for SQ infusions, so long as they are compatible with one another in solution (Table A2.1).

TABLE A2.1   Drugs that May Be Combined in a Syringe Driver

	Metoclopramide	Morphine	Methotrimeprazine	Midazolam	Dexamethasone	Ranitidine	Haloperidol	Promethazine	Octreotide
Metoclopramide	C	C	C	C		N	C	C	
Morphine	C	C	C	C	C	C	C	C	C
Methotrimeprazine	C	C	C	C			N		
Midazolam	C	C	C	C	N	N	C	C	
Dexamethasone		C		N	C	C	N		C
Ranitidine	C	C		N	C	C			
Haloperidol	C	C	N	C	N	N	C		
Promethazine	C	C	C	C			C	C	
Octreotide		C			C				C

The letter *C* indicates that the two drugs are *compatible*. The letter *N* indicates that the two drugs are *not compatible*. If the entry is blank, it means that we have no experience in combining the two drugs and their compatibility is therefore not known to us. If you need to combine more than two drugs in an infusion, use the table to check the compatibilities of each pair of drugs separately. For example, if the patient needs to receive metoclopramide, morphine, and midazolam, check the compatibility of

Metoclopramide with morphine (= C)
Metoclopramide with midazolam (= C)
Morphine with midazolam (= C)

In the example cited, each pair is compatible, so the combination of all three drugs is compatible.

Methods of Subcutaneous Drug Infusion

Syringe Driver (Fig. A2.1)

- Lightweight, battery-operated infusion pump (Graseby, Infumed).
- Most syringe drivers are designed to accommodate 10- or 20-ml syringes.
- Calibrated in mm/hr or mm/24 hr.
- Some models have a boost button, allowing the patient to receive an added bolus of medication on demand (patient-controlled analgesia).
- Need to be checked periodically for battery status and infusion rate.

Infusors

- Portable, disposable infusors developed for outpatient chemotherapy can be used for drug delivery in palliative care.
- Travenol-Baxter infusors (Fig. A2.2) have a capacity of 65 ml and weigh 90 gm when filled; different models can infuse at 0.5, 2, or 5 ml/hr (therefore can deliver medications for 12, 32, and 130 hours).

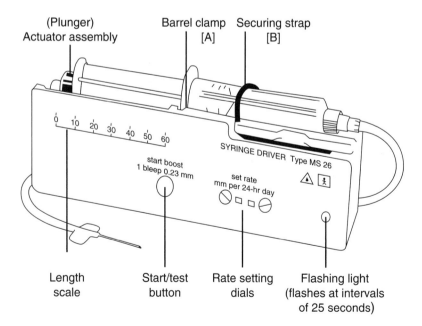

FIGURE A2.1 Graseby Syringe Driver, Model MS26. Drawing courtesy of Graseby Medical, Watford, United Kingdom.

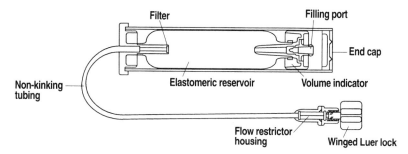

FIGURE A2.2 Baxter infusor. Drawing courtesy of Baxter Healthcare Corporation, Round Lake, Illinois.

- Infusors must be filled by a pharmacy under a sterile hood.
- Infusors are disposable.
- Cost per infusor is approximately $16 to $35. (Nondisposable boost button is available for $10.)

Simple Syringe and Subcutaneous Needle

- A 20- to 50-ml syringe can be prepared daily with the patient's 24-hour medication requirements.
- The syringe is attached to an indwelling SQ needle.
- The patient or caregiver injects a specified volume every 4 hours.

Hypodermoclysis

- An intravenous infusion apparatus is used to infuse medications SQ in up to 1.5 L/day of infusion fluid.
- The carrier fluid should be saline or a 2 : 1 mixture of dextrose–normal saline, as plain dextrose solutions may cause pain and swelling.
- In some centers, 500 to 750 U of hyaluronidase is added to each liter of infusion fluid to speed diffusion and absorption.

Steps in Initiating Subcutaneous Drug Infusion

1. **Explain** the procedure to the patient.
    - Many patients are wary of being "hooked up to a machine."

- Emphasize that continuous infusion will smooth out the peaks and troughs of intermittent dosing.
2. Prime the patient with an **intramuscular loading dose** of the medication to enable rapid achievement of therapeutic plasma levels.
3. **Calculate** the **24-hour medication requirements**, and draw up the desired dose into the syringe or infusion bag (disposable infusors will be loaded in the pharmacy):

Drug	Priming Dose (IM)	Start SQ Infusion with
Morphine	⅙–¼ the patient's previous 24-hour oral morphine requirement	⅓ the patient's previous 24-hour oral morphine requirement/24 hr
Haloperidol	0.5 mg	1.5 mg/24 hr
Metoclopramide	10 mg	30-60 mg/24 hr
Octreotide	100 μg	300 μg/24 hr
Midazolam	2.5 mg	5-30 mg/24 hr
Promethazine	6.25 mg	12.5-25 mg/24 hr
Atropine	1 mg	2-3 mg/24 hr

4. Prepare the **skin site** by swabbing with povidone-iodine, then alcohol:
   - For ambulatory patients:
     - Abdomen.
     - Upper chest, above breast, over intercostal space (not for cachectic patients, in whom the SQ needle may cause pneumothorax).
   - For bedridden patients:
     - Thighs.
     - Abdomen.
     - Outer aspect of upper arm.
5. **Insert the needle**:
   - Use a 25-gauge butterfly needle.
   - Insert needle into the subcutaneous tissue at an angle of 45 degrees (shallower angle shortens the viability of the injection site).
   - Secure the needle under an Omiderm or OpSite dressing.
6. **Connect the needle** to the infusion device (syringe driver, infusor, regular syringe, or infusion bag).
7. **Start the infusion**. If using a syringe driver, follow the manufacturer's instructions for operating the device.

Care of Subcutaneous Infusions

- The **site** must be **inspected daily.**
  - Stop the infusion at the first sign of local inflammation, and change to another site.
  - The frequency with which site changes are necessary depends on the drug(s) infused.
    - Some drugs are more irritating than others (e.g., dexamethasone) and shorten the lifetime of the infusion.
    - Average lifetime of an infusion site = 2 to 3 days (with morphine alone, site may remain uninflamed for 2 weeks).
- If using a **syringe driver,** check daily to make sure the device is infusing at the intended rate.
  - If infusing too slowly, check for kinks in the cannula tubing, local inflammatory reaction, or battery failure.
  - If infusing too rapidly, recheck rate calculations and settings.

References and Further Reading

Berger E. Nutrition by hypodermoclysis. *J Am Geriatr Soc* 32:199, 1984.

Bruera E. Ambulatory infusion devices in the continuing care of patients with advanced diseases. *J Pain Symptom Manage* 5:287, 1990.

Bruera E, Brenneis M, Michaud M, MacDonald N. Continuous SC infusion of metoclopramide for treatment of narcotic bowel syndrome. *Cancer Treat Rep* 71:1121, 1987.

Bruera E, Chadwick S, Bacovsky R, MacDonald N. Continuous subcutaneous infusion of narcotics using a portable disposable pump. *J Palliative Care* 1:46, 1985.

Bruera E, Legris MA, Kuehn N, Miller MJ. Hypodermoclysis for the administration of fluids and narcotic analgesics in patients with advanced cancer. *J Natl Cancer Inst* 81:1198, 1989.

Bruera E, MacDonald N, Brenneis C, et al. Metoclopramide infusion with a disposable portable pump (letter). *Ann Intern Med* 104:896, 1986.

Campbell CF, Mason JB, Weiler JM. Continuous subcutaneous infusion of morphine for the pain of terminal malignancy. *Ann Intern Med* 98:51, 1983.

Dover SB. Syringe driver in terminal care. *Br Med J* 294:553, 1987.

Ingham JM, Cooney NJ. Pneumothorax following insertion of subcutaneous needle. *Palliative Med* 6:343, 1992.

Johnson I, Patterson S. Drugs used in combination in the syringe driver—a survey of hospice practice. *Palliative Med* 6:125, 1992.

Lipschitz S, Campbell AJ, Roberts MS, et al. Subcutaneous fluid administration in elderly subjects: Validation of an under-used technique. *J Am Geriatr Soc* 30:6, 1991.

MacMillan K, Bruera E, Kuehn N, et al. A prospective comparison study between a butterfly needle and a Teflon cannula for subcutaneous narcotic administration. *J Pain Symptom Manage* 2:82, 1994.

Oliver DJ. Syringe drivers in palliative care: a review. *Palliative Med* 2:21, 1988.

Schen R, Arieli S. Administration of potassium by subcutaneous infusion in elderly patients (letter). *Br Med J* 285:1167, 1982.

Schen R, Singer-Edelstein M. Subcutaneous infusions in the elderly. *J Am Geriatr Soc* 29:583, 1981.

Storey P, Hill H, St. Louis R, Tarver E. Subcutaneous infusions for control of cancer symptoms. *J Pain Symptom Manage* 5:33, 1990.

Walsh TD, Smyth EM, Currie K, et al. A pilot study, review of the literature, and dosing guidelines for patient-controlled analgesia using subcutaneous morphine sulphate for chronic cancer pain. *Palliative Med* 6:217, 1992.

Appendix 3
Transcutaneous Electrical Nerve Stimulation (TENS)

What Is TENS?

- The use of electricity to relieve pain is recorded in Egyptian wall paintings of 2500 B.C. and in the Hippocratic writings of 400 B.C. (the electrical sources were biologic: electric ray, eel).
- In the eighteenth and nineteenth century, galvanic currents produced by hand-cranked magnetos were used for the same purpose.
- Transcutaneous electrical nerve stimulation (TENS) is a more recent and more precise technique for stimulating nerves in the skin and subcutaneous tissues, via electrodes placed on the body surface and connected to a battery-powered electrical pulse generator.

How Does TENS Work?

- The precise mechanism of action by which TENS relieves *pain* is not known.
  - The impetus for development of TENS came from the **Gate Control Theory** of pain (Melzack and Wall, 1965):
    - According to the Gate Control Theory, selective stimulation of cuta-

neous afferent large-diameter fibers might "close the gate" in the dorsal horn of the spinal cord and thereby inhibit pain perception.
- The Gate Control Theory is most applicable to *high*-frequency (>10 Hz) TENS.
- *Low*-frequency (<10 Hz) TENS ("acupuncture-like TENS") may trigger release of **endorphins**, for its effects can be blocked by naloxone.
- The mechanism by which TENS relieves some cases of *lymphedema* is entirely unknown.
- TENS may stimulate local microcirculation → more efficient removal of excess fluid.

Indications for TENS in Advanced Cancer

- **Pain**:
  - Types of pain particularly amenable to treatment with TENS:
    - Pain in the **head and neck** regions.
    - Pain due to **nerve compression** or nerve infiltration by tumor.
    - **Postherpetic** neuralgia.
    - **Bone** pain from metastases or multiple myeloma.
  - Patient selection criteria:
    - Any cancer patient with pain *may* benefit from TENS; the only way to know *which* patients will benefit is via therapeutic trial.
    - Patient must be *receptive to the idea*, and the patient or his caregiver must be capable of carrying out the treatments after appropriate instruction.
      - **Careful explanation** to the patient and caregivers is **essential**.
      - Many people fear electricity and need reassurance that electrocution cannot occur.
  - Advantages of TENS:
    - Virtually no adverse side effects.
    - TENS gives patients a sense of control that is otherwise mostly lacking in their care.
- **Lymphedema** (investigational).

Contraindications to TENS in Terminally Ill Cancer Patients

- Do not use TENS in patients with a cardiac **pacemaker** (especially demand pacemaker).
- Do not apply TENS electrodes
  - Onto damaged, irritated, infected, or irradiated skin.
  - Over the carotid sinus.

Electrode Placement

- The success of TENS treatment depends significantly on optimal electrode placement.
- There are several **systems for choosing electrode sites**; each system has its proponents:
  - Research has not yet established whether any system of electrode placement is superior.
  - Trial and error are usually necessary to establish which electrode placement gives the best results in any particular patient.

System for Electrode Siting	Comments
Dermatomes	Dermatome = cutaneous region innervated by a spinal nerve (refer to dermatome chart in Figure A3.1). Dual-channel electrodes enable stimulation of both anterior and posterior aspects of a dermatome.
Within or around the painful area	Placing electrodes on either side of a **surgical incision** or on either side of **herpetic lesions** has been effective in relieving pain.
Acupuncture points/ meridians	Probably the method of choice when using low-frequency, "acupuncture-like" TENS; may also be effective with conventional TENS.
Trigger points	A trigger point is a focus of hyperirritability in a tissue that is tender to palpation and, when compressed, produces referred pain and tenderness. When a trigger point for a given pain can be located and injection of local anesthesia is for some reason not feasible, TENS stimulation of the trigger point may be tried.
Spinal cord segments	Beside the vertebrae or between spinous processes of the spinal cord segment that gives rise to the nerve root involved. Electrodes may be placed on either side of the vertebrae; or one electrode beside the vertebra and its pair within the corresponding dermatome distal to the extent of pain radiation. May be especially effective for sciatic pain.
Peripheral nerves	For pain due to **peripheral nerve injury**. Electrodes should be *proximal* to the nerve lesion. The ulnar nerve, e.g., can be stimulated proximally at the axilla and distally at the olecranon groove or at the lateral wrist.
Brachial plexus	For **diffuse upper extremity pain**. Place the proximal electrode at Erb's point (2-3 cm above the clavicle at the level of C6 transverse process).

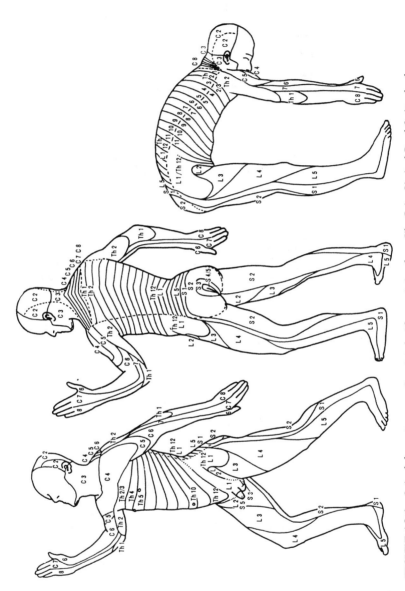

FIGURE A3.1   Spinal dermatomes.   Reprinted with permission from Ciba-Geigy Limited, Basel, Switzerland.

- Suggested initial electrode placements for various conditions are shown in Figure A3.2 and may serve as a guide for starting therapy. If initial electrode sites do not produce results, try another system.
- Electrodes should be placed on a clean, dry, relatively hairless skin surface.
  - Do not place electrodes over damaged skin.
  - Self-adhering carbon silicone electrodes are preferred; they do not require electrode gel or tape.
  - For rubber electrodes, apply electrode gel to the electrode surface; secure electrode to the skin with Velcro straps or hypoallergenic tape.
- For treatment of **lymphedema**, place one electrode from the electrode pair on the proximal limb and the other electrode on the distal limb. (If using a dual-channel machine, electrode pairs may be crossed on the same limb.)

Settings for TENS Treatments

1. Set the **pulse rate**:
   - For conventional TENS, aim to *maximize the rate*: Setting should be from **70 to 150 Hz**.
   - For "acupuncture-like" TENS, set the rate from 2 to 6 Hz.
2. Set the **pulse width** to a *minimum*: **130 μsec or less**.
3. Set the **pulse amplitude** (intensity) to the patient's level of comfort:
   - Slowly increase intensity until the patient reports a comfortable, deep tingling sensation beneath the electrodes.
   - For conventional TENS, muscle contractions should *not* occur.
   - For "acupuncture-like" TENS, some authorities recommend increasing amplitude until twitch is seen, but in any event, **TENS should not cause pain**.
4. Choose the pulse **mode**:
   - For conventional TENS, start with the **C** (conventional) **mode** → switch to **M** (modulated) **mode** after 5 minutes, to minimize habituation.
   - For "acupuncture-like" TENS, use the **B** (burst) **mode**.

Duration of Treatment

- Conventional TENS:
  - First treatment: 20 to 30 minutes.
  - Thereafter: 20 minutes tid to 24 hr/day, as required.
- "Acupuncture-like" TENS: 20 to 30 min/treatment q2-6h, as needed.

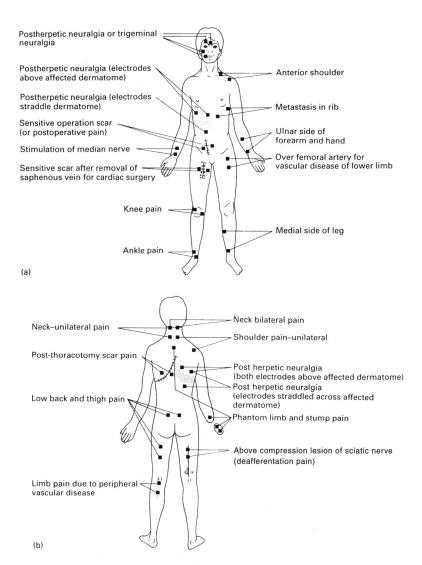

Postherpetic neuralgia or trigeminal neuralgia

Postherpetic neuralgia (electrodes above affected dermatome)

Postherpetic neuralgia (electrodes straddle dermatome)

Sensitive operation scar (or postoperative pain)

Stimulation of median nerve

Sensitive scar after removal of saphenous vein for cardiac surgery

Anterior shoulder

Metastasis in rib

Ulnar side of forearm and hand

Over femoral artery for vascular disease of lower limb

Knee pain

Medial side of leg

Ankle pain

(a)

Neck–unilateral pain

Post-thoracotomy scar pain

Low back and thigh pain

Limb pain due to peripheral vascular disease

Neck bilateral pain

Shoulder pain–unilateral

Post herpetic neuralgia (both electrodes above affected dermatome)

Post herpetic neuralgia (electrodes straddled across affected dermatome)

Phantom limb and stump pain

Above compression lesion of sciatic nerve (deafferentation pain)

(b)

FIGURE A3.2   Electrode positions commonly used for TENS. (a) Anterior aspect. (b) Posterior aspect.   Reprinted with permission from publisher and Thompson JW, Filshie J. Transcutaneous Electrical Nerve Stimulation (TENS) and Acupuncture. In Doyle D, Hanks GWC, MacDonald N (eds). *Oxford Textbook of Palliative Medicine*. Oxford: Oxford University Press, 1993, p. 232.

After Starting TENS Treatment

- TENS may enable reduction in analgesic dosage.
- Combination of TENS with an antidepressant may be especially effective in neuropathic pain syndromes.

Summary: Conventional TENS Treatment

1. Select electrode sites on undamaged skin. Change sites until optimal pain relief is obtained.
2. Set rate to 70-150 Hz.
3. Set pulse width to <130 μsec.
4. Set amplitude to level of comfortable paresthesias.

References and Further Reading

Avellanosa AM, West CR. Experience with transcutaneous nerve stimulation for relief of intractable pain in cancer patients. *J Med* 13:203, 1982.

Johnson MI, Ashton CH, Thompson JW. An in-depth study of long-term users of transcutaneous electrical nerve stimulation (TENS): Implications for clinical use of TENS. *Pain* 44:221, 1991.

Lampe GN. Introduction to the use of transcutaneous electrical nerve stimulation devices. *Phys Ther* 58:1450, 1978.

Librach SI, Rapson IM. The use of transcutaneous electrical nerve stimulation (TENS) for the relief of pain in palliative care. *Palliative Med* 2:15, 1988.

Mannheimer JS. Electrode placements for transcutaneous electrical nerve stimulation. *Phys Ther* 58:1455, 1978.

Melzack R, Wall PD. Pain mechanisms: A new theory. *Science* 150:971, 1965.

Ordog GJ. Transcutaneous electrical nerve stimulation versus oral analgesic: A randomized double-blind controlled study in acute traumatic pain. *Am J Emerg Med* 5:6, 1987.

Thompson J, Regnard CFB. Managing pain in advanced cancer—a flow diagram. *Palliative Med* 6:329, 1992.

Ventafridda V, Sganzerla EP, Fochi C, et al. Transcutaneous Nerve Stimulation in Cancer Pain. In Bonica JJ, Ventafridda V (eds). *Advances in Pain Research and Therapy*, Vol 2. New York: Raven Press, 1979, pp. 509–515.

Index

---

*Page numbers given in **boldface** indicate a principal presentation of the subject.